Conserving health in early modern culture

Manchester University Press

SOCIAL HISTORIES OF MEDICINE

Series editors: *David Cantor* and *Keir Waddington*

Social Histories of Medicine is concerned with all aspects of health, illness and medicine, from prehistory to the present, in every part of the world. The series covers the circumstances that promote health or illness, the ways in which people experience and explain such conditions, and what, practically, they do about them. Practitioners of all approaches to health and healing come within its scope, as do their ideas, beliefs, and practices, and the social, economic and cultural contexts in which they operate. Methodologically, the series welcomes relevant studies in social, economic, cultural, and intellectual history, as well as approaches derived from other disciplines in the arts, sciences, social sciences and humanities. The series is a collaboration between Manchester University Press and the Society for the Social History of Medicine.

Previously published

The metamorphosis of autism: A history of child development in Britain *Bonnie Evans*

The politics of vaccination: A global history *Edited by Christine Holmberg, Stuart Blume* and *Paul Greenough*

Payment and philanthropy in British healthcare, 1918–48 *George Campbell Gosling*

Conserving health in early modern culture

Bodies and environments in Italy and England

Edited by Sandra Cavallo and Tessa Storey

Manchester University Press

Published by Manchester University Press
Oxford Road, Manchester M13 9PL

www.manchesteruniversitypress.co.uk

British Library Cataloguing-in-Publication Data
A catalogue record for this book is available from the British Library

ISBN 978 1 5261 1347 4 hardback

First published 2017

Typeset
by Toppan Best-set Premedia Limited

Contents

Plates

The plate section can be found between pages xvi and 1

Figures

Contributors

Marta Ajmar (PhD Warburg Institute) is Deputy Director V&A Research Institute (VARI), Research Department, Victoria and Albert Museum. Between 2002 and 2006 she directed the research project, funded by the Getty Foundation and the AHRC, for the major V&A exhibition 'At Home in Renaissance Italy'. She was CI and consultant on the research project 'Healthy Homes, Healthy Bodies. Domestic Culture and the Prevention of Disease in Renaissance and Early Modern Italy', led by Sandra Cavallo and supported by the Wellcome Trust. Her research interests lie in the material culture of Early Modern Italy and the Mediterranean world. She has published on the domestic interior, gender, eroticism and the material culture of the family and childhood. Her publications include the edited volumes *At Home in Renaissance Italy* (London, 2006); *Approaching the Italian Renaissance Interior: Sources, Methodologies, Debates* (Oxford, 2007); *Approaches to Renaissance Consumption* (Oxford, 2002). Her current book project explores questions of artisanal practice, technology and materiality.

Leah Astbury completed her PhD at the Department of History and Philosophy of Science, University of Cambridge in 2015, funded by the Wellcome Trust. She is the 2017–18 Molina Fellow in the History of

Medicine at the Huntington Library, San Marino. From 2018 she will begin a research project on marriage and health in Cambridge, funded by a Wellcome Trust Medical Humanities Fellowship. Between February and May 2016, she held an AHRC Cultural Engagement Award to conduct a public engagement collaboration with the artist Emma Smith.

Caroline Castiglione is a historian in the departments of Italian Studies and History at Brown University. Her research interests are political, cultural, gender and medical history in Italy between 1500–1800. Her first book, *Patrons and Adversaries: Nobles and Villagers in Italian Politics, 1640–1760* (Oxford, 2005) won the Helen and Howard R. Marraro Prize from the Society for Italian Historical Studies in 2005. Her last book, *Accounting for Affection: Mothering and Politics in Rome, 1630–1730* (Basingstoke, 2015) examines the symbiotic evolution of politics and mothering in early modern Rome, where mothers did not hesitate to turn to the expanding judicial system if the future of their children were at stake. The study analyses the intersection of maternal affection, female advocacy and family conflict in the papal city. Articles related to this research have also appeared in *Historical Reflexions / Réflexions Historiques*, *Viator* and the *Journal of Social History*.

Sandra Cavallo is Professor of Early Modern History and co-director of the Centre for the Study of the Body and Material Culture at Royal Holloway University of London. She specialises in the history of medicine, gender and the home. Her publications include the monographs *Charity and Power in Early Modern Italy* (Cambridge, 1995), *Artisans of the Body in Early Modern Italy. Identities, Families, Masculinities* (Manchester, 2007) and *Healthy Living in Late Renaissance Italy* (Oxford, 2013), co-authored with Tessa Storey and awarded the R.H. Bainton prize for History 2014. She has co-edited the volumes *Widowhood in Medieval and Early Modern Europe* (Longman, 1999), *Spaces, Objects and Identities in Early Modern Italian Medicine* (Blackwell, 2008), *Domestic Institutional Interiors in Early Modern Europe* (Ashgate, 2009) and *A Cultural History of Childhood and the Family* vol. 3, *The Early Modern Age* (Oxford, 2010).

Maria Conforti is Associate Professor of the History of Medicine at the Unità di Storia della Medicina e Bioetica, La Sapienza, University of Rome. Her research interests focus on early modern Italy, especially on Rome and Naples, with a special interest in forms and structures of scientific communication (academies, learned journals) and medical practice (surgery, anatomy, women's medicine). She has also worked on medical historiography in Italy. She is currently writing a book on medicine in Naples in the seventeenth century. Among her recent publications, *Interpetare e curare. Medicina e salute nel Rinascimento* (Rome, 2013), co-edited with A. Carlino and A. Clericuzio.

Maria Pia Donato is Associate Professor in Early Modern History at the University of Cagliari, Italy, and *chargée de recherche* at the Centre National de la Recherche Scientifique, Institut d'Histoire moderne et contemporaine of Paris, France. She is the author of four monographs, the most recent being *Sudden Death. Medicine and Religion in Eighteenth-Century Rome* (Ashgate, 2014), and of many essays on the political, social and cultural life of early modern Rome, the history of medicine and the history of science. She has also co-edited, with J. Kraye, the volume Conflicting Duties. Science, Medicine and Religion in Rome, 1550–1750 (Warburg Institute, 2009).

Frances Gage is Associate Professor of Art History at Buffalo State, New York. She specialises in the history of collecting and the history, theory and criticism of Italian art, particularly the artistic production and reception of the Carracci, their pupils, and Caravaggio and his followers. She has investigated the intersections between art and medicine in early modern Italy in her book *Painting as Medicine in Early Modern Rome: Giulio Mancini and the Efficacy of Art* (Philadelphia, 2016) and in various articles. Her articles on the art criticism of the Sienese physician Giulio Mancini include 'Exercise for Mind and Body: Giulio Mancini, Collecting and the Beholding of Landscape Painting in the Seventeenth Century', which won the William Nelson award from the Renaissance Society of America in 2009.

Sasha Handley is Senior Lecturer in Early Modern History at the University of Manchester, specialising in aspects of social and cultural history. Her first monograph, Visions of an Unseen World: Ghost Beliefs and Ghost Stories in Eighteenth Century England (London, 2007), examined the meaning and vitality of ghost beliefs and ghost stories. Her current research focuses on the cultural history of sleeping practices in English domestic households from *c.*1660 to 1760. She is completing a monograph on this subject and has published articles on this theme in *History: The Journal of the Historical Association* (2013), *Journal for Eighteenth-Century Studies* (2012) and *Cultural and Social History* (2012).

Hannah Newton is a social and cultural historian of early modern England, specialising in medicine, emotion and childhood. Her first book, *The Sick Child in Early Modern England* (Oxford University Press, 2012), which is based on her PhD thesis, won the European Association for the History of Medicine and Health 2015 Book Prize. In 2011–14 she undertook a Wellcome Trust Fellowship at the University of Cambridge and researched her second monograph, *Misery to Mirth: Recovery from Illness in Early Modern England* (forthcoming). The aim of this book is to rebalance our overall picture of early modern health, which hitherto has focused almost exclusively on disease and death. Since 2014 Hannah has been based at the University of Reading, lecturing in History, where she has been granted a Wellcome Trust University Award (2016–21) investigating the senses in the early modern sickchamber.

Tessa Storey is Honorary Research Associate at Royal Holloway University of London. She completed her PhD at the EUI in Florence and her thesis on prostitution was subsequently developed into the monograph *Carnal Commerce in Counter-Reformation Rome* (Cambridge, 2008). She has published extensively on material culture and on masculinity. She has been a Leverhulme Research Fellow and research associate on a Wellcome Trust funded project on Italian recipe books at the University of Leicester. Her most recent book, the award-winning *Healthy Living in Late Renaissance Italy* (Oxford, 2013), co-authored with Sandra Cavallo, is the result of the Wellcome-funded research project 'Healthy Homes, Healthy Bodies in Renaissance and Early Modern Italy'. She is currently researching lay practices of medicine in early modern Rome.

Acknowledgements

This book originates from the conference 'Healthy living in pre-modern Europe: the theory and practice of the six Non-Naturals (*c*.1400–*c*.1700)', which was held in London, at the Centre for the Study of the Body and material Culture (CSBMC), Royal Holloway, in September 2013. We would like to thank the Wellcome Trust for the generous conference grant which made this event possible and the CSBMC for additional financial support. For the purposes of publication it was deemed necessary to shift the chronological frame of reference to after 1500, and to make this a volume with a comparative perspective. As a result, not all the papers from the conference, particularly those dealing with the medieval period, could be included in this volume, but we would like to acknowledge and thank all the participants in the conference for their thoughtful contributions and comments, which ultimately helped us to shape this collection. Moreover, we owe particular thanks to the external readers for their insightful and constructive comments on the volume proposal and earlier drafts of some chapters, and on the 'shape' of the whole book, which resulted in our adding a comparative chapter as a 'frame' for the collection of essays. We are also indebted to Elaine Leong for her encouragement and precious bibliographical references.

We would not have been able to include any of the colour images without a generous subvention from the Isobel Thornley Trust at the

University of London towards the costs of reproducing the images, permission rights, and the costs of publication, for which we are extremely grateful.

In the course of this book our original publisher was taken over, resulting in difficult and changing circumstances, and we would like to thank David Cantor for his tireless support of this volume and its images, from its inception. More recently Emma Brennan must be thanked for her patient help with all our queries. Finally we would like to thank all the contributors who have waited so patiently for this volume to appear.

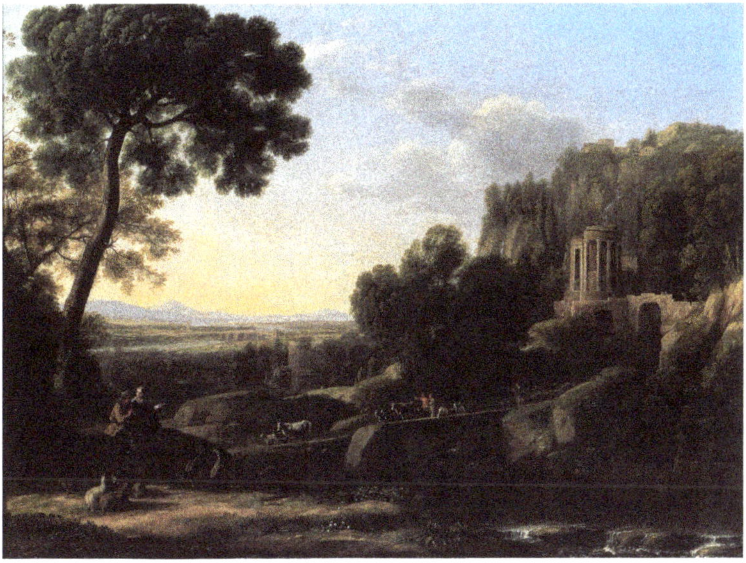

Plate 1 Claude Lorrain, *Pastoral Landscape*, 1644

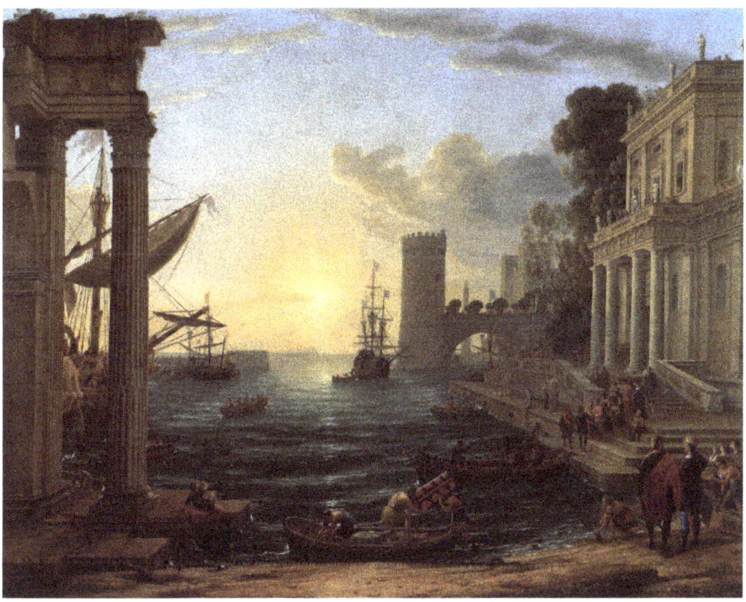

Plate 2 Claude Lorrain, *Seaport with the Embarkation of the Queen of Sheba*, 1648

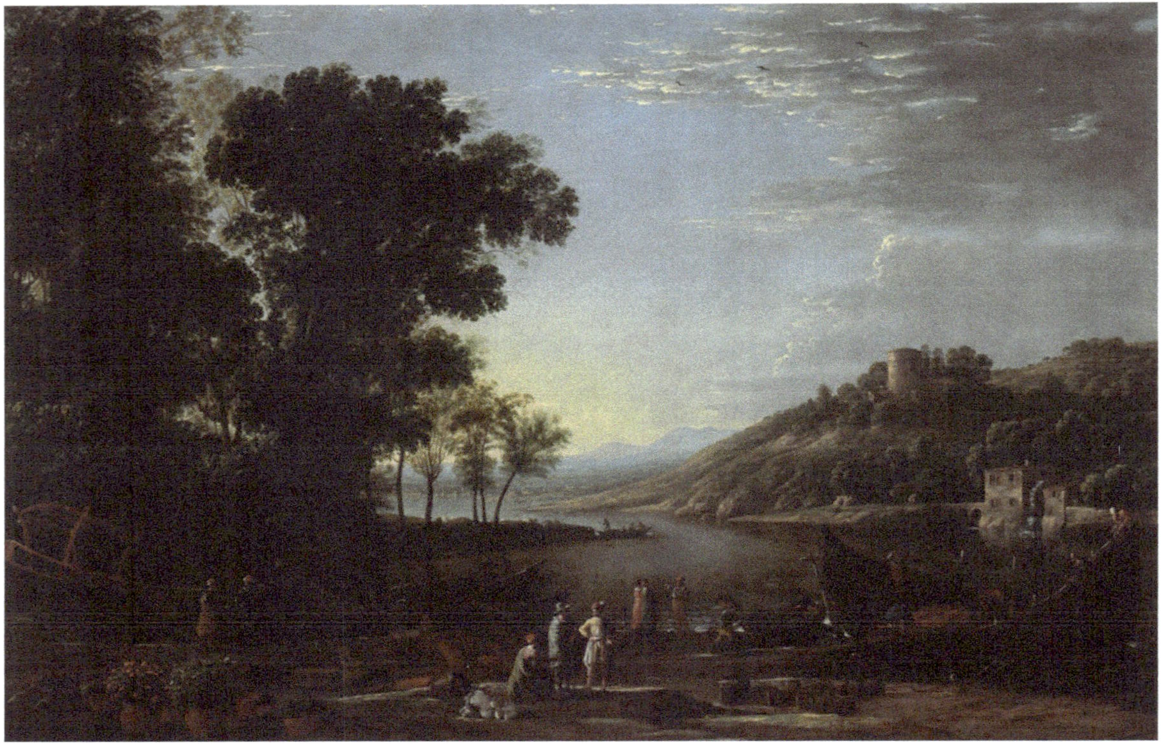

Plate 3 Claude Lorrain, *Landscape with Merchants*, 1629

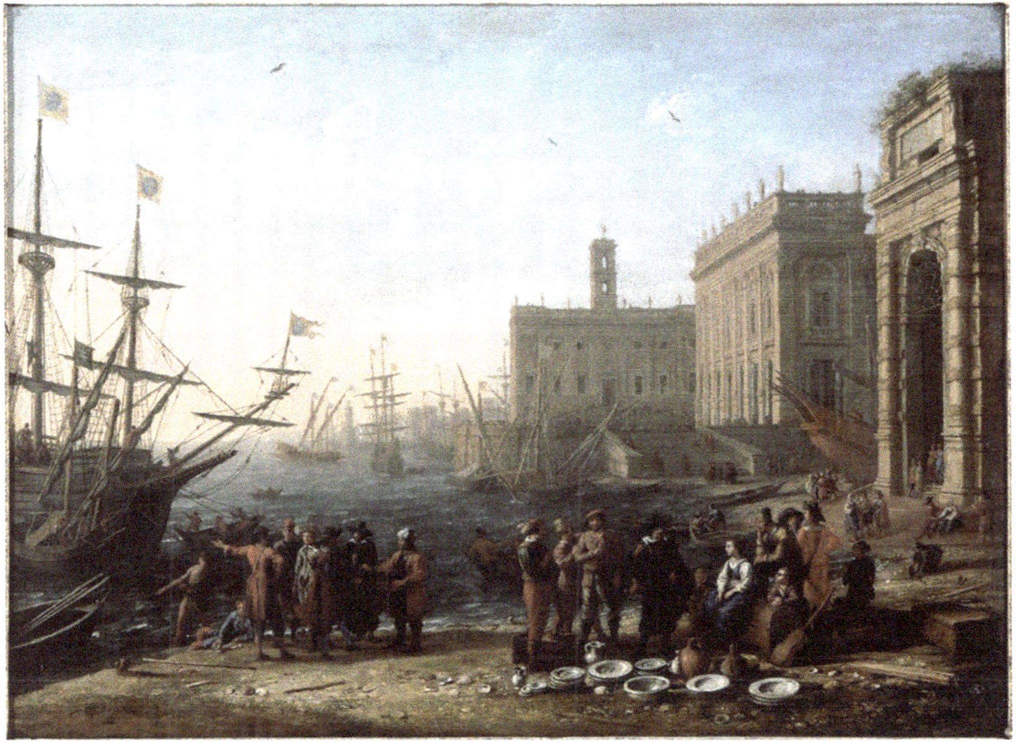

Plate 4 Claude Lorrain, *View of a Port with the Capitol*, 1636[?]

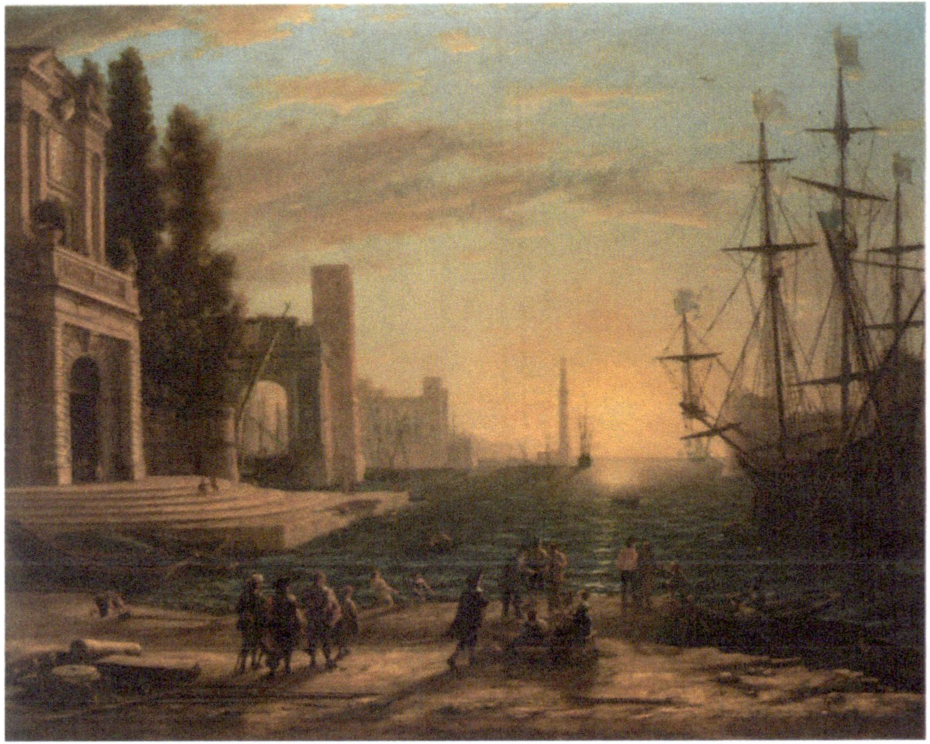

Plate 5 Claude Lorrain, *A Seaport*, 1644

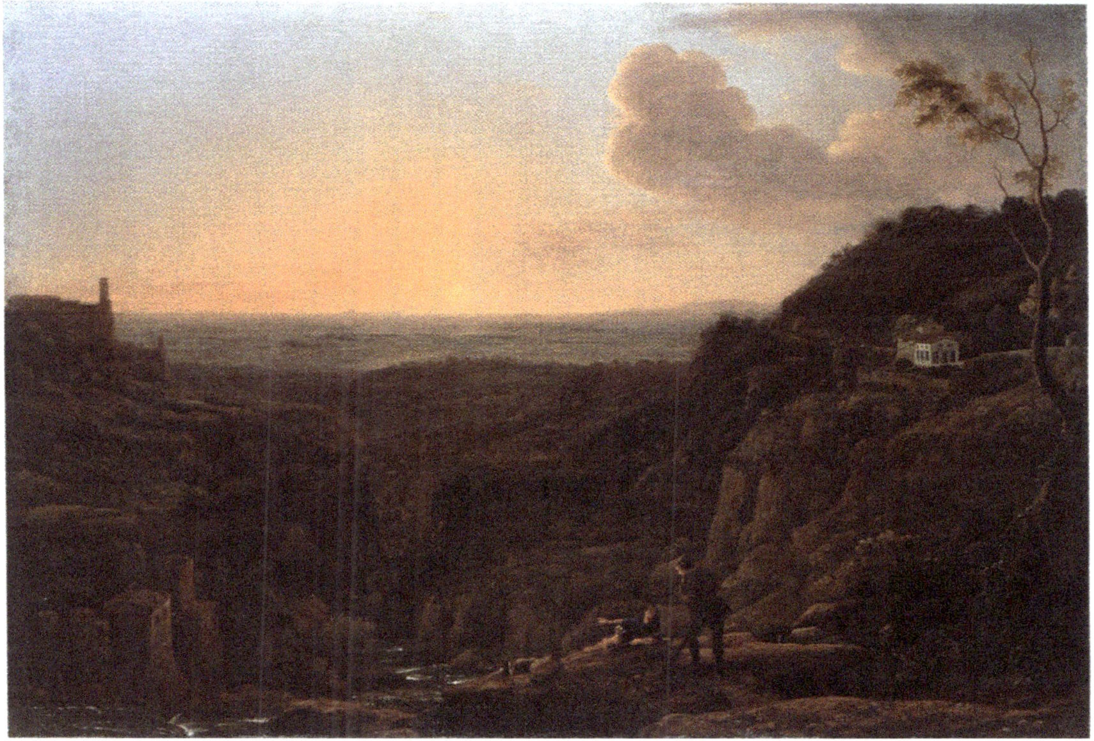

Plate 6 Claude Lorrain, *A View of the Campagna from Tivoli*, 1645

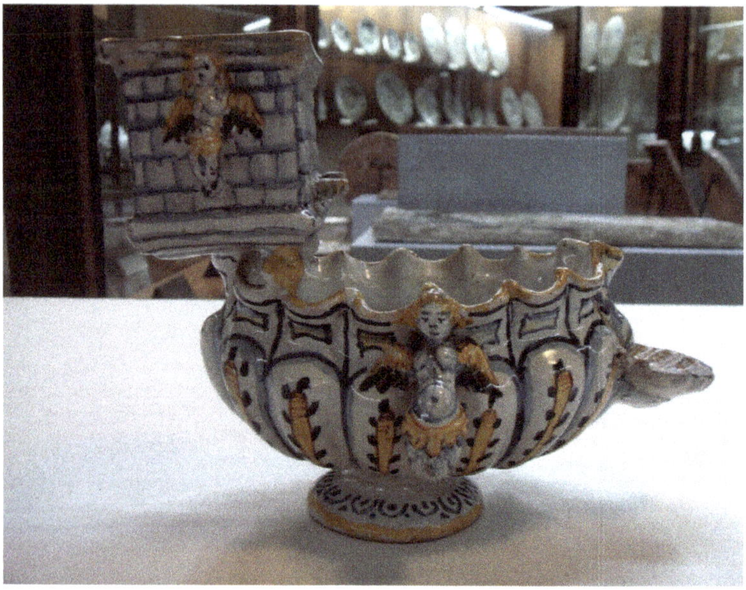

Plate 7 Pouring vessel, tin-glazed earthenware, Castelli (Italy), 1575–1600

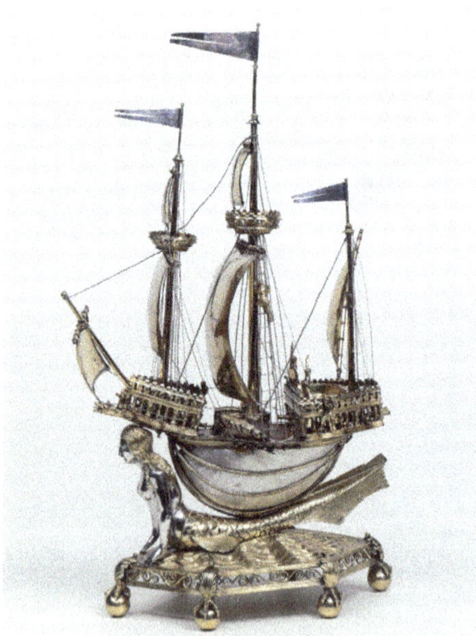

Plate 8 'Burghley Nef', Saltcellar, Nautilus shell with parcel-gilt silver mounts, raised, chased, engraved and cast, and pearls, Paris (France), 1527–28

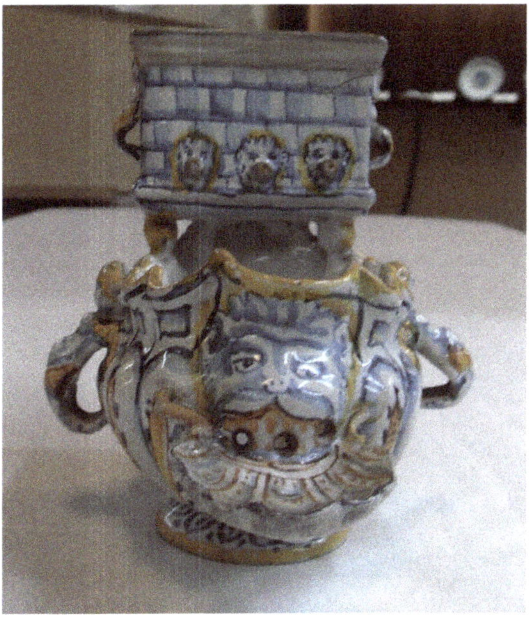

Plate 9 Detail of pouring vessel, Raccolte d'Arte Applicata, Castello Sforzesco, Milano

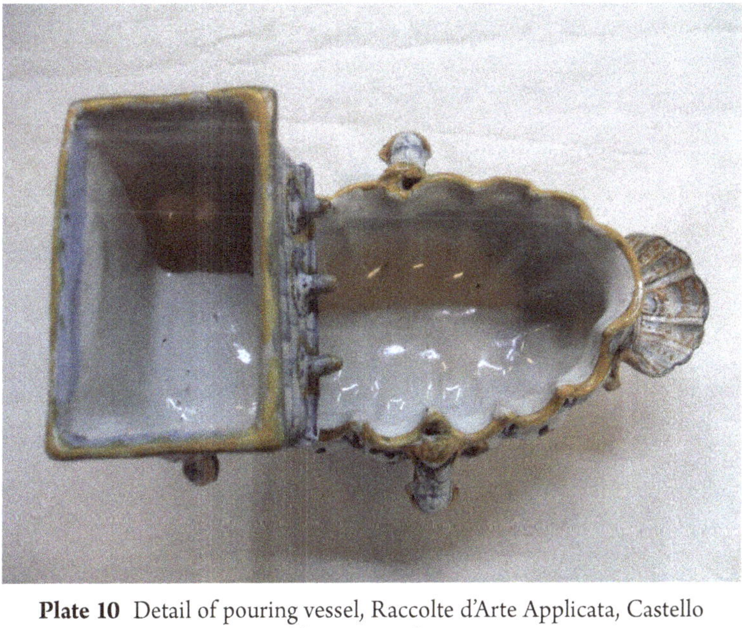

Plate 10 Detail of pouring vessel, Raccolte d'Arte Applicata, Castello Sforzesco, Milano

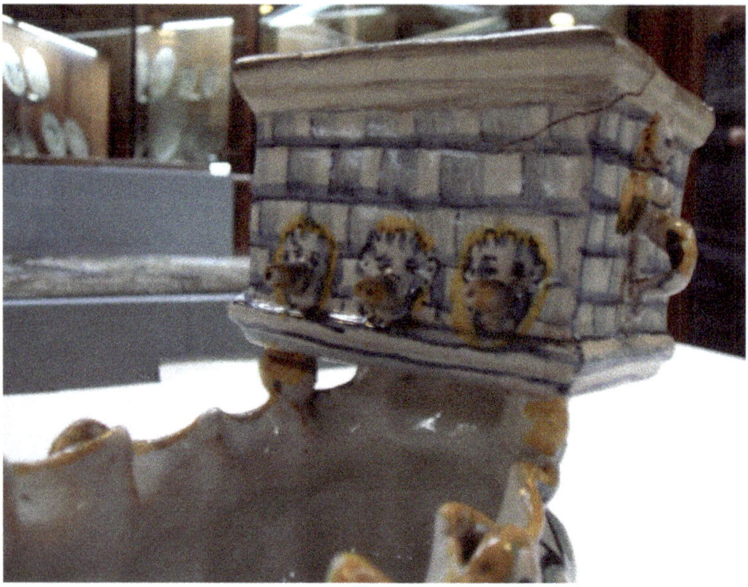

Plate 11 Detail of pouring vessel, Raccolte d'Arte Applicata, Castello Sforzesco, Milano

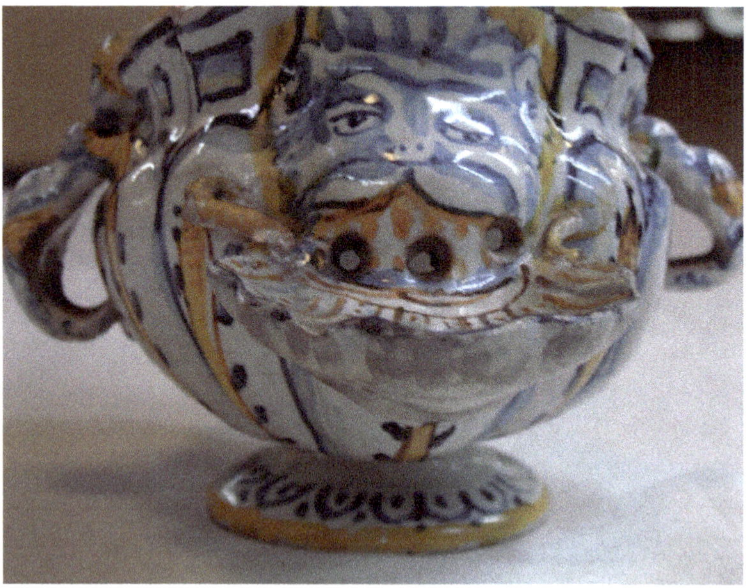

Plate 12 Detail of pouring vessel, Raccolte d'Arte Applicata, Castello Sforzesco, Milano

Introduction
Conserving health: the Non-Naturals in early modern culture and society

Sandra Cavallo

The study of early modern preventive medicine

According to the Galenic-Hippocratic tradition, 'preservative' medicine, that is the management of the body in health, was one of the three central pillars of the physician's art (*practica*), as important as therapeutics and surgery. With very few exceptions, however, until recently the history of medicine has concentrated on the study of illness, treatment and medicinal remedies, whilst the efforts made by our predecessors to keep in good health by adopting a healthy lifestyle have received scant attention. The few works that have focused on prophylactic medicine have addressed the topic almost exclusively from the perspective of the history of medical ideas.[1] There has been very little interest in the impact of these ideas on lay practice and even less in their reception and integration in non-medical intellectual and professional genres and disciplines. While the experience of illness from the patient's perspective has attracted much attention and has recently stimulated important new works from a variety of innovative angles, we still await the development of a patient-based history of prevention that focuses on what people actually did to prevent illness.[2]

Existing studies on prevention also tend to be very general; little attention is given to the specific recommendations concerning the spheres of life (the six Non-Naturals) which were seen as key to the maintenance of health. Some authors have provided more detailed accounts of medical preventive advice but in relation to only one of the Non-Naturals: hygiene, exercise, sleep or emotions, and especially food.[3] Very rarely is the whole set of recommendations concerning healthy living taken into account. This literature tends also to pay scarce attention to change, the preventive discourse is seen as remarkably stable over time or subject to alterations only in relation to the major turning points advocated by the traditional medical and philosophical periodisations. With few exceptions, the influence of specific political discourses and shifting sociocultural values on attitudes to health maintenance has been neglected.[4] The predominance of the intellectual perspective in most studies on prevention also stems from their tendency to adopt a pan-European viewpoint and, irrespective of the geographical specificity of their sources, draw indistinctly on texts published in different European countries and hence belonging to different cultural, political and religious contexts.[5] Normally, moreover, no distinction is made between texts published in Latin and in vernacular and directed therefore to different audiences, that is to the medical professionals and learned readership or to the wider public.[6] An exception to this trend is represented by the work of Andrew Wear, who has dedicated an important chapter and a number of articles to the popularisation of ideals of healthy living in England and its American colonies, focusing specifically on the rise of vernacular medical advice directed to lay people in these geographical contexts.[7] Here too, however, evidence about practice remains marginal, and the discussion is largely limited to the advice literature.

In their recently published monograph, *Healthy Living in Late Renaissance Italy*, the co-editors of this volume have attempted to correct these imbalances, first by charting the translation of health advice into practice in sixteenth- and seventeenth-century Italy, and second by paying considerable attention to the specific cultural and social conditions which encouraged the development of both a didactic preventive literature and an everyday and home-based culture of prevention in this part of Europe. Moreover, the study has showed that far from being stable, both the recommendations and the daily practices aimed at preserving health were reshaped, over the two centuries considered, not so much by new medical philosophies but under the influence of trends such as the rise of ideals of civility, new definitions of masculinity and gentility, and the increased importance that the domestic sphere acquired in certifying the status and virtue of householders in parts of the Italian peninsula.

A similar effort to place medical advice in broader sociocultural and geographically specific settings characterises the essays in this collection. The volume arises from the wish to explore further the forms through which preventive ideas were disseminated in different local contexts – whether through oral, written, medical and non-medical channels. It asks which areas of behaviour and which categories of patients were touched by these preoccupations, and whether preventive concerns varied in relation to gender and age, whether they changed over time and were different in different countries.

Central to the early modern preventive discourse were the spheres of life that the medical tradition saw as key to health, 'the six Non-Naturals': eating and drinking, sleeping, exercising, breathing, cleansing the body and managing the passions of the soul. The importance of paying attention to the way of life in order to preserve one's well-being has deep roots in ancient medicine. It was discussed in Hippocratic works and in many of Galen's writings, though the factors seen to have an impact on physical and mental health varied over time: in some periods they were limited to three categories, other times to four, five or more. In addition, the regulation of such activities and the control over the quality of food, drink and the air one breaths were encouraged but not yet presented as a permanent necessity in classical medicine. Only later did a standardisation of the areas of life relevant to health occur: in the works of the first Arabic medical authors, heavily influenced by Galenism, these elements came to be strictly organised in six categories (with sex and baths being sometimes subsumed under exercise, more frequently under evacuations); they were labelled 'the six Non-Natural things' or causes and were now regarded as necessary to a healthy life.[8] Since then the concept of 'the six Non-Naturals' gained currency in Europe, being propagated by the translations of Arabic medical texts undertaken in Italy and Spain in the eleventh and twelfth centuries (including the highly influential Avicenna's Canon), and by the centrality that this concept acquires in the numerous regimens of health compiled in Europe in the thirteenth and fourteenth centuries.[9] Whilst the timing of the development of this doctrine has therefore been fully addressed by historians, much less is known about the specific measures recommended to correctly manage the Non-Naturals, let alone those actually adopted.[10]

This volume begins to fill this gap by providing a wealth of evidence about the form taken by daily preventive practices. Using diaries and letters between members of the family, our authors (namely Newton, Gage, Handley, Castiglione) show that the preventive discourse pervaded everyday experience and had a real influence on key moments of life: their findings challenge therefore the scepticism often embedded in comments about the real impact of preventive concerns.[11] By focusing attention on the strategies devised by ordinary people to preserve their health, the analysis in these chapters also allows a rare insight into shared ideas of healthy and unhealthy and contemporary views of the functioning of the body. Moreover, it offers an opportunity for examining the relationship between the authority and discourse of medical practitioners and the practices of laypeople.

Some contributions to this volume demonstrate the pervasive presence of preventive ideas, and the Non-Naturals in particular, not just in people's actions but in various strands of early modern cultural production. Gage and Ajmar explore how these concerns were embedded in material elements of the living environment like paintings and domestic objects. Moreover, rather than considering the medical tradition in isolation, a number of chapters show that medical ideas about preserving health closely interacted with change in religious thought and practices (Handley) and were in turn affected by developments in other disciplinary fields such as geology and natural philosophy (Conforti, Donato).[12]

By its very nature therefore this is an interdisciplinary volume, which draws on the expertise of scholars who are not simply medical historians but contribute to medical history from a range of perspectives: art history, history of material culture, of philosophy and ideas, and religious discourse. Reflecting this variety of viewpoints, essays in this collection also rely on a broad range of sources: from landscape painting to surviving ceramics, from religious tracts and sermons to personal correspondence and diaries, and to debates on aspects of natural philosophy. The volume thus significantly expands the range of media which in one way or another appear to have contributed to promote health. As far as textual culture is concerned it goes well beyond the evidence provided by the learned medical literature: some chapters certainly also draw on scholarly medical texts but, with the exception of Donato's, it is the vernacular literature that flourished in this period and which populated the home that is the object of their analysis. Moreover, letters and diaries make it possible to illustrate the appropriation of the preventive medical discourse by categories of patients (e.g. women) whose active participation in healthy living may be obscured by the scarce attention they receive in general health advice texts.[13] On the other hand, some chapters in this collection prioritise the evidence obtainable from the close analysis of surviving artefacts and paintings over that drawn from texts.

Ajmar focuses on a single artefact – a puzzling sixteenth-century *maiolica* 'pouring vessel', of unknown use – to speculate on whether or not the object alone (its design, form, materiality and antecedents) might reveal its role in the recommended drinking practices of the time. Indeed, the question of whether hot liquids could be drunk as part of a healthy daily regimen was a subject of lively debate in the late sixteenth and early seventeenth centuries. Rather than suggesting a simple alignment between material features and textual advice, this chapter offers an example of the ambiguities inherent in the relationship between material and textual evidence. Moreover, it highlights how difficult the task of identifying with certainty the health function of domestic objects – extricating it from the 'multiple, interwoven meanings embedded' within them – could be.

Likewise, Gage is able to tease out the links between medical notions of healthy air and works of art through a close analysis of seventeenth-century *prospettive* paintings. She shows that in a period in which doctors were paying increased attention to climate as a major agent affecting health, artists such as Lorrain, active in seventeenth-century Rome, specialised in representing with unparalleled subtlety the observable signs of temperature and humidity in the air. His paintings acted at the same time as channels of information about the supposed effects on health of different types of air and as actual vehicles of health benefits for viewers. Indeed, visual representations of air were not understood as inert but as having somatic and mental effects on beholders; through the view of open, airy spaces and of great distances through which air may travel, being purified and cooled by this mobility, viewers could in fact experience the sensation of breathing more easily and inhaling salubrious air, and divert their mind from stifling rooms. Landscape paintings can therefore be seen as sources documenting the intense preoccupations about air that characterise the period.

A comparative perspective

Some authors in this volume also engage with variation, showing that the doctrine of the Non-Naturals was malleable and adapted to different circumstances: hence the comparative significance of individual Non-Naturals not only changed over time but presented specific characteristics in different geographical contexts.

Indeed, by concentrating on just two countries, this book emphasises the importance of comparison. The focus on Italy and England is partly motivated by the presence of ongoing research on the Non-Naturals in studies of these geographical areas; moreover, it is particularly helpful to compare Italy and England not only because they identify with different religious confessions but because, as we will see, the North–South divide becomes increasingly relevant in the perception of national differences in sixteenth-century Europe. Italy and England are also representative of regions unequally touched by humanism and the rediscovery of ancient medical and non-medical texts propagating the preventive paradigm; they are characterised by a different presence and significance of medical institutions, and their medical professions enjoy a different status. Leaving aside these specific contrasts, our main purpose in comparing the reception and appropriation of a common medical tradition in these two areas was to make a methodological point and show that we cannot generalise findings related to one country to the rest of Europe, nor can we use sources produced in different national contexts to provide a European synthesis.

The adoption of a comparative approach, even if just between two distinct geographical areas, allows us to explore the important question of the transnational extension of preventive health ideas. To date, little or no critical attention has been paid to this issue; rather, it is often implicitly assumed that health recommendations had a universal value, at least within the European or Western contexts. The frequent references to a Galenic-Hippocratic paradigm in the scholarly literature on prevention suggest that European countries relied on a singular and uniform classical tradition, a stance that implicitly justifies drawing on texts produced in and for different national and religious contexts as if they were offering a common picture.[14] In reality, the health advice texts (regimens) published in different parts of Europe may appear similar at a superficial glance but upon closer scrutiny they present significant specificities, as demonstrated in particular by two of the chapters, both in terms of content and in the dynamics which led to their publication.

The comparison between regimens of health in Italy and England is first developed in Chapter 1 (Cavallo and Storey). Surely this genre was not the only medium for the dissemination of precepts of healthy living. As documented in later chapters by Newton, Astbury and Handley, a range of printed sources provided advice about healthy living, and the transmission of preventive ideas also occurred by word of mouth, as the case of Roman noblewomen studied by Castiglione demonstrates. Regimens, however, unquestionably represented a key source of information for people of the time. Indeed the surge of this specific genre of preventive advice literature may explain, and at the same time mirrors, the increased attention to healthy living and the correct management of the Non-Naturals in the sixteenth century.[15] It makes sense therefore to dedicate a chapter to the forms that this so far neglected literature assumed in the two countries.

As we will see, in both contexts the print industry was the driving force in the establishment and rise of this genre. The authors suggest that the role of publishers, professional writers, printers and typographers in stimulating a demand for preventive advice deserves to be taken into greater account than has been previously. But along with similarities, the popularisation of medical preventive advice presents striking differences in the two countries, in terms of authorship, in the chronology followed by the development of the healthy living literature and in the ways in which the aims of the publication were framed. Also as a consequence of the entirely secular identity of authors, Italian regimens are much less imbibed with religious concerns than the English ones and health consciousness is presented as a sign of civility and rationality rather than piety. The more elevated status of the medical profession also gives Italian doctors a virtual monopoly on written preventive advice, though due to a reluctance to embrace the vernacular and abandon Latin as the medium of medical communication, new regimens replace translations of classical and medieval regimens later than in England. In England by contrast, the wish to empower the common people is framed in terms of patriotism and charity, and this drives many learned non-professionals to contribute to the vernacularisation of healthy living advice.

The comparative study carried out by Storey in Chapter 6 also highlights considerable differences, this time between the contents of Italian and English regimens, especially in relation to the effects of climate, food and venery on health. This additionally suggests that, even if Italian medicine was seen as a model, health advice was not passively received in England; only some elements are similar and there are even instances of explicit rejection of healthy living in the Italian way.

The influence of the specific cultural framework – in this case the religious landscape of seventeenth-century England – on health prescriptions is also stressed by Handley in relation to sleep. In Italy, sleep was addressed in a much more secular way, and sensitively to class issues, new models of masculinity and changing generational habits.[16] Another significant national difference concerns the extent to which vernacular regimens provided health advice about pregnancy and infant care. Although the prime concern of these texts remains the health of men and children, in England a certain number of preventive handbooks include post-partum regimes and lifestyle recommendations aimed to encourage the conception of healthy babies. Moreover, as Astbury demonstrates, the English health advice literature places considerable emphasis on the cautions required in managing the newborn.[17] In Italy, by contrast, only obstetrical vernacular texts explicitly directed to midwives and women address these preventive concerns, and even there in a rather cursory way.[18] These texts are much more concerned with pregnancy-related health complaints and therapies than with the precautionary measures pregnant women and mothers should adopt.

These findings clearly demonstrate the need for more comparative work and an in-depth exploration of the reasons for these divergences. It is hoped that they will stimulate discussion on the question of similarities and differences between various medical traditions within Europe. The multifarious discrepancies – in contents, authorships, chronology and motivations – between Italian and English texts also lead one to question the idea of an unrestrained circulation of medical ideas in the Renaissance and early modern age. Although communication among the learned increased through letters and printed texts in this period, there were also barriers, frictions and resistances, which impeded the movement and reception of information.[19] These limitations deserve recognition and invite us to reconsider the idea of a Europe-wide, overarching republic of letters.[20]

The role of the Non-Naturals

The essays in this volume seek to display the unexpectedly wide range of fields in which the Non-Naturals came into play. Chapters 2–4 provide fresh evidence about the centrality of the Non-Naturals in relation to groups whose health has not yet been investigated in works about prevention: babies, women and convalescents. Castiglione and Astbury show that the correct management of the Non-Naturals was regarded as absolutely crucial to guarantee a healthy pregnancy, and to overcome the well-known risks associated with the first months of life. Focusing on the epistolary exchange between Roman noblewomen, Castiglione demonstrates that even in the late seventeenth century – a period which saw the decline of a specific literature on healthy living in Italy – prevention, more than medicines, was still regarded as the key to conceiving and then to the health of the pregnant woman. In different ways both Castiglione and Astbury also shift scholarly attention away from an exclusive focus on childbirth in England, as in Italy, childbirth was not the only or prime preoccupation of mothers to be. Castiglione shows that while giving birth was medicalised, pregnancy and the ability to conceive were regarded very much as the responsibility of the mother and depended on her commitment to a healthy diet, frequent exercise and emotional balance, in other words on her ability to discipline herself. In spite of the disparaging comments occasionally found in preventive literature about the alleged carelessness of women in health matters, prospective mothers were in reality very aware of the need to pay particular attention to their lifestyle both during pregnancy and when wishing to conceive.[21] Similarly, as Astbury demonstrates, in a period in which babies were increasingly nursed in the home, and no longer sent to external mercenary wet-nurses, a mother was invested with considerable responsibilities regarding the maintenance of the baby's health in the first months of life.

The attention to prevention adds therefore new dimensions to the way in which we conceptualise the relationship between medicine and pregnancy. Moreover, by concentrating on the health of these still under-investigated age groups these chapters uncover important details about how the physiology of the infant's body was understood for example, Astbury shows that the crying of babies was perceived as a form of excretion of the harmful liquid that clogged in the lungs and as a way of cleansing the brain, as well as a form of exercise. She also brings to light specific hygienic practices aimed to clear the conduits and enable the infant body to regularly rid itself of any potentially damaging waste.

Preventive advice was not undifferentiated, nor simply articulated by individual complexion, as often assumed. Specific recommendations were aimed at pregnant women and newborn infants. Moreover, as Newton (Chapter 4) demonstrates, particular measures in the management of the Non-Naturals were reserved for those recovering from illness, a group who until now have received only scant scholarly attention. Understood as occupying a liminal (or 'neutral') state between health and sickness, the convalescents were seen as a separate category of patients and were given specific advice especially in relation to purging the body and to diet. This chapter highlights therefore the importance, for medical historians, of expanding the repertory of patients they ought to consider.

A distinctive trait of this volume is the attention it devotes to the role that *each* Non-Natural was seen to play in guaranteeing a healthy life. The food one eats has received disproportionate attention in the historiography on prevention. Here the emphasis moves instead away from the often exclusive focus on diet and precious detail is uncovered to illustrate the understanding, management and inherent reciprocity of all the Non-Naturals. For example, the importance of the emotional state (the 'passions') to the preservation of health is a motif which recurs through several of the chapters, but it often appears interwoven with discussions of the other Non-Naturals. Handley, for instance, points to the link between healthy sleep and happiness, and, conversely, to people's attempts to calm their passions in order to procure sleep. Gage notes the role that certain passions could play in resisting the effects of bad air, as well as the beneficial impact of good air on the emotional balance. The current interest in the history of the emotions has somehow obscured the holistic quality of early modern preventive health advice and the fact that the effects of the Non-Naturals on the body were in reality interdependent on one another.

However, a number of chapters also highlight that some Non-Naturals were regarded as less important than others in relation to the health of specific groups. Interestingly, for example, diet is mentioned only rarely in discussions between female members of the family concerning health in pregnancy – as if women were already quite disciplined in this respect. The frequent references to the disorderly eating habits of pregnant women found in the Italian obstetrical literature in the vernacular do not find any echo in women's correspondence, where gluttony is systematically presented as a typically male vice (Castiglione).[22] This reveals an interesting gender difference in the perceived hierarchy of the Non-Naturals, a completely unknown territory so far, which deserves further attention.

Air is another Non-Natural whose significance for health is subject to variation in relation to different groups. Newton, who focuses on the early part of the period (sixteenth and early seventeenth centuries), suggests that all six of the Non-Naturals were taken into account in defining a regimen for the convalescent but the advice about air appears rather cursory. It mainly concerns temperature and is seen as an element to consider principally in relation to exercise. This contrasts greatly with the evidence from Rome and Naples, where, as Gage and Conforti document, convalescents were often moved to other localities or urban districts, or at least taken to more elevated parts of the city for promenades by coach or litter, to benefit from the good air that was seen as key to their recovery. Air is also marginal in prescriptions to promote the health of infants in England (Astbury) and in recommendations to pregnant women in Rome later in the century. Here four Non-Naturals prevail: adequate movement, rest, the moderate purging of the body, and the mental and spiritual state of the pregnant woman seem to be the most important preconditions for a healthy pregnancy. Less attention is given to the quality of the air, possibly because this is less controllable by pregnant women, who were in any case discouraged from travelling and therefore could not easily relocate.[23] Apart from generic references to the benefits of the fresh air, we find that only the deleterious effects of strong smells, including that of tobacco, were mentioned with preoccupation in relation to expecting mothers.[24]

By contrast, air occupies central stage in the chapters by Gage and Conforti. Here we find confirmation of the suggestion put forward in previous work, that the role of this element grows, at least in Italy, in the definition of causes of bad health in the early modern period.[25] These authors demonstrate how the qualities of the local air are the object of both heated intellectual controversy and constant debate among lay people. Indeed Gage shows that often people changed their location or lodgings, precisely because they were chasing good air. The fear of the dangerous effects of bad air even justified turning down prestigious offices that involved moving to another part of the country.

Change over time

Chapters in this volume also show that ways of ascertaining the quality of the air varied over time, reflecting broader social trends. By the late sixteenth century the fertility of the soil, made visible by the abundance of its agricultural produce, acquired increased importance in Italy as an unquestionable sign of healthfulness of the locality. The new value placed on agriculture in the Italian peninsula, where expert management of the land had become a new field of interest and active involvement of the Italian nobility, and one less and less regarded with disapproval, was clearly a factor in this development.

This increased attention to the local ecology also means that, in Italy at least, the quality of the air was perceived as more and more localised, a point stressed by both Storey and Conforti. This tendency was certainly influenced by the dissemination of Hippocratic ideas but also by exploration in the sixteenth century. The experience of travelling and settling in distant countries made the variety of climates present in the world and the seriousness of their effects on the health of those not used to certain ecological characteristics more tangible. Conforti highlights the role of the local environment in emphasising certain preoccupations related to health: she focuses on the geological specificity of Naples, showing how the frequency of disruptive natural phenomena encouraged a consideration of the relationship between the earth and the environment, subterranean fires and air, and contributed to establish particularly close links between medical, chemical and geological thinking in the region. She emphasises therefore how health threats were increasingly conceptualised in a framework of medical micro-topography.

However, these discussions also have a national basis. Storey finds that the way in which the quality and effects of air were understood reflected a North–South divide and the varied political configurations of different countries. As she demonstrates, there was much less emphasis on the regional characteristics of the air in England than in Italy, and the local mutations of the air did not engage physicians, natural philosophers and laypeople in a comparable way in the two countries.

The space that various sources devoted to individual Non-Naturals also changed over time. Attention to sleep becomes prominent in England after 1650 and acquires spiritual undertones (Handley), while Donato notices the increased importance attributed to food and the air one breaths in early eighteenth-century Italy and the parallel decline in the attention granted to other activities previously seen as relevant to preserving health. The way in which the characteristics of the Non-Natural things and the way in which they operated were conceptualised was also redefined. Conforti finds that interpretations of the appearance of epidemic disease no longer blame the local putrid air but rather see it as being transmitted through contagion or by mineral particles in the air.

These changes in the value and meaning attributed to certain Non-Naturals were only to a degree linked to a medical periodisation. Handley shows that the new emphasis on healthy sleep in England was only in part a reflection of new neurological theories that saw well-regulated sleep as key to the health of the brain and the nervous system. These developments were largely related to religious trends: that is to the fragmentation of religious identities and the decline of public worshipping in favour of domestic devotion that characterise England after 1650. These shifts led to a confessionalisation of domestic practices and transformed healthy sleep into a pious activity. Meanwhile both Conforti and Donato see major philosophical shifts, such as the rise of chemical theories and corpuscularism, as affecting thinking about healthy living in subtle and gradual ways rather than representing radical turning points. Donato observes how chemical and mechanistic ideas of the body led to the attribution of new powers to certain Non-Naturals, those which could be understood through a material lens, rather than undermining their significance for health altogether. Conforti illustrates how in Naples the creation of a 'bricolage' of old and new ideas and theories produced diverse and inconsistent results. She argues that we cannot understand changing ideas about the Non-Naturals by looking only at the evolution of medical thought. Rather, as she shows, new trends in the understanding of nature, and in particular in meteorological, geological and chemical knowledge, had a bearing on how health hazards were defined over time. And in different ways both authors show how broader intellectual developments in the late seventeenth century led to the enhancement of the collective aspect of preventive health care, with a focus on improving the environment for the benefit of the wider public.

Medical authority and preventive lay practice

Chapters in this volume also throw some light on the important issue of the autonomy of the patient in preventive behaviour. While Newton and Astbury point to the similarities between medical advice and the practices adopted by laypeople in their lives, Gage shows that although aware of medical opinions, people put these views to the test and eventually did what, on the basis of their experience, proved to work for them. This independence is particularly noticeable with regard to the air one breathed, since, as the author demonstrates, considerable uncertainty surrounded the possibility of ascertaining whether a certain air was good or bad. At the end of the day therefore, it was individual experience that counted most and dictated for example where people thought it was best for them to live, independently from, or even in contrast with, doctors' advice. This observation provides a balanced answer to the somehow simplistic question, Did people follow medical advice or ignore it? They seem to have taken it very seriously but, precisely as they did with medicinal remedies, they then established what was best for themselves through an empiric approach, by a process of 'trial and error'.

In the case studied by Castiglione the thick circulation of knowledge about healthy pregnancy taking place among wealthy Roman women seems to make doctors' advice superfluous. Indeed the confidence about the soundness of their medical opinions that transpires from these women's letters is striking. And in fact, to judge from a comment by Mercurio in *Errori Popolari*, in Italy 'very rarely, if ever did physicians seek to advise on the care of pregnant women'.[26] These findings and remarks also tie in with the already noted lack, or very limited presence, of specific health advice for pregnant women and for those who wish to conceive in the Italian advice literature of the period.[27] At first sight the suggestion of an absence of actual involvement of medical practitioners in these matters may appear at odds with the picture drawn by

Katharine Park, Monica Green and others: according to these authors women's medicine undergoes a process of masculinisation already in the fifteenth century.[28] The evidence in these studies, however, largely concerns the engagement of male practitioners in gynaecological anomalies, such as menstrual irregularities and infertility, in pregnancy-related ailments and in difficult childbirths. Indeed, these are also the themes extensively covered in the texts by Marinello and Mercurio, the most popular among the few obstetrical treatises published in vernacular in early modern Italy. If we shift attention – as some chapters in this volume do – to other stages of the reproductive process, such as conception, the daily management of pregnancy and the tending of the newborn, we may find that these areas of health concern were not yet medicalised or 'made masculine'. These phases, it was maintained, required a careful regulation of the six Non-Natural spheres of life from which health depends; grounded in daily, domestic routines these activities were controlled by women's networks according to the evidence provided by Castiglione and Astbury, and only benefited from the occasional input of female health professionals – midwives and wet-nurses.

Taken as a whole the essays in this volume heighten our awareness of the crucial, but so far overlooked, role played by the Non-Naturals in the intellectual and social life of the period comprised between the sixteenth and the early eighteenth centuries. They identify territories of health practice that have not received sufficient attention and in which the input of medical practitioners was perhaps particularly marginal and subject to negotiation with the accumulated experience of laypeople. At the same time, by reducing the focus to only two European countries, the volume gives particular emphasis to the neglected question of difference: the comparative lens allows contributors and, we hope, readers, to tease out sometimes subtle, sometimes quite striking differences in approaches to health between different groups, periods and countries.

Notes

1 H. Mikkeli, *Hygiene in the Early Modern Medical Tradition* (Helsinki: Finnish Academy of Science and Letters, 1999); K. Bergdolt, *Wellbeing: A Cultural History of Healthy Living* (Cambridge: Polity Press, 2008).

2 New important works on the experience of illness include H. Newton, *The Sick Child in Early Modern England, 1580–1720* (Oxford: Oxford University Press, 2012); M. Stolberg, *Experiencing Illness and the Sick Body in Early Modern Europe* (London: Palgrave Macmillan, 2011); and O. Weisser, *Ill Composed. Sickness, Gender, and Belief in Early Modern England* (New Haven: Yale University Press, 2015).

3 See for example V.S. Smith, *Clean. A History of Personal Hygiene and Purity* (Oxford: Oxford University Press, 2007); A. Arcangeli, 'Del moto e della quiete. Esercizio e igiene nella prima età moderna', *Medicina e Storia*, 8:1 (2004), pp. 35–55; K. Albala, *Eating Right in the Renaissance* (Berkeley: University of California Press, 2002); D. Gentilcore, *Food and Health in Early Modern Europe. Diet, Medicine and Society 1450–1800* (London: Bloomsbury, 2015); K.H. Dannenfeldt, 'Sleep: theory and practice in the late Renaissance', *The Journal of the History of Medicine and Allied Sciences*, 41:4 (1986), pp. 415–41; E. Carrera (ed.), *Emotions and Health 1200–1700* (Leiden: Brill, 2013).

4 Exceptions to this self-referential approach include S. Shapin, 'How to eat like a gentleman: dietetics and ethics in Early Modern England', in C.E. Rosenberg (ed.), *Right Living: An Anglo-American Tradition of Self-Help Medicine and Hygiene* (Baltimore: Johns Hopkins University Press, 2003), pp. 21–58; A. Wear, 'Making sense of health and the environment in Early Modern England', in A. Wear (ed.), *Medicine in Society: Historical Essays* (Cambridge: Cambridge University Press, 1992), pp. 119–47; idem, 'Place, health and disease: the airs, waters, places tradition in Early Modern England and North America', *Journal of Medieval and Early Modern Studies*, 38 (2008), pp. 443–65; A. Guerrini, 'Health, national character and the English diet in 1700', *Studies in History and Philosophy of Biological and Biomedical Sciences*, 43:2 (2012), pp. 349–56.

5 Mikkeli, *Hygiene*; Bergtold, *Wellbeing*. This approach also characterises more socially oriented works such as Gentilcore, *Food and Health*.

6 See also Arcangeli, 'Del moto'; Carrera, *Emotions*.

7 A. Wear, *Knowledge and Practice in English Medicine* (Cambridge: Cambridge University Press, 2000); idem, 'The prospective colonist and strange environments: advice on health and prosperity', in K. Oslund et al. (eds), *Cultivating the Colony: Colonial States and their Environmental Legacies* (Athens, OH: Ohio University Press, 2011), pp. 19–46; and articles cited in note 4.

8 L. García Ballester, 'On the origins of the "six non-natural things" in Galen', in his *Galen and Galenism* (Aldershot: Ashgate, 2002), pp. 105–15, esp. 107.

9 *Ibid.*; L.J. Rather, 'The "six things non naturals". A note on the origins and fate of a doctrine and a phrase', *Clio Medica*, 3 (1968), pp. 337–47; P.H.

Niebyl, 'The Non-Naturals', *Bulletin of the History of Medicine*, 45 (1971), pp. 486–92; and more recently M. Nicoud, *Les régimes de santé au Moyen Âge: naissance et diffusion d'une écriture médicale (XIIIe–XVe siècle)* (Rome: Ecole Francaise de Rome, 2007).

10 Random examples of their contents are found in P. Gil-Sotres, 'The regimens of health', in M.D. Grmek (ed.), *Western Medical Thought from Antiquity to the Middle Ages* (Cambridge MA: Harvard University Press, 1998), pp. 291–396.

11 See for example, Wear, *Knowledge and Practice*, especially p. 154; P. Slack, 'Mirrors of health and treasures of poor men: the uses of the vernacular medical literature of Tudor England', in C. Webster (ed.), *Health Medicine and Mortality in the Sixteenth Century* (Cambridge: Cambridge University Press, 1979), pp. 238–73, on p. 261; Gentilcore, *Food and Health*, p. 26.

12 For the dissemination of prophylactic concerns in a number of non-medical textual genres (architectural writings, household management handbooks and treatises on children's education or gentlemen's conduct) and their impact on domestic material culture see also S. Cavallo and T. Storey, *Healthy Living in Late Renaissance Italy* (Oxford: Oxford University Press, 2013).

13 This is the case particularly in Italy, where regimens of health are ostensibly directed to the adult male. See Chapter 1 in this collection for a discussion of the gender of readers.

14 The existence of a single humoral understanding of the body in Greek-Roman medicine has recently been challenged by H. King in her 'Female fluids in the Hippocratic corpus. How solid was the humoral body?' in P. Horden and E. Hsu (eds), *The Body in Balance* (New York, Oxford: Berghan, 2013), pp. 25–52.

15 On this literature see, for England, C.A. Bonfield, 'The Regimen Sanitatis and its dissemination in England c. 1348–1550', PhD Thesis, University of East Anglia, 2006; on Italy, Cavallo and Storey, *Healthy Living*, chapter 1.

16 Cavallo and Storey, *Healthy Living*, ch. 4.

17 For England see for example John Jones, *The Arte and Science of Preserving Bodie and Soule in Healthe* (London: Henrie Bynneman, 1579), chapters II–VII, IX; John Ghesel, *Rule of Health* (Cambridge: Printers to the Universitie, 1633), p. 9; H. Brooke, *Ugieine: or Conservatory of Health* (London: R.W., 1650), pp. 143ff.; Thomas Tryon, *A Treatise of Cleanness in Meats and Drinks* (London: Printed for the Author, 1682), p. 13, and texts cited in Chapter 3.

18 Scipione Mercurio, *La Commare o Raccoglitrice* (Milan: G.B. Bidelli, 1618, first. ed. 1595) devotes only four pages (pp. 117–20) to how to preserve the health of a pregnant woman and the foetus before birth. Likewise, Giovanni Marinello's *Le Medicine Partenenti alle Infermitá delle Donne*

(Venice: G. Bonadio, 1563) has three pages on preventive advice (see cc. 214–16). For another text touching on issues of women's health, though in highly disparaging terms, see n. 21 of this chapter. On the marginal remarks on these matters in Italian regimens see Cavallo and Storey, *Healthy Living*, pp. 152–53.

19 For example, in relation to the development of observational practices Pomata talks of the formation of a European scholarly culture in the mid-sixteenth century, made possible by the development of horizontal networks of exchange among scholars based in different countries and engaged with a variety of disciplines. G. Pomata, 'Observation rising: birth of an epistemic genre, 1500–1650', in L. Daston and E. Lunbeck (eds), Histories of Scientific Observation (Chicago: University of Chicago Press, 2011), pp. 45–79; Ian Maclean highlights geographical variation in participation in these networks and the growing importance of confessional divides in the late sixteenth century in his 'The medical republic of letters before the Thirty Years War', *Intellectual History Review*, 18: 1 (2008), pp. 15–30.

20 On this point we are grateful to L. Dacome's enlightening comments to our panel 'Regimens of Health in Early Modern Europe', at Scientiae 2015, Toronto.

21 See the disparaging comments in S. Mercurio, *De gli Errori Popolari d'Italia* (Venice: G.B. Ciotti, 1603), pp. 229–35, 239, 245.

22 Mercurio, *La Commare*, p. 77. See also Mercurio, *De gli Errori Popolari*, pp. 229, 231, 235.

23 On the restrictions on pregnant women's travelling and movement in general see Cavallo and Storey, *Healthy Living*, pp. 153, 169, 173.

24 Indeed mention of the sensitivity of mothers-to-be to smells is also found in written health advice and deserves further attention: for example the use of perfume to conceive male children, to keep the womb and foetus healthy during pregnancy and childbirth is mentioned in Italian treatises. Marinello, *Le Medicine*, pp. 247–48; Mercurio, *La Commare*, pp. 237–38.

25 Cavallo and Storey, *Healthy Living*, ch. 3.

26 '[R]arissime volte, o non mai s'adoprano i medici per consigliar quanto si debba far nella cura delle Donne gravide'; Mercurio, *De gli Errori Popolari*, p. 230.

27 It should be noted that this advice was somehow removed from these kinds of texts precisely in the early modern period. The second book of Michele Savonarola's unpublished manuscript 'De Regimine pregnantium', written in vernacular in the 1460s, was entirely occupied by a 'regimen for pregnant women regarding the six Non-Natural things' – these recommendations occupy more than 20 pages in the modern edition of the text: *Il Trattato Ginecologico-Pediatrico in Volgare: ad Mulieres Ferrarienses de*

Regimine Pregnantium et Noviter Natorum usque ad Septennium, ed. L. Belloni (Milan: Industrie Grafiche Italiane Stucchi, 1952), pp. 65–87. This detailed advice was reduced to two or three pages in later similar treatises.

28 K. Park, *Secrets of Women: Gender, Generation, and the Origins of Human Dissection* (New York: Zone Books, 2006); M. Green, *Making Women's Medicine Masculine: The Rise of Male Authority in Pre-Modern Gynaecology* (Oxford: Oxford University Press, 2008).

I

A comparative perspective on preventive literature

1

Regimens, authors and readers: Italy and England compared

Sandra Cavallo and Tessa Storey

Just as prevention has not been recognised as an important field of medical history, so the specific textual genre that disseminated preventive advice, the vernacular regimen, has attracted little interest. This neglect is an aspect of a more general trend. The focused study of individual forms of early modern medical writing is still in its infancy, especially as works in the vernacular are concerned. While specific typologies of learned and Latinate medical outputs are attracting increasing attention, the distinctive characteristics of various forms of popular medical literature have not yet received the attention they deserve.[1] Certainly the process of popularisation of medicine set in motion by the introduction of print and by an ever-increasing market for vernacular publications has been at the centre of scholarly attention since the 1980s.[2] In this important strand of research, however, a tendency to consider various types of texts all together has prevailed: hence collections of remedies and herbals, midwifery tracts and compilations about specific diseases (plague, venereal, etc.), general self-help books and regimens have been taken as a single object of study, on the grounds that they were all directed to the wider public, rather than exclusively to medical practitioners. Some more specific information about the distinctive characteristics of different forms of vernacular medical literature has emerged from a second strand of research, which looks at these various genres in a comparative perspective.[3] Yet we still lack dedicated studies which engage with the precise chronology, contents and features of each individual genre.[4] In spite of the considerable attention that scholars have paid to recipe books for example, the focus of research has been on their manuscript form, and the study of the printed exemplars on which these often drew has been neglected.[5] This pattern also applies to regimens. Even though prevention is starting to be recognised as an important field of medical history, and these texts are increasingly identified as a precious source, the focus has primarily been on handwritten, personalised regimens rather than on their printed counterparts.[6] Moreover, they are examined for the information they provide about specific dietetic advice rather than for their distinctive characteristics as a genre.[7]

In what follows we would like to apply Pomata's concept of epistemic genre and consider regimens as a discreet form of medical advice literature whose goal is the popularisation of expert recommendations about how to preserve health in everyday life through the correct management of one's lifestyle and, more precisely, of the spheres of activity that medical theory defined as the six Non-Naturals.[8] As Nicoud has demonstrated by reconstructing the formation of the genre over the Middle Ages, when this still took both Latinate and vernacular forms, medieval regimens certainly present distinctive characteristics within the vast field of medical writing.[9] Even if much less is known about the features the genre assumes following the advent of print and the subsequent process of vernacularisation, regimens do maintain a separate identity also in the early modern period. This is especially so by comparison with other vernacular medical genres. For example there is minimal overlap between printed regimens and recipe books, especially in Italy. For example, Ficino's Latin regimen, published in Italian as *De le tre vite* in 1548, is unusual in that it includes a few recipes; likewise the best-selling *Tesoro* by Durante, whilst Auda's very popular *Breve Compendio* contains both a regimen and a collection of recipes, but, significantly, these are presented in two entirely independent sections.[10] In England it was more common to print a regimen with recipes or other medical information appended but, as in Italy, these were generally clearly separated.[11] Moreover, regimens are a genre that looks at the conservation of health not in emergencies but under normal circumstances. They are therefore distinct from plague tracts, a more hybrid genre directed at both protecting the body from an ongoing epidemic and curing the first manifestations of the disease.

In what follows we propose to sketch a first, tentative profile of this genre of health advice literature, with the aim of defining the timeline of the emergence of regimens in printed, vernacular form in Italy and England and of identifying the driving forces behind their rise. Was the popularisation of healthy living advice a product of medical culture or was it rather due to the initiative of printers, translators and professional writers? Do we encounter different patterns in different periods in this respect? We will also pay attention to the social and intellectual profiles of medical authors and to the aims and ambitions which, at some point, turned them into agents of this dissemination of preventive awareness. Finally, we will address the question of who these texts were directed to, both in gender and social terms, and of whether the declared intended readership can be taken as an indication of actual readership. Our underlying question throughout this investigation concerns the extent to which we can identify similar patterns in the chronology, authorship, aims and readerships of regimens in Italy and England. To what extent was the popularisation of preventive advice drawing on a common preventive paradigm in the two countries? In other words, can we talk of shared models of healthy living, at the European level, and of an unrestrained circulation of ideas of healthy conduct?

Translations, adaptations and the role of the print industry: the first phase of publishing

Striking similarities characterise the first wave of publications of vernacular regimens in England and Italy. In both countries these first appeared in print in the 1480s, while others followed in the first decade of the sixteenth century. But the analogies are not limited to chronology. They extend to the nature of these publications and the agents behind them. The print industry had a key role in the process, as they capitalised on a ready-formed readership avid for preventive health advice in the local language well before any physicians were involved.[12] For example in England the earliest printed vernacular advice books on healthy living, *The Governayle of Helth* and *Dyctary of Ghostly Helth*, had already been circulating in manuscript form before being printed by Caxton and Wynkyn de Worde between 1498 and 1530, and appeared with no attributions of authorship or claims to medical authority amongst them.[13] Moreover, in both countries publishing was dominated by translations or new editions of classical and medieval health advice texts in this phase, possibly because, as has been suggested, it was far cheaper than commissioning new books.[14]

The role played by publishers and translators is clarified for us in the account of an exchange between the publisher Thomas Berthelet, and the translator Thomas Paynell. Paynell reports that Berthelet had asked him to translate Von Hutton's treatise on the French Disease for him, on the grounds that it was 'nedefull and now beneficiall to the common welth' at a time when the disease was ravaging Europe.[15] Berthelet also told Paynell that his 1528 translation of the *Regimen Sanitatis* had been selling well, and that 'in his mynde it was a boke moche necessarye, and very profitable', suggesting that Berthelet was keeping his eye firmly on the market and may well have prompted Paynell to translate the *Regimen Sanitatis Salerni* in the first place.

In Italy too, the establishment of this distinct medical genre is not to be seen as an expression of professional medical culture but as the results of the efforts of a range of commercial agents who sensed the existence of a receptive terrain for preventive writing in the vernacular, and pursued well-thought-out publishing strategies. However, things were slightly more complicated than in England since the trend for translations and adaptations of ancient and medieval regimens does seem in reality to have been triggered by a doctor, Girolamo Manfredi, whose text *Il Perché* (1474) went through twenty-seven Italian editions between 1474 and 1678 as well as five in Catalan and Spanish.[16]

This said, the immediate popularity of Manfredi's text was certainly boosted by his fame as an astrologer and author of prognostications as well as his name as a doctor. Moreover, the fact that the book catered for a range of interests was certainly a selling point: Book I was a didactic compendium on the preservation of health, Book II included curiosities such as the humoral characteristics of various foodstuffs, climates, the physiology of various parts of the body, physiognomy and palmistry. Undoubtedly however, the success of the text also derived from being presented as a translation of what was regarded at the time as an Aristotelian text, the *Problemata*.

In this and other respects Book I of Manfredi's compendium represented a prototype for the publications that followed. These continued to exploit the appeal of celebrity names of the past to impress and attract readers, sometimes even resorting to false attributions. Hence the second regimen to be published in the vernacular, the *Tractato Utilissimo* (1481), was attributed to the renowned doctor Ugo Benzi, university professor and personal physician of the Este family, although in reality it was the translation of a Latin regimen by Benedetto Reguardati, a less distinguished physician, slightly older than Benzi.[17] The trick was repeated in 1549, when a regimen written in the fourteenth century by doctor Maino de' Maineri appeared in Italian as the work of the better-known, to the wider public, Arnald of Villanova.[18] Similar strategies were used in England too. Berthelet's 1528 edition of the *Regimen Sanitatis* is attributed to Joannes of Milan and the commentary on it to Arnald of Villanova.

In Italy, Arnald's fame was also exploited in publications which, following again in Manfredi's footsteps, combined two texts either on adjacent topics or directed to slightly different readerships. In 1550, the translation of the regimen by the German doctor Pictorius, presented in the learned form of the dialogue, was printed together with a plain and more widely accessible treatise on how to prolong life, attributed precisely to Arnald of Villanova.[19]

The policy of capitalising on the celebrity status of prominent figures of the past is also evident in the posthumous publication (1508) of a regimen by the renown fifteenth-century doctor Michele Savonarola, and then in the translation of the guide to healthy living written, also in the fifteenth century, by Marsilio Ficino, 'the principal philosopher of the time' – as the publisher Tramezzino boasted in the dedication (1548).[20] A year later the same publisher turned to an even more legendary medical authority, promoting the translation of Galen's *De Sanitate Tuenda*, under the title *Di Galeno*, while in 1538 the pseudo-Aristotelian text *Secreta Secretorum* had already appeared under the title *Col Nome di Dio*, translated and adapted by Giovanni Manente, a merchant and broker who described himself as 'a philosopher by inclination rather than training'.[21] A version of this text had also been printed in English in 1528 and English translations of Plutarch's *The Governaunce of Good Helth* appeared in the 1540s and 1555.[22] For several decades, therefore, preventive medical publishing was in the hands of printers, booksellers, and professional or even amateur translators such as Manente. Rather than simply rendering classical and late medieval texts in the vernacular these men often reduced, summarised and adapted the text to the modern reader.[23]

Newly authored regimens and the identity of medical authors

In Italy we have to wait until the 1550s to encounter the first newly authored regimen, written by doctor Tommaso Rangoni, a shrewd market operator in the publishing world.[24] A graduate in arts and medicine, Tommaso initially built a reputation for himself as an astrologer before refashioning himself as erudite natural philosopher, humanist scholar and physician. Already well acquainted with the Venetian print industry, which for years had published his predictions, he then turned to medical publishing.

He published two quite similar health guides, choosing titles which evoked the time-honoured textual traditions of *retardanda* and *consilia*: *De vita hominis ultra CXX annos protrahenda* (How men can live 120 years or more), a work with many Venetian references, which includes recipes as well as advice on how to prolong life, and *De vita principis et venetorum commoda semper consilium* on how Venetians, in particular, could for ever live healthy.[25] The novelty of the approach, that is the fact of focusing in particular on the health of the Venetians, clearly made his work more appealing to local readers than the existing good-for-all guides to healthy living, and was probably key to its success. Indeed each text had six Latin and vernacular re-editions, all during the life of the author, suggesting that Rangoni himself might have actively promoted his works.

To cater for a more varied audience the re-editions were drastically reduced versions of the original texts: for example the *De vita hominis*, initially a dense text in Latin in 4° and 120 pages long, was reduced to 8° format and to 80 pages in the first vernacular translation, and then further abbreviated to just sixteen pages in the subsequent editions.[26] So the role of publishers, and the importance of adopting shrewd marketing strategies was just as important even when it came to regimens published by doctors.

It was only after the publication of Rangoni's texts in 1556 that newly authored regimens completely took over from translations in Italy.[27] In England this shift to a second phase of publications, based on new regimens, emerged earlier, with the publication of Thomas Elyot's *The*

Castel of Helth in 1534.[28] Elyot was a government official, diplomat, humanist scholar and prolific translator. By 1546 he had published at least fourteen books with the astute publisher Thomas Berthelet and it is quite possible that the latter actively encouraged Elyot to write his *Castel of Helth,* since he went on to reprint it at least six times within the next thirty years.[29]

Judging from the attacks made on Elyot, physicians were clearly piqued that such a successful volume should have been written by a non-medical man and others soon started to capitalise on the success of the genre – even to the extent of printing collections of remedies but under the title of a regimen or dietary as if this would help sales.[30] By 1634 at least nine actual English regimens had appeared, overwhelmingly written by physicians, and one regimen by an exiled Italian Protestant physician, Guglielmo Grataroli, had been translated into English.[31] This appropriation of the genre by practising physicians was even more radical in Italy, where, after 1565, the close correspondence between authors and medical doctors persisted until the decline of the genre more than a century later.[32] This differs from England where, from the 1630s, a third phase of publications including several translations takes place and the identity of authors becomes again quite varied.

In both countries, however, what is striking is the large number of provincial doctors with a good local reputation amongst our authors. If we take the authors of these middle-period regimens in England we find that William Bullein practised medicine in Northumberland, Durham and only later in London. Thomas Cogan was a physician who practised in the Manchester area whilst Tobias Venner was a physician based at the fashionable spas in Bath and James Hart was a puritan physician who practised successfully in Northamptonshire. The exceptions were Christopher Langton and Thomas Moffett in that they were based in London, whilst Andrew Boorde lived in so many places in England and Europe that he defies categorisation.

In Italy, too, the protagonists of the popularisation of health advice are by and large modest figures like Boldo, a doctor in Pralboino, near Brescia, Camaffi in Perugia, Gallina in the little town of Carmagnola. Often, the vernacular regimen represents these physicians' only published work. Some authors had experience of publishing but, remarkably, not in the medical sector, rather it would seem that, as local erudites, these doctors constructed their intellectual status through a wide engagement with the humanities.[33] For others the regimen is one of two medical publications, the other being a plague tract, as in the case of Traffichetti, active in the Romagna region and Rimini, Viviano Viviani, in Venice, and Frediano, doctor in Lucca. By contrast, the most prominent and widely published physicians of the day, such as Gerolamo Cardano and Alessandro Petronio, were still hindered by the stigma attached to publishing in the vernacular and continued to compile their regimens in Latin.

The rise of the vernacular regimen as a printed genre seems therefore to offer locally known doctors an opportunity to fulfil their ambition to become a published medical author. However, as we will see later, their dedications also reveal their eagerness to cultivate a reputation as knowledgeable and disinterested advisors, promoting the well-being of the public. Significantly, a number of these authors (Camaffi, Durante, Bertaldi, Galeano, Ciccolini) were also counselors to local authorities in issues of public health, and were therefore particularly sensitive to the importance of preventive measures. Some clearly embraced the new fashion for environmental medicine and compiled specific studies of the air of the city in which they lived (Rangoni, Bruno).

It is worth underlining, therefore, that we do not owe the dissemination of healthy living principles among the population to men who enjoyed an international reputation through their works in Latin. Rather, it was the modest local doctor, strongly engaged with the medical and non-medical affairs of the community, and with local prestige to defend and boost who performed this role. The focus on regimens allows a rare insight into the neglected but important part played by practitioners who did not belong to the better-studied elite of the profession and did not leave significant medical writings.

In spite of the modest medical profile of these authors, some of their regimens enjoyed considerable publishing success. Not surprisingly, the texts most frequently re-edited were those which conveyed the information in the most accessible manner, not just in terms of prose and structure, but of layout of the page. In this endeavour the authors were assisted by creative printers who devised innovative typographical features for these texts, as in the cases of the bestselling treatise on healthy food by Pisanelli and of Durante's regimen.[34] This brings us back therefore to the role of the print industry, key not just to the establishment of the genre but to the extraordinary success of some of its later examples.

Among the strategies employed by English publishers and authors was that of publishing the regimen together with another medical text – often dedicated to the sick rather than the healthy. Presumably they were hoping thereby to extend their hold on the market, possibly also by imitating Elyot's example, given that he too had included similar extra sections in his *Castel*. Thus William Bullein placed a lengthy section on the use of medicinal plants in his *Government of Health* (1559) and his *Diet for Health* (1585) appeared in a volume primarily dedicated to the use of medicinal balsams, whilst in his *Bulwark* (1562) there are sections on anatomy, the treatment of wounds and on the making of medicinal compounds. Moreover, he generally adopted an accessible, usually dialogic format. Several decades later Ghesel's regimen was printed alongside a separate section on bloodletting, and James Hart's *Klinike* is actually composed of separate treatises, one being a regimen for the sick and another a lengthy section on bloodletting. The Italians were even more creative: in 1560, a short regimen by the Flemish doctor Robert Grospre', simplified in content and reduced to only seventeen pages of the original Latin version, was appended to a work on table service and the medicinal properties of different foodstuffs by the papal *scalco* (steward) Romoli.[35]

National differences

We find striking differences in the trajectories and character of the published preventive health advice between the two countries. In Italy, in the second half of the seventeenth century the genre seems to have been running out of steam as only one new tract was published after 1656 and after the 1670s re-editions of existing regimens were also very rare.[36] By contrast, the English public seems to have retained a keen interest in preventive approaches right up until the eighteenth century.[37] Four new regimens were published after 1650, two of which were reprinted several times; two new translations of older ones appeared, and many health advice tracts by Thomas Tyron were published.

Another distinctive characteristic of English regimens was that several were published by non-medical men, such as the philosopher Francis Bacon (1638), the priest Edmund Gayton (1659) and the mystic Thomas Tryon.[38] Indeed, a marked religious component appears to have found particular favour with English readers right from the early sixteenth century – and many of the authors or translators of regimens which were popular in England either had formal ties with the church at some point in their career, or were deeply religious men. Thomas Paynell had been Canon of Merton Priory; Boorde became a Carthusian monk; Bullein was a rector; Grataroli was an exiled convert to Protestantism and his translator, Newton, was also a rector whilst Hart was a staunch Puritan. Moreover two key translations, which appeared together in 1634, were of deeply moralising texts. And, as storey shows in her chapter, these proved to be particularly successful in England. These were: the *Hygiasticon* by the Flemish Jesuit Leonardo Lessius and *On the Sober Life*, by the Italian gentleman Alvise Cornaro. Moreover, Cogan authored devotional literature, William Vaughan was famed for his religious poetry and Thomas Tryon was a fervent religious mystic. In Italy, by contrast, the genre remained dominated by doctors until its decline, and we do not encounter non-professional authors or churchmen, except very marginally in the role of translators.[39] Presumably, only qualified, practising doctors are seen as authoritative enough to provide medical advice in Italy, a fact that is likely to reflect the higher professional status enjoyed by physicians in the peninsula, while in England medicine does not appear to be the domain of the specialist to the same extent.

Why the regimen should have declined so abruptly in Italy, however, has not yet been fully explained. Donato's chapter explores some of the circumstances surrounding this decline, in particular the lessening importance of the individual in medicine against the background of an increasing emphasis on the importance of public health measures, and the creation of a salubrious overall environment. We also offer some tentative explanations in our book: we attribute this trend to market saturation but also to a less preventive attitude to health maintenance. This is perhaps supported by the comments of the physician Bernardino Ramazzini (himself the author of a Latin regimen), that printers no longer wished to invest in these kinds of books, since doctors were mere inclined to cure rather than to prevent disease,[40] but also to a demise of the holistic idea of health. Regimens which covered all the six Non-Naturals were in fact replaced by works which explored the effects of single substances on health (water, tobacco, acquavite, coffee, etc.).[41]

One question which arises out of this comparative study is whether the regimen developed along similar lines in both Italy and England once the vernacular genre was established and to what extent, if any, there was a continued influence from Italy. We have already noted some variations in chronology and at the level of authors' professional and intellectual identity. As will appear evident in the chapter by Storey, there are also considerable differences in content in English regimens. These national differences may therefore go some way towards explaining why, apart from Cornaro's moralising tract, only one Italian regimen proper (the *Treasury of Health* by Castore Durante) was translated into English, a century after its original publication, and why relatively few regimens by Italians (whether in Latin or Italian) appear to have circulated in England. This is judging by the preliminary findings from the examination of a few extant inventories of a London bookseller and library catalogues.[42]

It would seem the principal explanation for the relative lack of interest in Italian regimens in England must lie partly with religious antipathy and partly with the continued importance of Latin as the language of medical authority at the same time as large numbers of Latin medical texts were being imported into the country.[43] Indeed, this impression of the relative insignificance of Italian authors in English vernacular discussions of dietetics is reinforced within the texts themselves, since we find barely any references to Italian doctors as against repeated citations of the French physician Jean Fernel (d. 1558), the German Leonard Fuchs (d. 1566) and the Swiss Conrad Gesner (d. 1565). Not by accident, the only significant references to Italian works were to the Latin regimens by Ficino, by Cardano and to Mercuriale's work on exercise.[44]

In any case the limited circulation of regimens between the two countries suggests that not all knowledge was exchanged in early modern Europe. As the chapter by Storey will further illustrate, environmental, cultural and religious factors meant that there were specific trajectories and pathways along which books and knowledge moved or did not move. We will see that priorities were different in the two countries with regard to how health should be maintained, and this made the advice literature produced in England and Italy largely incompatible.

Aims and intended readership

The declared aim of both Italian and English regimens was to popularise preventive advice and empower laypeople to 'learn the principles' of medicine, 'know about health ... and conserve it'.[45] The use of the vernacular, the simplified prose compared to that found in treatises directed to medical professionals and the clearly organised text were the means employed to reach this objective, though there were also national variations. We see these intentions expressed in prologues and dedications, which represent 'the book's presentation of itself' in Mary Fissell's words.[46]

Writing in the vernacular rather than in Latin was certainly central to Elyot's project. He defends his decision with an implicit challenge to other authors, when he notes that the 'panimes [Muslims] and Jewes' in ancient times had written in 'their own propre and own maternal tongues', thereby making their medical knowledge accessible to all. Compared to English physicians, who wrote in Latin, he declared that in 'this parte of charitye they farre surmountid us Christianes'.[47] However, it should also be noted that Elyot was not a physician. For medical authors, the shift from Latin to the vernacular was perhaps a more tortuous process, as it meant renouncing an important component of professional prestige. Indeed, extensive sections of the first edition of Thomas Cogan's *Haven of Health* were Latin citations of medical authorities – presumably left in Latin to demonstrate his medical authority. However, in the preface to the second edition (1589) he notes that he has now translated these into English at 'the importunate request of diverse of my frendes, which being no good latinists could not welle wade in the reading of my book, by reason of much Latin'.[48] The appropriateness of publishing a regimen in vernacular is also the key issue in the controversy which develops in print in 1565 between two minor Italian doctors.[49]

In the preface to the second edition of Elyot's *Castel* we find not only a defence of the vernacular form, but also evidence of 'the pastoral and charitable purposes of medical translation' that Faye Getz has already identified as integral to medieval English medical texts.[50] Indeed, Elyot declared that his 'labours' were 'without hope of temporall reward, onely for the fervent affection whyche I have ever borne toward the publikye weale of my countrey'.[51] Moreover the notion of serving the 'common-weal', rooted in Christian civic humanism, was seized upon by English Protestants and much used in subsequent regimens to justify their use of the vernacular in medical publishing.[52] These ideals were also a driving force for later authors and publishers. For example the preface to Bullein's 1562 *Bulwarke* reads, 'And I beyng a childe of the common wealthe, am bounde unto my mother, that is, the lande, in whom I am borne; to ... use his gifts not to instructe the learned but to helpe the ignoraunt, that thei meaie resort to this little Bulwarke.'[53]

These religious, charitable and political implications which are found also in Spanish vernacular health advice literature are by contrast completely absent from Italian regimens.[54] Here the value of the service these authors render to their patron and readers by summarising, reordering, correcting and updating ancient and modern medical opinions is articulated in secular terms. Traffichetti's regimen is dedicated to the local lord but inspired by the desire to 'donate to the world' a work, which, he hopes, will be useful to many, since no one else has 'treated these matters in such a clear, well-ordered and essential manner'.[55] Viviani observes that many texts are unnecessarily detailed, tedious and obscure for the non-professional and promises to avoid any academic disputes.[56] Similarly, the Italian translation of Fonseca's regimen stresses the accessibility of his text, which is written 'for those engaged in whatsoever profession'.[57] Razzi explains why his translation and reorganisation of the Schola salernitana is beneficial: the information related to the same matter is no longer scattered in various parts of the text but collated in one place; the book can now easily be searched thanks to the alphabetical index of matters and, as a result, it can now be accessed by all those who can read, including women, and not just by those who know Latin.[58] These texts are depicted as comprehensive but brief, cast in accessible prose and clearly organised.

In his preface Viviani also stresses the convenience of the portable format of his text, so small that it can be carried in one's pocket and be consulted in any circumstance. Indeed the 8° format, or even the smaller 12° or 16°, is a key feature of Italian vernacular regimens.[59] Many of them were also quite slim volumes. However, this is not quite as true for England as it was for Italy.[60] Whilst several regimens were printed in either 12° or 8°, all of Berthelet's editions of Paynell's *Regimen Sanitatis* were in 4°, editions of Elyot's *Castel* alternated between 8vo and 4°, and some such as Bullein's *Bulwarke* and Hart's *Klinike* were very long and in folio – suggesting quite a different readership. However, this starts changing in what we have defined as the 'third' phase of publishing in England (from the mid-1630s onwards), when regimens by all appeared in more truly 'pocket' editions in 8vo or 12°, suggesting that they were now aimed at a wider readerships.

In Italy the smaller size seems to have been thought more appropriate in particular to women readers. In 1556, the Italian edition of Rangoni's *De vita hominis* was said to be published in 8vo format precisely to appeal to women. Other regimens (Durante, Salando) were dedicated to women patrons and implied a female readership, an aspiration explained by Durante on the ground that women will in this way not only learn the rule of healthy living for their own sake but become capable of assisting physicians in maintaining the health of other members of the family.[61] The assumption that women would play a central role in overseeing the diet and health regimens not just of children but of men is made even clearer in some later English texts. Certainly it is women who are blamed for the ill health not just of infants but of adult men. Maynwaring argues that the 'tender bodies [of infants] are soon discomposed and disordered by bad nurses, their erroneaous customes and the ill properties of their milk', whilst Thomas Tryon states that 'The whole preservation of men's health and strength does chiefly reside in the wisdom and temperance of women.'[62] Indeed, he goes further, arguing that 'As women are our nurses for fifteen or sixteen years', it is they who establish the pattern for later life, and their fault if men develop bad habits subsequently.[63] Paradoxically therefore, it is implicitly expected that women will read these books, or at least will be aware of their contents for the preservation of the health of the family even though, to honour the gender hierarchy, the advice contained in regimens is not explicitly directed to women. One would expect that women were at least the main recipients of advice specifically concerning pregnancy and infant health. However, even texts which consider women's health among their topics, such as, in Italy, Mercurio's *Degli errori popolari* (which devotes an entire section, Book V, to it), is directed to men and heads of households 'who know how important it is and must with reason and persuasion make them [women] see the common danger they are running', since women, especially if young, 'lack good judgement and have little sense'.[64]

In sum, vernacular regimens imply that women are less competent readers than men, and in any case are in constant need of male supervision in their role as health-carers, but not that they cannot read. This raises the question of precisely who could and did read vernacular regimens. The social and gender composition of early modern readerships is, however, a puzzling issue which historians have confronted extensively.[65] Certainly severe class and gender biases affected levels of literacy and big discrepancies also existed between the situation in cities and in the countryside, so generalisations about levels of literacy are difficult. But literacy is also hard to ascertain since, among the lower classes, the ability to read was often independent from that of writing. Given that children in schools were first taught to read and only later to write those who stopped their education early never acquired writing skills. For some time, moreover, while reading skills were encouraged in girls also for devotional purposes the ability to write was deliberately seen as not desirable in a woman. These considerations shed considerable doubts on earlier attempts at assessing literacy based on the ability to sign, which have often provided a rather pessimistic picture.

The possibility of extracting helpful information from a text might also have been more widespread than previously believed. The opposition literate–illiterate now appears simplistic and it seems more appropriate to talk of levels of literacy. There were ways of accessing the contents of a text other than reading: texts were read aloud to groups made up of people with unequal literacy skills or even completely illiterate; the information then circulated orally and could be memorised also by those who could not read.[66] Many households did themselves encompass unequal reading skills, being made up of the better-educated masters and men, and of women, children and servants who had received a more patchy and basic education.

There were therefore several channels through which preventive advice could be disseminated, but certainly it was regarded as important to convey this to various categories of people. This included the younger generation, judging from the suggestion by the editor of the *Secrets of Secrets* (1528), that the text could be ideal for teaching children to learn to read.[67] Likewise, in Italy we find that conduct books for school pupils recommend that passages from Ficino's regimen be read every day – some even include a summary of the main precepts of healthy living. Clearly, these were regarded as useful to absorb from an early age.[68]

Insights into the social connotation of the readers of regimens can be also gleaned from the latter's declared intentions. While Italian regimens remain unspecific about their public, except for rare references to women, some English regimens explicitly address the issue. The subtitle of Paynell's 1528 translation of the *Regimen Sanitatis Salerni* reads, 'this boke techyng al people to Governe them in Helthe'. Half a century later Cogan points out that his approach will be easier for the 'dull' of understanding, although he notes subsequently, 'So I write not these precepts for laboring men, but for students, and such, as through they be no students, doe yet follow the order and diet of students.'[69] This exclusion of the lower orders seems to be re-proposed by Venner in the preface to the second part of his popular regimen *Via Recta* (1623). He addresses his

> generous and religious readers; to you have I heretofore written my Via Recta ... not to rustickes, or men of vile and rusticke quality, who ... respect nothing lesse than the welfare of their bodies; nor to any prophane or seeming religious patron ... but to you that are religious and truly generous, that maintaine your blood and reputations by your noble and vertuous lives.[70]

The references to generosity, religiosity and virtue show, however, that the quote is not to be read in exclusively social terms, as drawing an opposition between classes, but in moral terms: only the pious and civil man is regarded as being capable of taking care of his health. These moral overtones are even amplified in Italian texts, where health awareness is depicted as a sign of true 'nobility', an attribute not to be taken literally, as referring to a legal status defined by birth and pedigree, but as a civil way of life in which intelligence, rationality and the ability to control oneself and one's subordinates figure highly. Indeed conduct books for the correct management of the household increasingly portray the health of all its members as the responsibility of the head of household.[71] In Italy, however, these qualities are articulated in exclusively secular terms, with an additional emphasis both on the practical advantages for men who are expected to take part in the running of the city or state and on the savings made by a healthy family. Apart from the occasional comment that health is a gift of God and therefore is particularly worth preserving, no association is established between health and piety in Italian writings.

Actual readers

A more tangible indication of the social composition of readers of regimens is provided by their presence in private libraries and by the signatures of ownership found on some exemplars preserved in libraries. This is again an imperfect clue, since access to preventive vernacular texts and ownership often did not coincide: for example, various members of a household could access the same text; moreover, books were frequently exchanged, lent and even owned collectively.[72] Hence the social fruition of a book was much larger than what single ownership would suggest. Yet the evidence from these indicators is still useful since it dispels the idea, often found among commentators, that preventive concerns were limited to the elite. Andrew Wear, for example, talks of 'the luxury end of medicine' in relation to the fruition of printed health advice, re-proposing the often repeated argument that 'Choice of diet and lifestyle was restricted to those who had the means to make choices.'[73] This would imply that readers of this kind of texts were only the cultivated and the upper classes. In reality the evidence from Italy points to a large readership, which certainly includes the middling sort. For sure there is a strong urban connotation, as owners of regimens tend to be based in cities, but these can also be small provincial towns such as Saluzzo or Rivalta Scrivia. In terms of occupation, professionals (lawyers, notaries, physicians and apothecaries), local administrators, monks and parish priests are highly represented, though noblemen like members of the Giustiniani and Spada Roman families are also present.[74] But so are men who sign their name without adding any title or position; and given that it was customary to do so, we infer that they belonged to that multitude of shopkeepers, low traders or artisans that constituted the urban middling sort.[75] The well-developed system of primary schools in Northern and Central Italian city states and the consequent high level of literacy among the Italian urban classes in the Renaissance, may explain this phenomenon, which also accounts for the numerous diaries, chronicles and autobiographies authored by humble artisans already in the late fifteenth and early sixteenth centuries.[76] The early introduction of the vernacular as the language of administration and official deeds in these regions was another factor which contributed to promote popular literacy. Moreover, from the late sixteenth century, the diffusion of catechism schools made elementary education widespread, even for girls.[77]

In England we do not dispose of comparable evidence on the ownership of regimens in particular, as studies on the subject have focused on vernacular medical texts in a more undifferentiated way, with an emphasis on the early sixteenth century, certainly before 1560.[78] Like Wear, Slack postulates a readership of the 'leisured elite' for vernacular medical books in general, and considers it unlikely that readers included many of the 'middle sort', that is the increasingly literate tradesmen and yeomen.[79] Successive discussions of regimens have uncritically repeated these assumptions.[80] However, if the readership of regimens was limited to the upper ranks of society, why would there be so much insistence on reaching out to those with little education? The title of Bullein's *Governement of Health* (1559), for example, contains the words, 'Reduced into the forme of a dialogue for the better understanding of the unlearned'; where 'unlearned' may refer particularly to those who did not understand Latin, as in Cogan's friends cited above.[81] As we have seen, Italian regimens, although not explicitly mentioning those with low levels of education, also refer to the unprofessional and those who cannot read Latin.

As indirectly suggested by Bullein, the extent to which these texts could be considered 'popular' can also be inferred by the literary form chosen by the authors.[82] Certainly, the dialogue form used by Bullein in England and, in Italy, by the translation of Pictorius, and even more the question and answer format adopted by the highly successful *Il Perché* and in England by *A Help to Discourse*, denote texts that were trying to cater for a relatively wide audience, not used to reading long stretches of text but increasingly familiar with the concise, factual information contained in 'how-to' books on all sorts of subjects.[83] Indeed, the thirst for detailed advice about healthy living should be understood as an aspect of the changing purposes of reading, which increasingly included technical and practical instruction. This explains the popularity of texts such as *A Help to Discourse*, a publisher's compilation which included questions on preventive health conduct sandwiched between jokes, riddles, poetry, a yearly 'oracle', advice on farming and in later editions, advice on cookery.[84] The presence of quotations in Latin and references to famous doctors or philosophers could actually be seen as a device aimed at reinforcing the credentials of the author and the authority of the text rather than as a sign of a selected readership that could read Latin and had direct knowledge of the writings of Aristotle or Galen.[85] The regimen genre therefore consciously offered readers a range of choices tailored for people of different social background and education, acknowledging in this way the existence of a composite readership.

Physical characteristics such as the size and the typographical features of the book also deserve more attention as indications of an extending readership. The simplified paratextual apparatus employed by many texts, such as numbering the points within each chapter, and then discussing each of them in a very short paragraph, the inclusion of indexes and short subheadings in the margins to make the text searchable, and in general the structured narrative and clear layout of the page were another way of rendering the text accessible to many.[86] In both countries, however, the regimens more likely to appeal to the lower end of the social scale, and perhaps even to the illiterate, were those expressed in easy-to-memorise verses, like the various alleged translations of the *Regimen Sanitatis Salernitanum*. In other cases the rules of healthy living were in prose but condensed in a really short pamphlet, which, being only few sheets long, could also be bought and read unbound. These cheap texts adopt what looks to us like a truly 'popular' guise, presenting purely prescriptive instructions in no particular order and without offering any rationale for their precepts.[87]

However, short, oversimplified pamphlets, rarely stood alone, certainly in Italy. This phenomenon of appending regimens ostensibly suitable for basic levels of literacy or for reading aloud to others, to a more demanding text, suggests a multiple and mixed readership of the same volume, perhaps coexisting in the same household, and different reading practices.[88] Moreover, as Grendler has suggested, even more competent readers were avid consumers of 'popular' literature.[89]

These observations invite us to abstain from attempting to establish an exclusive social characterisation for readers of regimens. The number of editions of these texts speaks volumes of their unquestionably broad success: in Italy the bestsellers (Manfredi, Pisanelli and Durante) were reissued twenty-three, twenty-eight and thirty-four times, respectively, up to the 1670s. In England Elyot and the various versions of the Salernitan Rules and *A Help to Discourse* were the main medical bestsellers amongst popular books until the late seventeenth century, with seventeen editions for Elyot and at least nineteen for the other two.[90] The English 'bestsellers' therefore went through significantly fewer editions than their Italian counterparts but, by way of compensation, interest in the genre was longer lived than in Italy.

Conclusion

This comparative analysis of the vernacular regimen has revealed both similarities and differences in its development as a distinctive genre in England and Italy. We might consider the period between the 1470s and 1550s as being an 'emergent' phase for the printed regimen, not yet characterised by the 'standardized textual format' that Pomata posits as a characteristic in her description of the 'epistemic genre'.[91] However, once authorship by physicians had become the norm in the mid-sixteenth century, 'recognisable conventions' of format, style and content were established.[92] In addition to the distinctive focus on prevention and lifestyle, one of the most significant conventions was that generally each chapter or section of the regimen was devoted to one of the Non-Naturals. And despite the occasional discussion about which of these was most important (with Air generally winning the argument, at least in Italy), at the heart of the advice was an emphasis on how to ensure the correct interaction as well as balance of these different spheres of daily life so as to guarantee good health. In this context it should be noted that regimens are sometimes erroneously conflated by scholars with dietary tracts, perhaps because the section on eating and drinking is longer than those devoted to the other Non-Naturals.[93] However, this was not in itself a sign that diet was regarded as the most important element in a healthy life, simply another standard feature of the regimen was the tendency to include a catalogue-style assessment of the qualities of each foodstuff and this was inevitably lengthy. In reality the correct management of diet could hardly be disentangled from that of sleep, exercise and evacuations since a healthy diet depended not just on the quantity and quality of foodstuffs but on the timing of eating in relation precisely to these other activities and on their quality.

Whilst these formal conventions largely persist in Italy through the seventeenth century, in England after the 1630s a split developed, perhaps thanks to the success of Cornaro and Lessius's moralising tracts. Thus whilst some texts remained faithful to the conventions of the genre, others started to focus more or less exclusively on dietary advice – though these can no longer be considered as traditional 'regimens'.

Pomata also observed that the 'epistemic genre' should be seen as a 'social', collective scholarly endeavour to which different authors contributed and this was also true of many of the vernacular regimens penned by physicians.[94] Such authors often offered their own perspectives to this body of knowledge; adding nuance and new insights to what was recognised as a fairly standard series of topics and principles. They were updating these issues with reference to their own experience as practitioners, responding to contemporary, even local events (such as the death of a local notable induced by his or her unhealthy lifestyle), to fashionable trends but also incorporating new concerns in philosophical and medical inquiry, as we will see. This engagement and dialogue with the present presumably contributed to its wide appeal in both Italy and England.

In both countries the vernacular regimen was a genre produced largely by relatively obscure provincial physicians in tandem with a publishing industry eager to capitalise on a public hungry for information on preventive health. The contents of these texts circulated widely and were appropriated through a myriad of other oral or literary forms, thereby contributing to reinforce the culture of prevention that, as the remaining chapters in this volume document, pervaded many spheres of early modern life.

Notes

1 For examples of interest in specific forms of medical writing see G. Pomata's work on case histories, 'Sharing cases: the *Observationes* in Early Modern medicine', *Early Science and Medicine*, 15:3 (2010), pp. 193–236; on published collections of medical letters, N. Siraisi, *Communities of Learned Experience: Epistolary Medicine in the Renaissance* (Baltimore: Johns Hopkins University Press, 2014).

2 For discussions of vernacular medical publishing in England see P. Slack, 'Mirrors of health and treasures of poor men: the uses of the vernacular medical literature of Tudor England', in C. Webster (ed.), *Health Medicine and Mortality in the Sixteenth Century* (Cambridge: Cambridge University

Press, 1979), pp. 238–73; A. Wear, 'The popularization of medicine in Early Modern England', in R. Porter (ed.), *The Popularisation of Medicine 1650–1850* (London: Routledge, 1992), pp. 17–41; E. Lane Furdell, *Publishing and Medicine in Early Modern England* (Rochester, NY: University of Rochester Press, 2002), and works cited in note 3. For Spain, M. Solomon, *Fictions of Well-Being. Sickly Readers and Vernacular Medical Writing in Late Medieval and Early Modern Spain* (Philadelphia: Penn Press, 2010). For Italy we still miss similar analyses of vernacular medical writings.

3 In particular M. Fissell, 'The marketplace of print', in M.R.S. Jenner and P. Wallis (eds), *Medicine and the Market in England and Its Colonies* (Basingstoke: Palgrave Macmillan, 2007), pp. 108–32; 'Popular medical writing', in J. Raymond (ed.), *The Oxford History of Popular Print Culture*, vol. 1: *Cheap Print in Britain and Ireland to 1660* (Oxford: Oxford University Press, 2011), pp. 418–31; I. Taavitsainen and P. Pahta (eds), *Early Modern English Medical Texts: Corpus Description and Studies* (Amsterdam and Philadelphia: John Benjamins, 2010).

4 An exception is represented by work on herbals. See A. Arbor, *Herbals. Their Origin and Evolution. A Chapter in the History of Botany 1470–1670* (Cambridge: Cambridge University Press, 1986); R. Laroche, *Medical Authority and Englishwomen's Herbal Texts 1550–1650* (Aldershot: Ashgate, 2009); B. Elliott, 'The world of the Renaissance herbal', *Renaissance Studies*, 25:1 (2011). Work on Italian herbals has focused on individual examples rather than on the genre as a whole.

5 Printed recipe books tend to be discussed in the wider contexts of books of secrets: A. Kavey, *Books of Secrets: Natural Philosophy in England, 1550–1660* (Urbana and Chicago, IL: University of Illinois Press, 2007); W. Eamon, *Science and the Secrets of Nature. Books of Secrets in Medieval and Early Modern Culture* (Princeton: Princeton University Press, 1994); Meredith Ray, *Daughters of Alchemy. Women and Scientific Culture in Early Modern Italy* (Harvard: Harvard University Press, 2015), especially ch. 2; or in relation to manuscript collections: E. Leong, 'Medical recipe collections in seventeenth-century England: knowledge, gender and text', DPhil thesis, University of Oxford, 2005, pp. 37–67; T. Storey, 'Italian books of secrets database: study documentation', https://lra.le.ac.uk/handle/2381/4335.

6 See for example I. McCleery, 'Wine, women and song? Diet and regimen for royal well-being (King Duarte of Portugal, 1433–1438)', in S. Katajala-Peltomaa and S. Niiranen (eds), *Mental (Dis)Order in Later Medieval Europe* (Leiden: Brill, 2014), pp. 177–96; E. Hurren, 'Cultures of the body, medical regimen, and physic at the Tudor court', in T. Betteridge and S.

Lipscomb (eds), *Henry VIII and the Court: Art, Politics and Performance* (Farnham: Ashgate, 2013), pp. 65–90.

7 An exception is represented by J. Richards, 'Useful books: reading vernacular regimens in sixteenth-century England', *Journal of the History of Ideas*, 73:2 (2012), pp. 247–71, which focuses on the formal characteristics of regimens to chart their different uses. For a first exploration of this genre in Italy see S. Cavallo, 'Secrets of healthy living. The revival of the preventative paradigm in late Renaissance Italy', in E. Leong and A. Rankin (eds), *Secrets and Knowledge in Medicine* (Aldershot: Ashgate, 2011), pp. 191–212, and S. Cavallo and T. Storey, *Healthy Living in Late Renaissance Italy* (Oxford: Oxford University Press, 2013), ch.1.

8 G. Pomata, 'Observation rising: birth of an epistemic genre, ca. 1500–1650', in L. Daston and E. Lunbeck (eds), *Histories of Scientific Observation* (Chicago: University of Chicago Press, 2011), pp. 45–80.

9 M. Nicoud, *Les Régimes de Santé au Moyen Âge: Naissance et Diffusion d'une Écriture Médicale (XIIIe–XVe siècle)* (Rome: École Française de Rome, 2007).

10 M. Ficino, *De le tre vite, cioè, a qual guisa si possono le persone letterate mantenere in sanità* (Venice: Tramezzino, 1548); D. Auda, *Breue compendio di marauigliosi secreti rationali ... Con vn trattato ... per conseruarsi in sanità* (Rome: de' Lazari, 1652).

11 An important exception is W. Bullein's, *Bulwarke of defence: againste all sicknes, sornes and woundes, that dooe daily assaulte mankind* (London: John Kyngston, 1562). The advice on regimens is interwoven with other topics from fol. lxv.

12 On the continuities in reading practices from manuscript to print see M. Lane Ford, 'Importation of printed books into England and Scotland', in L. Hellinger and J.B. Trapp (eds), *The Cambridge History of the Book in Britain*, vol. 3, 1450–1557 (Cambridge: Cambridge University Press, 2008), pp. 179–201, 179–80, and P. Murray Jones, 'Medicine and science', in *ibid.*, pp. 433–48, 434, 447.

13 On their manuscript circulation see G.R. Keiser, 'Practical books for the gentleman', in Helliger and Trapp (eds), *Cambridge History*, pp. 470–94, 491.

14 H.S. Bennett, *English Books and Readers*, vol. 1, 1475–1557 (Cambridge: Cambridge University Press, 1969), pp. 42–43, 152.

15 Bennett cites Paynell's recollection of his exchange with Berthelet regarding Von Hutton's *De Morbo Gallico* (1533), in *ibid.*, pp. 43, 103.

16 The first three editions appeared under the title *Liber De homine*, with list of contents in Latin, the subsequent editions under the titles *Libro intitulato Il perché* or *Opera Nuova intitulata il perché*. On the characteristics and

fortune of this text A. Carré and L. Cifuentes, 'Girolamo Manfredi's *Il perché*: I. The *Problemata* and its Medieval tradition', *Medicina e storia*, 19/20 (2010), pp. 13–38, and 'Girolamo Manfredi's *Il perché*: II. The *Secretum secretorum* and the book's publishing success', *Medicina e storia*, 19/20 (2010), pp. 39–58.

17 U. Benzi, *Tractato utilissimo circa lo regimento et conservatione de la sanitade* (Milan: Petromartire, 1508). On this false attribution see J. Hill, Cotton, 'Benedetto Reguardati: author of Ugo Benzi's *Tractato de la conservatione de la sanitade*', *Medical History*, 12 (1968), pp. 175–89.

18 [Maino de Maineri], *Opera utilissima di Arnaldo da Villanova di conservare la sanità* (Venice: Tramezzino, 1549). On this text J.A. Paniagua, '*El regimen sanitatis ad regem Aragonorum* y otres presuntos regimens arnaldiana', in *Studia Arnaldiana. Trabajos en torno a la Obra Medica de Arnau de Vilanova s.1240–1311* (Barcelona: Uriach, 1994), pp. 335–84.

19 G. Pictorius, *Dialogi ... del modo del conseruare la sanitá* (Venice: Bottega d'Erasmo di Vincenzo Valgrisi, 1550).

20 This was the first book of his *De le tre vite*. Originally written in Latin, it was first published in the original language when the author was still alive (1489, 1498). M. Savonarola, *Libreto ... de tutte le cose che se manzano ... e de sei cose non natural* (Venice: Simone de Luere 1508). Michele Savonarola (c.1384–c.1464) was university and court physician in Ferrara, and the author of numerous medical treatises in the vernacular. On this figure see C. Crisciani and G. Zuccolin (eds), *Michele Savonarola: Medicina e Cultura di Corte, Micrologus 37* (Florence: SISMEL Edizioni del Galluzzo, 2011).

21 *Di Galeno. Delli mezzi, che si possono tenere per conseruarci la sanità* (Venice: Tramezzino, 1549); *Col nome de Dio. Il segreto de segreti* (Venice: Zuan Tacuino da Trino, 1538).

22 *The Governaunce of Good Helth by the moste excellent phylosopher Plutarche* (London: R. Wyer, 1549(?) and 1555). *The secrete of secretes of Arystotle ... with rules of helthe for body and soule* (London: R. Copland, 1528).

23 On the figure of the professional writer in Italy in this period, the 'polygraph', see the seminal work of C. Bareggi di Filippo, *Il Mestiere di Scrivere: Lavoro Intellettuale e Mercato Librario a Venezia nel Cinquecento* (Rome: Bulzoni, 1988).

24 On this figure see also the entry by F. Bacchelli in *Dizionario Biografico degli Italiani*, www.treccani.it/enciclopedia/tommaso-giannotti-rangoni_(Dizionario-Biografico); S. Minuzzi, 'Il medico Tommaso Giannotti Rangone (1493–1577) nell'economia della cura, ovvero un trionfo di libri, segreti e *regimen sanitatis*', *Medicina e Storia*, N.S., 1/2013, pp. 29–66.

25 The first Latin editions of *De Vita* and *Consilium* came out in 1550 and 1558, respectively. These were each followed by two further Latin editions (1553, 1560; 1570, 1577) and by two vernacular editions (1556, 1557; 1565, 1577).
26 Minuzzi, 'Il medico', pp. 58–9.
27 There are only two exceptions to this trend, over more than a century: the translation of Levinus Lemnius's *De habitu et constitutione corporis*: L. Lennio, *Della complessione del corpo humano* (Venice: Domenico Nicolino, 1564), and Giuseppe Galeano's translation and compendium of Galen's De Sanitate Tuenda: Del conseruar la sanitá libri sei di Galeno (Palermo: Nicoló Bua, 1650).
28 T. Elyot, *The Castel of Helth* (London: T. Berthelet, 1541, first ed. 1534).
29 Fissell notes that the first edition was published in either 1534 or 1536 but the earliest surviving edition is from 1539. Overall it went through at least seventeen editions; 'Popular medical writing', p. 420.
30 Elyot refers to these attacks in the preface to the second edition of his *Castel*. A. Boorde's 1547 *Breviary of Helthe* and Phaer's 1544 translation of Goeurot's *The Regiment of Life* are actually books of remedies. T. Moulton's *Myrrour or Glasse of Helth* (1539) contains specific advice and remedies against the plague.
31 The authors were Andrew Boorde (1542), Christopher Langton (1545), Henry Wingfield (1551), William Bullein (1559 and 1562), John Jones (1569), Thomas Cogan (1588), Nicholas Vaughan (1600) and Tobias Venner (1620 and 1623).
32 The following authors were all physicians (in brackets is the date when their regimen was published in vernacular): Traffichetti (1565), Bruni (1569), Durastante (1576), Boldo (1576), Pisanelli (1583), Durante (1586), Anguillara (1589), Gallina (1589), Petronio (1592), Rosaccio (1594), Paschetti (1602), Fonseca (1603), Salando (1607), Camaffi (1610), Bertaldi (1618), Viviani (1626), Panaroli (1642), Pietragrassa (1649), Frediano (1656), Galeano (1650), Ciccolini (1697). Auda (1652) was a pharmacist.
33 Paschetti for example also wrote a dialogue in praise of Genova; a tract on jealousy and one discussing 'moral and natural' questions.
34 B. Pisanelli, *Trattato della natura de' cibi* (Bergamo: Comino Ventura & C., 1587); C. Durante, *Il tesoro della sanità* (Venice: Andrea Muschio, 1586). On the page layout and other visual features of these texts see Cavallo and Storey, *Healthy Living*, pp. 27–30.
35 R. Gropretio, *Un breue et notabile trattato del reggimento della Sanità* in D.Romoli, *La singolar dottrina* (Venice: Tramezzino, 1560).
36 The last regimen was B. Ciccolini, *L'oro della sanità ritrovato nel clima romano* (Rome: Vannacci, 1697). The latest re-edition was probably

Rangoni's Consilium, now titled *Svegliarino alli signori veneziani* (Venice: L. Pittoni 1691).

37 Brook (1650) Culpeper (1656 with five re-editions), Gayton (1659), Maynwaring (1663 with three re-editions) and translations of Durante (1586) and Flamant (1697). For Tryon's many tracts see below. This contrasts with the views of D. Gentilcore in *Food and Health In Early Modern Europe. Diet, Medicine and Society, 1450–1800* (London: Bloomsbury, 2016). He maintains that 'during the seventeenth century preventive medicine gave way to an emphasis on therapeutics', only becoming popular once more in the eighteenth century (p. 29, and pp. 11, 15).

38 J. Ghesel, *Rule of Health* (Cambridge: Printers to the Universitie, 1633); F. Bacon, Viscount St Albans, *History Naturall and Experimentall of Life and Death, or of the Prolongation of Life* (London: Lee and Mosely, 1651); E. Gayton, *The Art of longevity or a Diaeteticall Institution* (London: printed for the author, 1659); T. Tryon, *A Treatise of Cleanness in Meats and Drinks* (London: Printed for the author, 1682), *A Way to Health, Long Life and Happiness* (London: Andrew Sowle, 1683), and *Monthly Observations for the Preserving of Health* (London: Andrew Sowle, 1688).

39 Fonseca's regimen was translated by the young priest Poliziano Mancini da Montepulciano; the Dominican father Serafino Razzi translated and edited the Scuola Salernitana.

40 See Donato in this volume, p. 158–82.

41 For example, on chocolate, A. Colmenero, *Della cioccolata discorso* (Rome: RCA, 1667), trans. from Spanish; on coffee, G.Galeano, *Il caffé con piú diligenza esaminato in ordine al conservamento della salute* (Palermo: D. D'Anselmo, 1674).

42 Although the presence of Italian medical texts overall ranged from about two to eighteen per cent of their holdings. J.L. Lievsay, *The Englishman's Italian Books 1550–1700* (Philadelphia: University of Pennsylvania Press, 1969), on the Bodleian, p. 26, on Sir Edward Coke's library, pp. 48–49, and on Lord Lumley's, p. 53.

43 Ian MacClean argues that Latin remains the language of international intellectual communication until the 1630s. *Scholarship, Commerce, Religion: The Learned Book in the Age of Confessions, 1560–1630* (Cambridge, MA: Harvard University Press, 2012), p. 56.

44 Particularly R. Mulcaster, *Positions wherin those primitive circumstances be examined which are necessarie for the training up of children, either for skill in their booke or health in their bodie* (London: Thomas Vautrollier, 1581).

45 'Imparare i suoi principi, conoscere la sanitá ... e conservarla' (our translation). B. Traffichetti, *L'arte di conservare la salute tutta intiera* (Pesaro: Girolamo Concordia, 1565), preface.

46 Fissell, 'Popular medical writing', p. 18.
47 Elyot, *Castel*, pp. 2–3.
48 T. Cogan, *The Haven of Health* (London: Thomas Orwin, 1589), 'To the Reader'.
49 The debate can be followed in M. Bruno, *Discorsi ... sopra gli errori fatti dall'eccell.te M. Bartolomeo Traffichetti da Bertinoro. Nell'arte sua di conseruar la sanità tutt'intiera* (Venice: Andrea Arrivabene, 1569); B. Traffichetti, *Idea dell'arte di conseruare la sanità ... et hora per il medesmo diffesa dalle false oppositioni di M. Matteo Bruni* (Venice: Bindoni & fratelli, 1572).
50 F.M. Getz, 'Charity, translation and the language of medical learning in medieval England', *Bulletin of the History of Medicine*, 64 (1990), pp. 1–17, on p. 11.
51 Elyot, *Castel*, preface.
52 On Elyot's Catholic sympathies and former friendships see S. Lehmberg in the *ODNB* http://0-www.oxforddnb.com/view/article/8782. According to Andrew Wear the 'commonwealth' becomes a 'particularly Protestant notion'. 'The popularisation', pp. 24–6. On the link between Puritanism and the good of the 'commonwealth' see J.H. Cook, 'Institutional structures and personal belief', in A. Cunningham and O.P. Grell (eds), *Religio Medici. Medicine and Religion in Seventeenth Century England* (London: Scholar Press, 1996), pp. 91–114, on pp. 99–100. For other declarations of the 'common weal' see for example the prefaces to *Bullein's Bulwarke*, p. 163 and to Ghesel, *Rule of Health*.
53 *Bullein's Bulwarke*, preface. See also G. Grataroli, *A Direction for the Health of Magistrates and students* (London, William How, 1574, first publ. Latin 1555), preface. On the charitable drive in seventeenth-century regimens see Wear, 'The popularisation', p. 29. The theme of the commonwealth is discussed at length in Storey's contribution to this volume.
54 Solomon, *Fictions of Well-Being*, p. 5.
55 'Giovevoli a molti, non avendo veduto fin qui chi abbia trattato quest'arte con ordine cosí essenziale e facile come io mi proposi. Onde mi son risoluto ... donargli al mondo' (our translation). Traffichetti, *L'arte di Conservare*, preface.
56 V. Viviani, *Trattato del Custodire la Sanità* (Venice: Girolamo Piuti, 1626), preface.
57 'Per quelli che a qualsiasi professione attendono'. Fonseca, *Del Conservare*, p. 2.
58 *Scuola salernitana del modo di conseruarsi in sanità* (Perugia: Petrucci, 1587), ed. and trans. S. Razzi, preface.
59 Viviani, *Trattato*, p. 2, copy of letter of Cardinal Orsini, commissioner of the work, 29 July 1626.

60 It is not until a 1557 edition by Abraham Vele that the *Regimen* goes into 8vo.

61 See Durante's dedication to the Pope's niece Camilla Peretta in Durante, *Il Tesoro* and Salando's dedication to the Duchess of Mantua. F. Salando, *Trattato sopra la Regola del vivere* (Verona: Angelo Tamo, 1607).

62 E. Maynwaring, *Vita Sanae Longa* (London: J. D., 1669) p. 22.

63 Tryon, *A Treatise of Cleanness*, p. 13.

64 '[L]e donne gravide gioveni hano poca prudenza e manco cervelo, nodimeno gli huomini, e padri di famiglia, chesanno quanto cio importi, devono con ragione, e persuasioni farli veder il pericolo comune'. S. Mercurio, *De gli errori popolari* (Venice: Gio Battista Ciotti, 1603), p. 231.

65 Recent works discussing female literacy and readership include H. Brayman Hackel, *Reading Material in Early Modern England: Print, Gender and Literacy* (Cambridge: Cambridge University Press, 2005); W. Sherman, *Used Books: Marking Readers in Renaissance England* (Philadelphia: University of Pennsylvania Press, 2009), chapter 3. For Italy see X. Von Tippelskirch, *Letture Femminili in Italia nella Prima Età Moderna* (Rome: Viella 2011); M. Roggero, 'L'alphabétisation en Italie: une conquête féminine', *Annales Histoire, Sciences Sociales*, 55 (2001), pp. 903–26; T. Plebani, *Il Genere dei Libri. Storie e Rappresentazioni della Lettura al Femminile e al Maschile tra Mediovevo e Etá Moderna* (Milan: Franco Angeli, 2001). On social access to medical texts, in particular: P. Murray Jones, 'Medical literacies and medical culture in early modern England', in Taavitsainen and P. Pahta (eds), *Medical Writing in Early Modern English* (Cambridge: Cambridge University Press, 2011), pp. 30–43. M. Fissell, 'Readers, texts and contexts. Vernacular medical works in early modern England', in Porter (ed.), *The Popularisation of Medicine*, pp. 72–96.

66 C. Jones, 'Discourse communities and medical texts', in P. Pahta and I. Taavitsainen (eds), *Medical and Scientific Writing in Late Medieval English* (Cambridge: Cambridge University Press, 2003), pp. 23–36; Fissell, 'Readers, texts and contexts', for a wide coverage of reading practices.

67 'The rules of helthe for body and soul very proffytable for every man, and also veray good to teche children to lerne to rede Englysshe.' Cited in C.A. Bonfield, 'The Regimen Sanitatis and its dissemination in England c. 1348–55', PhD thesis, University of East Anglia, 2006, p. 26.

68 See for example O. Lombardelli, *Il giovane studente* (Venice: Francsco Uscio, 1594) and B. Meduna, *Lo scolare* (Venezia: Pietro Fachinetti, 1588).

69 Cogan, *Haven*, p. 9.

70 T. Venner, *Via Recta ad Vitam Longan Pars Secunda* (London: G.Eld, 1623). The text was actually written in 1603 and was amongst the most popular English regimens in the seventeenth century.

71 This literature greatly develops after 1550. D. Frigo, *Il Padre di Famiglia: Governo della Casa e Governo Civile nella Tradizione della 'Economica' tra Cinque e Seicento* (Rome: Bulzoni, 1985).
72 For Italy see Cavallo and Storey, *Healthy Living*, pp. 31–7.
73 Wear, *Knowledge and Practice*, p. 154; Slack, 'Mirrors', p. 258.
74 See the evidence in Cavallo and Storey, *Healthy Living*, pp. 33–6.
75 See the examples in *ibid.*, note 73 p. 34 and figs 1.5, 1.6, pp. 35–6. For definitions of 'middling sort' see M. Hunt, *The Middling Sort: Commerce, Gender, and the Family in England, 1680–1780* (Berkeley: University of California Press, 1996), p. 1.
76 P. Grendler, *Schooling in Renaissance Italy: Literacy and Learning, 1300–1600* (Baltimore: Johns Hopkins University Press, 1989); A.S. Zmora, 'Schooling in Renaissance Pistoia: community and civic humanism in small-town Tuscany', *The Sixteenth Century Journal*, 34:3 (2003), pp. 761–77.
77 G. Pelliccia, 'Scuole di catechismo e scuole rionali per fanciulle nella Roma del seicento', *Ricerche per la Storia Religiosa di Roma*, 4 (1980), pp. 237–68; Roggero, 'L'alphabetisation en Italie'; A. Petrucci, *Scrittura e Popolo nella Roma Barocca, 1585–1721* (Rome: Quasar, 1982), pp. 9–10, 17.
78 Or on book ownership generally, as in M. Lane Ford, 'Private ownership of printed books', in Helliger and Trapp (eds), *Cambridge History*, vol. 3, pp. 205–28.
79 See Slack's discussion on readership, in 'Mirrors', esp. pp. 256–61.
80 C. Suhr, 'Regimens and health guides', in Taavitsainen and Pahta (eds), *Early Modern English Medical Texts*, pp. 111–18, on p. 116.
81 W. Bullein, *A newe boke of phisicke called ye government of health* (London: John Day, 1559). See also prefaces to Brooke, *Ugieine*, p. 8; *Bullein's Bulwarke of Defence* and W. Vaughan's, *Directions for Health, naturall and artificial* (London: Bradock, 1602), 'conceived of for the health of all'.
82 On the term popular in relation to texts see the considerations by Fissell, 'Popular medical writing', pp. 417–18.
83 On the diffusion of technical literature in this period N. Glayser and S. Pennell (eds), *Didactic Literature in England 1500–1800: Expertise Constructed* (Aldershot: Ashgate, 2003); P. Smith, 'Making Things: techniques and books in Early Modern Europe', in P. Findlen (ed.), *Early Modern* Things 1500–1800 (London: Routledge, 2012), pp. 173–203.
84 W. Basse, E. Philips and E. Pond, *A Helpe to discourse: or, More merriment mixt with serious matters* (London: Nicholas Vavasour, 1635); nineteen editions of this book were published between 1619 and 1632.
85 Likewise, the dialogue form had of course classical roots but could be adapted to convey easily accessible information.

86 For an example see N. Culpeper, *Health for the Rich and poor by Dyet without physic* (London: Peter Cole, 1656). On paratextual devices see also the discussion in Storey's chapter and our *Healthy Living*, pp. 24–9.

87 Two examples from Italy would be L. Tartaglini, *Opera nuoua nella quale se contiene la natura dil sonno cioé come l'Huomo debbe dormire per mantenersi sano* (Venice: Tartaglini, 1551), and G. Rosaccio, *Avvertimenti a tutti quelli che desiderano regolatamente vivere* (Florence: G. Caneo, 1594).

88 See above pp. 29, 34, 45 and notes 19, 35 for the examples of Pictorius and Grospré (Gropretius). The Scola Salernitana is another case: it occupied only sixteen to forty pages in the various editions and was always associated to a longer text in prose: in 1587 to the commentaries attributed to Arnald, in 1630, 1666, 1677 and 1712 to Cornaro's *Discorsi della vita sobria*, and in 1677 and 1712 also to the short *Altre regole per conservare la sanitá* by Pictorius.

89 P. Grendler, 'Form and function in Italian Renaissance popular books', *Renaissance Quarterly*, 46 (1993), pp. 451–85, here p. 453.

90 Fissell, 'Popular medical writing', pp. 425–6. It is not clear when the first edition of *A Help of Discourse* was printed. The 1635 edition states that it is the eleventh edition, but we cannot trace any earlier surviving examples.

91 Pomata, 'Observation rising', p. 48.

92 *Ibid.*

93 As for example at times in D. Gentilcore, *Food and Health*.

94 *Ibid.*

II

The Non-Naturals and the vulnerable body

2

'What to expect when you're always expecting': frequent childbirth and female health in early modern Italy

Caroline Castiglione

Pregnancy constituted a frequent physical state for many women of the early modern European aristocracy.[1] In an age of high child mortality, the practice was considered laudable for the continuation of the aristocratic lineage. The rapidity of procreation required the sharing of knowledge among women regarding how to survive the physiological and psychological demands of frequent pregnancy and childbearing. Occasionally catastrophic events necessitated extreme interventions by medical practitioners or the ingestion of remedies prescribed by physicians. But success in frequent childbearing relied upon close attention to the Non-Naturals through the adoption of specific practices believed to be most conducive to successful pregnancy and good health in newborns. From proper rest and moderate exercise to limiting exposure to noxious fumes, purging the body and attending to the emotions of melancholy and anxiety, the pregnant woman was believed to have some control over her fertility and the positive outcome of her pregnancies.

Among Roman aristocratic women, attention to the ideal everyday regime was thought to be essential for the 'trade' (*mestiere*) of frequent childbearing in service to their marital dynasties.[2] As was the case with all trades, it had traditions and knowledge shared among its practitioners. It did not evolve in an isolated periphery of medical hearsay, but rather among women with frequent access to the trained care of professionals, and to information passed from mothers to daughters, and among sisters, midwives and wet nurses. How did aristocratic women envision the daily health habits that they believed most conducive to the survival of the mother in this aristocratic female occupation? An extensive corpus of epistolary evidence by one Roman aristocratic woman, Eleonora Boncompagni Borghese (1642–95) provides precious insights into the thoughts of women on the place of the Non-Naturals in the healthy female body and in particular, the frequently pregnant and childbearing aristocratic mother.[3]

Eleonora's hundreds of letters sketch the panorama of seventeenth-century Roman life. She reflected openly on the religious controversies over quietism, the dilemmas of wayward aristocratic men and rebellious children, the challenges of aging and the ubiquity of illness. Above all she preferred issues related to health – there was little in that vast domain that escaped her scrutiny. Eleonora's medical perspective was clearly informed by the tenets of Galenic medicine, especially its emphasis on the centrality of balancing the body's humours and its attention to the Non-Naturals. The Non-Naturals emphasised that good health was linked to an individual's attention to movement, rest, bodily evacuations, air, diet and mental states that could enhance her or his health. Although recent scholarship has begun to recover the significance of the Non-naturals to early modern medical practice and to theories of human health, much less is known about how individuals without formal medical training factored them into their thinking on health and illness.[4] Eleonora did not employ the term Non-Naturals, but the practices associated with them were critical to the way she thought about health in pregnancy. She placed the greatest emphasis on four of the Non-Naturals: adequate movement, rest, the moderate purging of the body, and the mental and spiritual state of the pregnant woman. She devoted less attention to the quality of the air, although she mentioned it occasionally and, as we shall see, in dire terms. Men (in her view) had much more trouble with proper diet than did women, so it received only occasional treatment in her letters regarding women's health.[5]

Eleonora's attention to the Non-Naturals echoes a similar focus in several popular and oft-reprinted early modern texts, including those by Scipione Mercurio and Giovanni Marinello. Eleonora never specifically referenced such works nor did she attend (as such manuals did) to the physiological elements of procreation and fertility. Vernacular texts offered readers explicit information on the sexual organs, the act of intercourse, and the techniques believed efficacious for impregnation and the production of boys in particular.[6] From the perspective of twenty-first-century readers, Eleonora's perspective may seem less compelling, since she omitted such topics in her writing. Whether she did so for reasons of decorum (but might have discussed them in person) or whether she judged such information not the relevant issue for the recipient of her letters has not come to light in the extant letters of the noblewoman. Eleonora's imperative that good health derived from the practice of good habits is the recurring and consistent theme of her correspondence. She considered such attention the key variables for fertility, pregnancy and the successful delivery of offspring.

To grasp the relevance of the Non-Naturals for the health of mothers in particular, this article will attend first to the familial context that required a life of nearly continuous pregnancy for aristocratic women. Women's focus on good health habits has to be located in the challenging physical demands the aristocratic family regime made upon some women's bodies. Eleonora's emphasis on four Non-naturals as the foundation for the fecund female body illuminates the central place they held in her understanding of health and fertility. How each should be practised by women of childbearing age will thus be examined in detail.

The aristocratic 'trade' of frequent childbirth

A key reason why aristocratic women needed to be particularly attuned to the health demands of pregnancy was that they were pregnant so often. The aristocratic Boncompagni family illustrates this trend well. Beginning in the last years of the fifteenth century, through to the last years of the seventeenth century, each generation of the family had as many as eight to thirteen children. In each generation, the children were borne by a single woman who had married into the Boncompagni dynasty. Many other noble family trees testify to the fertility and the labour of their women, whose activity could occur over a long span of time, sometimes almost two decades of childbearing.

A close look at the implications for specific Roman aristocratic women illustrates the demands these practices made upon them. Boncompagni mothers, for instance, bore children at the rate of almost one per year, as did Leonor Zapata y Brancia (1593–1679) whose nine children came into the world in the space of just twelve years. This relentless efficiency was surpassed by her daughter-in-law Maria Ruffo (1620–1705), who added thirteen souls to the ranks of the dynasty during a sixteen-year span, by the end of which time she was 38 years old. Bearing two sets of twins added to the fecundity of her enterprise. It was Maria Ruffo's daughter, Eleonora Boncompagni Borghese, who left behind the voluminous ruminations on the necessity and the difficulties of frequent childbirth. Eleonora was Maria Ruffo's firstborn girl, so she observed both her mother's experiences and knew well and admired her long-lived grandmother.

While Eleonora herself had only four children who lived to adulthood, she accepted that her grandmother's and her mother's trajectory was the typical lot of a noblewoman. Eleonora communicated her observations to her younger sister-in-law, Ippolita Ludovisi Boncompagni (1663–1733), at the beginning of her childbearing years. It was the fecund path that she wished for Ippolita. She should 'fill the Casa with children', which was 'the principal good fortune that a woman could create' for her marital family.[7] There was a special urgency to Ippolita's task, for her husband, Gregorio (Eleonora's twin brother) was 39 years old at the time of his marriage to Ippolita. It was his second marriage and he had no legitimate surviving heirs from his first matrimony, and only one daughter, born out of wedlock.

The limited fertility of Gregorio's first marriage aside, aristocratic women could bear large numbers of offspring because they did not breastfeed their children, which can lower fertility. The aristocratic familial system required a sharp division of labour – since most of the girls (willingly or unwillingly) were consigned to religious life – the one or two who did marry were likely to experience childbearing and childrearing of the intensity just described. As Eleonora framed the life of women, 'God willed that to me would fall such sorrows and [to my sisters in the convent] peaceful repose.'[8] Aristocratic female experience also contrasted sharply with the pattern of childbearing among the lower classes, whose later marriage age and tendency to breastfeed their own children limited the number of offspring during their childbearing years.

Since sexual activity or pregnancy was believed to ruin the milk for the infant,[9] the hiring of wet nurses allowed aristocratic women to give birth, take a series of steps to cause the cessation of the milk flow, and within a short time, return to sexual relations with their spouses.[10] The demands of the aristocratic mother's pregnancies had to be managed alongside the close care of the mother's other offspring.[11] The whole production, even with the assistance of midwives for the mother and wet nurses for the children, could be daunting. Illnesses could be mysterious, especially in children. Good daily habits were essential to maintain health and build up the body to meet the adversities of illness and the physical demands of pregnancy. Emotional states, especially worry and melancholy, could have deleterious impact on the mother's fertility and ability to give birth to healthy children. These perils, too, had to be contained, but how could they be?

In her more realistic moments, Eleonora acknowledged that there were certain aspects of pregnancy that were beyond the control of aristocratic women. Which women would succeed in bearing large numbers of offspring was not always predictable, even with the best of practice. Eleonora had high praise for her sister-in-law, Maria Virginia Borghese Chigi, who bore twelve children. Yet, Maria Virginia had confessed to Eleonora that she had scarcely been convinced that it would be her destiny. She had begun married life with the more modest hope of three or four children.[12] A series of mysterious maladies and gynaecological complications substantially reduced Eleonora's fertility by comparison with her Chigi sister-in-law.[13] A comment on Eleonora's own daughter, whose first child had been rapidly followed with another pregnancy suggested an ambivalence on the noblewoman's part about the whole fertility regime: her daughter and her husband, she predicted, would breed 'like rabbits'.[14] So childbearing could even be too rapid, in Eleonora's view, crossing the divide between the ideals of human procreation and the fertility of animals in the fields. Nonetheless, Eleonora's wish for her beloved Ippolita was that she could make a dozen babies, as had Maria Virginia Borghese Chigi, and that Ippolita would prove to be 'good at making boy and girl babies'.[15] Both genders, she reminded the young mother, were essential to the aristocratic family's strategy.[16]

Since Eleonora was also on hand for some of Ippolita's births, the epistolary exchange between them on this subject is thinner, although childbirth itself put the woman's life in great peril. Eleonora was pleased with the midwife employed by Ippolita for her deliveries, and had sent the same midwife to her own daughter during her confinement.[17] Confidence in the midwife perhaps mitigated some of Eleonora's concerns about the considerable risks of childbirth. Because childbirth was unpredictable (Eleonora observed that no two births were the same), Eleonora was more reticent on this subject. She issued, however, multiple cautions about Ippolita's preparations for childbirth and the postpartum period, but she assured the young mother that the second birth would not be as difficult as the first (which it was not). But she acknowledged the perils of childbirth.[18] She cautioned Ippolita that what went wrong in childbirth could have an impact on her for the rest of her life, including her ability to have other children. If matters were grave enough, the repercussions could lead to her death.[19] Maintaining one's health during pregnancy was the best contribution a mother could make to a successful childbirth and for this reason, the dilemmas of becoming pregnant and being healthy during pregnancy received far more attention from the older mother than the risks of childbirth itself, which were best managed by a competent midwife.

The dialogue among women on healthy pregnancy and the Non-Naturals

Much of the information and advice regarding frequent pregnancy and childbirth remained within the realm of oral culture and direct observation among aristocratic women. Eleonora Boncompagni, for instance, would have mostly known her own mother in a state of pregnancy until Eleonora was 16 years old, at which point Eleonora left the Boncompagni household to begin her own married and childbearing life. It can be difficult to know how women faced its challenges, learned its practices and survived its potentially deadly outcomes. Such information was derived by watching and by listening, by conversation with female relatives, midwives and wet nurses.

Occasionally, however, the distance between two women could create a context in which such information was exchanged in writing, and we catch a glimpse of this aristocratic 'trade' from the perspective of its practitioners. Eleonora, for instance, resided in Rome, about seventy miles distant from the Boncompagni family estate of Sora, where Ippolita and Gregorio began their married life. Between visits, she offered epistolary advice on how the couple (but particularly Ippolita) might meet the goal of frequent pregnancies. Her extensive correspondence in the 1680s captures the difficulties and identifies the particular solutions that a mother might bring to bear on the problem of producing as many children as possible, and especially male children. Through epistolary mentoring between visits with her sister-in-law, Eleonora hoped to help a younger mother succeed in these goals.

Eleonora Boncompagni's correspondence to Ippolita Ludovisi is but one aspect of the larger ongoing dialogue among the Boncompagni and Ludovisi regarding matters of health. Their frequent talk on health spilled over into their epistolary exchanges, which preserved their medical knowledge, especially in times of illness.[20] For Eleonora, family letters were especially valuable because of the medical secrets they might divulge, which included medical practices as well as recommendations about medical practitioners.[21] In their epistolary circulation of medical advice it is clear that family members were assiduous in their attention to personal health as well as to the health of their kin. The exchange extended across generations and among lay and clerical family members. One of the Boncompagni women who became a nun in the convent of Santa Marta was admired and remembered for her cures.[22] Ippolita Ludovisi carried on her own medical exchange with relatives beyond Eleonora. She extolled the virtues of walking and pondered the limitations of the Lenten diet with her brother-in-law, Cardinal Giacomo Boncompagni.[23] Epistolary communiqués transmitted shared family medical knowledge in writing.

Such letters also testify to the aristocratic families' easy and frequent access to physicians. Eleonora consulted with them regularly in her lifetime and she knew and admired four of them enough to remember them in her will with cash bequests.[24] She had so much confidence in the medical expertise of some trained professionals that she forwarded descriptions of Ippolita's son's symptoms to physicians in Rome to secure their opinion.[25] Since medical professionals could disagree on diagnosis and treatment, family members debated their relative merits in their correspondence. Eleonora was dubious of their knowledge in what she considered female areas of expertise, especially the health of women and the care of infants.[26] In such domains physicians could not match the collected wisdom of medically informed women[27] nor women's skills in the observation of 'trifles' (*bagatelle*) necessary to diagnose a woman or child, individuals with whom physicians had less experience.[28] The gynaecological care of women provided by midwives was mostly outside the purview of doctors because it involved menstrual blood, a problematic substance whose bearers were therefore left to the care of midwives, the only licensed female medical practitioners of the early modern era.[29]

The perils of a woman in childbearing years were especially anxiety provoking, and a frequent inspiration for Eleonora Boncompagni to write to her young sister-in-law. Doctor's reports sought near and far, and familial discussions were also resources to determine treatment for a family member whose health was faltering or whose last hours seemed to be at hand. The health of a childbearing mother could be particularly fraught with concern. If she could not successfully bear children healthy enough to survive the dangers of infancy, the survival of an entire dynasty could be at stake, since the practice of primogeniture had reduced the future of great families to the procreative success of a single couple. The combination of restricting marriage to one male heir and the high mortality of children necessitated a fecund marriage for that designated heir and his spouse(s). This high stakes scenario was precisely the context in which Eleonora attempted to advise Ippolita, encouraging her to adopt the best strategies for her pregnancies.

In addressing the trade of frequent childbearing, Eleonora's focus was almost entirely on the Non-Naturals. Her specific concerns centred closely on the balance between moderate exercise and rest, the appropriate cleansing of the body, and (most importantly) the health impact of a person's mental and spiritual state. Even in the face of illness, Eleonora remained sceptical about the value of medications. 'Have more faith in good living than in medicines, which, the more you use them, the worse off you are', was an adage of the older mother.[30] She believed that the surest remedy to good health was not found in the prescriptions of physicians, but rather in the individual's close attention to diet and moderation in all activities,[31] or 'la buona regola', the just measure in all things: eating, sleeping, exercise and medications, when used, had to be used in moderation.[32] This counsel she extended from cradle to grave. For infants, she noted, milk was the best remedy for their maladies, and sure to restore their health more quickly than the medicines of doctors, replete with side effects, and frequently prescribed in a quantity that could harm or even kill a young child.[33] Men's ill health resulted from their failure to attend to the Non-Naturals: their excessive eating and drinking led to their ruin.[34] Maternal health also originated in habits. Doctors were unlikely to be successful in restoring health through medicines in the childbearing woman if they did not attend to the Non-naturals.

Pregnancy could be an unpleasant state, even if a highly desirable one for women hoping to reproduce an entire generation. She acknowledged its many inconveniences and difficulties, but noted that 'it was an evil that brought good'. Fatigue, Eleonora acknowledged, was simply an outcome of 'the unique trade of making children'. Vomiting was another unavoidable feature of pregnancy. Fainting was not an unusual or a particularly worrisome symptom. Women were also more prone to colds and to upper respiratory congestion during pregnancy. 'More pregnancies', Eleonora observed, 'were more bad than good', and she noted that for her 'one pregnancy was worse than the other'. While the mother had to assiduously monitor and modify her mental state, pregnancy itself could bring on melancholy.[35] Its dilemmas were further exacerbated by other contexts beyond the woman's control. The heat of summer, for instance, made pregnancies during that season the worst to endure.[36] One wished for it to be over and done with, she noted, even if one feared the death that could occur in childbirth.

Yet, Eleonora refused to pathologise these problems: they were part of the natural course of procreation and they rarely required medication. In pregnancy as in childrearing, Eleonora discouraged making too much of minor discomforts or even comparing one pregnancy to another. When at last Ippolita became pregnant with her second child, Eleonora reminded her that with each pregnancy she would recognise individual differences in the way she carried the child. Such discrepancies should not worry her.

Balancing motion, rest and airborne risks

Despite the physical demands of pregnancy, there were steps that an aristocratic woman could take to help her pass successfully through pregnancy to childbirth, to the next pregnancy. From the very earliest weeks of pregnancy, a woman had to attend to details, including her clothing. Restrictive clothing and corsets could harm the child and the mother, as the mother's waistline expanded. Eleonora counselled corsets that were loose and short in the front and the back, a style Ippolita preferred anyway, the older mother noted approvingly.

Such clothing was conducive to the key activity during pregnancy, which was motion. Movement, Eleonora believed, could correct many dilemmas of the pregnant woman. Ippolita worried about weight gain during and between pregnancies, but Eleonora underscored its obvious necessity and inevitability during pregnancy. The problem was instead excessive weight gain, and while Eleonora acknowledged the deleterious effects of excessive eating, movement was the best counterbalancing activity for women. Staying in bed during pregnancy was not a good idea. She reported with disillusionment and concern that her own daughter, Anna Camilla, spent far too much time in bed early in pregnancy. It could lead to difficulty in pregnancy and in the delivery of the child. A lack of movement also exacerbated her daughter's melancholy, a state already likely to be brought on by the pregnancy itself.

For Eleonora, motion never lost its value for any individual, especially a pregnant woman. The key variable for motion and motherhood was timing. Certainly the heat of summer made it impossible for some women to move about with ease, but the mother simply had to shift her walking routine until after sunset. Both the walk and the fresh air were critical in the latter part of pregnancy, in preparation for childbirth. While ambulatory exercise was necessary, Eleonora cautioned against excessive activity early in pregnancy. In the initial months of pregnancy, Eleonora was opposed to travel by carriage, too much walking, and above all the use of the stairs.[37] Later in pregnancy she encouraged walking, and as the birth neared, she encouraged Ippolita to move as much as possible.[38] Life, in Ippolita's view, would come to be a long perambulatory exercise and she would later admonish herself for her own sedentary lapses.[39] Motion for pregnant women, Eleonora had taught her, might make the difference between health and illness for mother and unborn child.

To some extent, exertion was unavoidable for Roman aristocratic women during pregnancy, since they were expected to carry on with their diplomatic duties, which included serving as ambassadors for their families' interests; as intermediaries between cardinal brothers-in-law and husbands; as advocates for their children in the domestic and the judicial realms of Rome.[40] They did all these activities while continuing to tend to the childrearing needs of their growing families. While aristocratic women could rely on the labour of wet nurses to succour their children and servants and some relatives to assist in the care of older children, the ultimate responsibility for the organisation of the childcare fell to the mother. Wet nurses in particular could be difficult to retain, and the large number of children under the age of three (the typical age of weaning) necessitated that the aristocratic woman remain in a constant search for such women. The mother's success or failure in choosing the wet nurse could mean the life or death of her child. When combined with the plethora of ailments and physical and psychological transitions of children, the aristocratic woman's work was continuous. She could wear herself out with supervising the care of her children, and the outcomes might not always be positive or within her control.[41] Ippolita was intensely involved with the care of her children, sometimes, according to Eleonora, to a fault. Her resulting fatigue could jeopardise her health as well as that of her child in utero. Activity was necessary, but in excess could pose a peril.

Children could present other dilemmas to the pregnant mother. Their frequent illnesses added to the mother's exertions and risks. Eleonora recalled a grave illness of one of her sons. Since she was pregnant at that time, she confessed that she simply avoided him, entrusting his care to her grandmother-in-law (who co-resided with her) and her husband, even though the child was deathly ill.[42] A suitable protection for the pregnant mother's well-being was simply to remove herself from the presence of sick people, but especially sick children, even her own. In addition to reducing the mother's risk of infection, the distance between the mother and her offspring acted to reduce her activity as well as limit her worry, since she could not track the inevitable ups and downs of their daily life. This allowed the pregnant mother to rest and contributed to the calm necessary to maintain the health and well-being of the mother.

The combined exertions of pregnancy and childbirth necessitated rest especially in the aftermath of the latter. The absolute minimum for bed rest was fifteen days, according to Eleonora. She was dismayed to learn that Ippolita was up and about so quickly after the birth of her third child, Costanza. She pointed out to Ippolita that Ippolita's mother had followed a similar pattern of early postpartum exertion and (she implied) had died as a result at a relatively young age, 38 years old, when Ippolita herself was about 2 years old. Fifteen days of bed rest was necessary because 'the trade of bearing children was fatiguing'. Although Ippolita could rely on her youthful energy, she had to pace herself for the many years of childbirth ahead of her. Forty days was the full period of restricted activity recommended by the older mother. After forty days, a woman could begin 'a little exercise', but Eleonora confessed that she herself would not rest easy until she knew that Ippolita had passed the forty-day mark, was out of bed and, in her view, out of danger.[43] Shorter periods of rest and premature return to too much activity could be dangerous. She counselled Ippolita against 'showing off' by getting up too soon or writing too many letters.[44] Due to the use of quills and ink wells, writing had to be done upright and required more physical exertion than such an activity would today.[45] Even worse, in Eleonora's view, was Ippolita standing on her feet in the days following the birth.[46] For Eleonora, the consequences of excessive activity were multiple. It deprived the mother of oxygen and potentially damaged her kidneys. Any blood built up in her system under the circumstances of such strain would leave her weak in the future. The results of such overexertion following childbirth would be long-lasting, in the older mother's view. Ippolita's rising too early from bed rest compromised subsequent pregnancies, successful childbirth and the health of future children.[47] If these dire warnings were not enough, Eleonora added pragmatically that Ippolita would suffer more frequently from fainting as a result of her fatigue. Any such outcome that could be avoided should be.

The mother's attention to rest indoors could also protect her from the ill effects of cold wind that might make her ill. Rest in isolation from other people could further protect the mother from the risks of noxious odours, to which the fatigued body of a woman after childbirth was particularly vulnerable. To reinforce her point, Eleonora recounted the sad death of a young woman who had 'given birth many days before, and was up and about and who died in a few hours after smelling an odour in some papers'. There are few instances in which Eleonora focused on the quality of the air, one of the Non-Naturals critical to good health. Yet the risks of bad air profoundly disturbed her, especially noxious fumes in the immediate aftermath of her delivery. She praised God that Ippolita had dodged an odour that could have killed her. The older mother advised that after childbirth she eliminate all strong odours (especially Gregorio's tobacco) since such smells were believed to be deadly to the recently delivered women.[48]

In addition to enhancing the postpartum woman's survival, rest was also the critical component for the return to fecundity, since the overly fatigued woman was not likely to conceive,[49] and even less likely to become pregnant with a boy.[50] It was the responsibility of the child-bearing mother to bring herself back to the level of health that made pregnancy more likely.[51] Motion and rest in the proper balance were the keys to a woman's well-being and her resumption of the aristocratic woman's trade.

Cleansing and the fecundity of the ageing female body

Eleonora acknowledged that sometimes the pregnant woman's health might require the use of a purgative or bloodletting to restore the proper balance between blood, phlegm, black bile and yellow bile. She fully accepted the theory that each person had a particular complexion, or balance of these humours,[52] and she thought it likely that these combinations ran in families.[53] She further believed that the age of the individual shaped the equilibrium between the humours. Ippolita, to whom she referred early in their correspondence as a 'giovinetta' (young thing), tended to have too much blood and needed to be bled periodically.[54]

This excess of blood could negatively impact her health during pregnancy, and if she did not address it, such problems could continue after pregnancy, decreasing her fertility. Eleonora recommended bloodletting in the sixth month of the pregnancy, but not before, to address this potential compromise to Ippolita's health. 'Many women', she observed, 'had tried it to good effect.' Ippolita's situation was complicated by the fact that she had not lost enough blood during her first two childbirths, further exacerbating her condition. Bloodletting at the right moment in pregnancy could set the mother right again, according to Eleonora.

Bloodletting, however, had to be used with caution. Eleonora believed that an excessive recourse to bloodletting over a long period of time could lead in later years to 'incurable illnesses'. A purge might balance Ippolita's system just as well. Purgatives were believed to increase the chance of conceiving a boy.[55] Flushing the body through the use of waters was another sound practice, in Eleonora's view.[56] She sent particular waters to Ippolita, including a miracle-working water that was supposed to help overcome the potential procreative deficiencies even in an 'old, unhealthy spouse, crippled by gout', as Eleonora was sometimes wont to describe her brother.[57] She included details on the way Ippolita should use the water and in what quantity. The remedy would purge her kidneys, refresh her uterus, improve her stomach and liver function, and restart her menstrual cycle.[58] She pronounced herself more knowledgeable than a local physician regarding its efficacy.[59]

Childbearing women had to be especially attentive to an aspect of their bodies that physicians generally hoped to avoid: their menstrual blood and the postpartum discharge. Ippolita worried that if the latter were not profuse, she might suffer from a blockage.[60] Later, she worried about its lengthy duration.[61] Typically Eleonora discouraged Ippolita from fretting about such developments, since time, in her view, would take care of most things. Context made a difference, however – her recommendation of specific waters emerged in the aftermath of the death of Ippolita's son and a subsequent miscarriage experienced by Ippolita herself. These two events heightened Ippolita's anxiety over conceiving again. Even under less fraught circumstances, Ippolita would have attended to the return of her menstrual cycle, which signified the recovery of her fertility. Ippolita was anxious about its delay.[62] Her husband monitored such issues as well. Eleonora reported her relief learning from him that Ippolita 'was well and that [her] period had also come'.[63] Ippolita studied the colour and quantity of her menstruation to assess her fertility, and she once worried about both in a letter to Eleonora.[64] Eleonora attributed its light colour to the effects of the miracle water, but urged its continued use since it produced 'favourable ... evacuations'.[65]

Such signs were valuable clues to achieving a large family, since that goal necessitated a short time limit between births, especially in the early years of childbearing. The case of Maria Ruffo is instructive in this regard. She had about one birth every fourteen months until she approached 30. Then in her thirties, the space between children was closer to two years. Early in Ippolita's childbearing years, Eleonora urged her to keep to the one-year schedule. When another pregnancy did not follow the birth of Ippolita's firstborn son, Eleonora accused her of wanting to raise Ugo to manhood before she had another child. He was but four months old at the time, but Ippolita should have already been expecting another child, by Eleonora's calculations, an expectation that suggests she assumed the couple would resume sexual relations about three months after Ippolita's delivery.[66]

Seven years later, Ippolita and Gregorio were even more pressed for time, due to Gregorio's advancing age, the loss of their first son and a period of over four years in which no pregnancy led to successful childbirth. What could cause such a negative outcome? In previous pauses between pregnancies, the young woman had expressed her theories, but the older mother was sceptical of her reasoning. Eleonora doubted that Ippolita's headaches could point to infertility, but if headaches continued, Ippolita would have to be bled. Early in her childbearing years, Ippolita had noted the post-pregnancy changes in her body, and worried that they could be a factor in limiting her fertility. She found her weight gain and her haemorrhoids particularly disturbing. Eleonora dismissed these issues, and advised against Ippolita paying too much attention to her body and its changes over time. A little rotundity in Ippolita was 'not a fault'. After Ippolita's first birth, the older mother suggested that she was bloated and a remedy for gas could be the solution. Bitter wine was the remedy for the haemorrhoids. Later, Eleonora admitted that bodily changes were annoying (especially the weight gain and the haemorrhoids) but a part of the ageing process – one was bound to have something wrong when one passed a certain age.[67] Purges and bloodletting were the best recourse for the return of the menstrual cycle and the fecundity of the mother. The other physical issues marked the passage of time, but did not limit Ippolita's chances of becoming pregnant again.

The mental and spiritual states of the healthy mother

No factor impinged more greatly upon a person's health, in Eleonora's view, than the mental and spiritual state of the individual. She acknowledged this for herself, as well as for others, readily admitting that the source of her own illness was her spiritual state: 'The illness of my body is that of my soul.'[68] The converse was also true: the joys of childrearing could enhance the mother's health. The presence of robust and lively children, even if labour-intensive, testified to a mother's success both in pregnancy and childrearing, and provided positive feedback likely to lead to further pregnancy. 'These girls are your only pastime', Eleonora observed, 'and truly when children grow up healthy and spirited, one is happy, and it is all a mother and a father could wish for and there is no pleasure like this one.' Ippolita evidently experienced delight in some aspects of mothering and shared them with Eleonora, who praised their benefit.

Yet, such outcomes were scarcely guaranteed in the perilous world of the nursery, where as many as half the children died before they reached adulthood. Even children who lived were frequently ill, but the fecund mother had to respond with stoic calm. 'After good things, you must be prepared for bad ones', she reminded the younger mother. Ippolita had the misfortune to lose early in her childbearing years the only male child that she bore, Ugo, who passed away at about two-and-a-half years old. Prior to his passing, both Ippolita and her husband Gregorio agonised about the mystery of their son's maladies and struggled with the difficulty of finding a cure for them. At his death the couple were plunged into a long period of mourning and intense worry about the fate of their surviving daughter and the likelihood that they would ever have another boy to carry on the lineage. Eleonora remained convinced that Ippolita's grief for her dead son represented the greatest risk to her, greater than any other health problems she discussed in her correspondence with Ippolita.

Ippolita's pregnancy immediately following her son's death was marred by anxiety and sorrow. In the view of Eleonora, a mother who experienced both apprehension and melancholy was likely harming her own health and the health of her future child.[69] The older mother acknowledged that some people were, because of their humoral balance, melancholic.[70] By contrast, Eleonora knew Ippolita to be happy by nature and so 'giving herself over to melancholy ... was not her duty but rather she had to content herself with what God sent her', including the death of her son.[71] It was in Ippolita's power to change her emotional state. While Eleonora condemned her brother for his extended sorrow after the loss of the child, she observed that the impact on the procreative future of the family rested upon Ippolita's ability to resign herself to the will of God, accept the death of her son, console the rest of the *casa* and focus on becoming pregnant as soon as possible.[72] A relentless forward motion had to propel the aristocratic mother into the next phase. Melancholy and anxiety could lower the mother's fertility, decrease her health during pregnancy and harm her unborn child.[73]

In the aftermath of Ippolita's protest that Eleonora was insensitive to her grief, the older mother acknowledged 'that you consider me cruel and little sympathetic to what has happened'.[74] Eleonora attempted to soften, but did not really modify her view though she acknowledged her own grief over the loss of Ugo.[75] But against such deleterious states of mind and soul, everyone (especially the pregnant mother) had to struggle successfully – by appealing to God for help and resigning oneself to his will; by movement and exercise; by a change of scenery and the distractions of entertainment, if everything else failed.[76] She clearly expected more from Ippolita than she did from her own daughter, who, in her own childbearing difficulties had dissolved into inconsolable grief. Eleonora, physically and emotionally distant from her daughter, thought that chocolate could be her only consolation, and sent it to her.[77] Her counsel instead for Ippolita incorporated the religious surrender of quietism (declared heretical in 1685, but still followed by many Roman noblewomen thereafter).[78] Resignation to God's will dovetailed with the noblewoman's duty to serve the aristocratic dynasty by tending first to her own physical and mental well-being.[79]

The only other possibility, to which Eleonora also devoted considerable examples and rhetorical flourish, was to convince a mother to develop an unflappable approach to the daily and repetitive difficulties of her young children. Not only was it best for the children themselves, but also the tranquillity of the mother improved her health. Certainly calm in the face of children's difficulties was what Eleonora praised most in her own mother. Through many years of epistolary and in-person mentoring, she hoped to train Ippolita to achieve the same state, even in the face of her children's mostly minor illnesses as well as during the more serious and finally fatal condition of her son.

Eleonora's repeated attention to the mental and spiritual state of the mother became a sore point between the two women. Ippolita could initially find little consolation in Eleonora's observation that God would make Ugo a greater prince in heaven than he could ever be on earth. Ippolita and Gregorio, by contrast, clung mistakenly to the 'mirage' of wishing for the return of their ill and departed son, rather than asking God for more and healthier children, and returning to the conjugal activities necessary to make such an outcome possible, most likely an oblique reference to their resumption of sexual intercourse. For Eleonora, the connection between mind, soul and body were so powerful that they were the driving consideration for fertility. She critiqued Ippolita for excessive concern for the minor ailments of her children.

These were useless worries that would limit her ability to become pregnant and carry pregnancies to term.[80]

However, Eleonora also faulted her own mother for a lack of attachment to her daughters.[81] By contrast, Eleonora stressed the value of Ippolita's affection for her children of both genders. She had high praise for Ippolita's passion (*passione*) for Ugo.[82] Yet, she never connected the contradictory implications of all of her recommendations. Ippolita engaged in co-sleeping with her offspring, which together with other physical demonstrations of her affection won her praise from Eleonora.[83] Unfortunately, the same level of engagement undermined Ippolita's ability to separate herself from her offspring when one died (in the case of Ugo) or to relax her concerns for her remaining children when they were ill. Ippolita had difficulty regulating her mental state due to her affections, Eleonora observed, probably leading to her decreased fertility. Paradoxically, these were the very emotions Eleonora counselled her to have as a good mother.[84]

Conclusion

Even in the face of these irreconcilable contradictions, Eleonora's approach to achieving frequent pregnancies rested on the maintenance of health through the proper choice of behaviours and attitudes on the part of the mother. Eleonora assumed that both were within an individual's control, or at least under the control of women, if not always for men, with their disorderly lifestyles.[85] The Non-Naturals placed high value on human agency – what was not beyond the control of the individual should be controlled. A good example of this, in Eleonora's view, was that since Ippolita was not, by the balance of her humours, melancholic, she had therefore the capacity (and therefore the duty) to return herself to a contented and stable mental and spiritual state.

Pregnancy, even at a rapid pace of procreation, was not a malady, and should not be treated as such. Only in the circumstances of lowered fertility, miscarriage or the failure to produce male offspring did Eleonora counsel more complex remedies. Otherwise the best choice was to allow the body's own capacities for healing and for achieving what it was designed to do to happen in due course. But most importantly, health in the frequently pregnant woman followed from good habits and from good habits followed frequent pregnancies. Without mastery of these practices, the trade of frequent childbearing would be fraught with failure and anxiety, which would further undermine the woman's task of bearing a generation for her marital family, and especially procreating its male heirs. The foundation for such success was the Non-Naturals, especially their emphasis on motion and rest, cleansing the body at appropriate times, and improving the mental and spiritual state of the person. While positive additions to the health of most people, such practices made all the difference for the aristocratic woman's success in the trade of frequent pregnancy and childbirth.

Notes

1 For a recent survey on the history of motherhood, with particular emphasis on childbirth, see L. McTavish, 'Maternity', in A.M. Paska and K.A. McIver (eds), *Ashgate Research Companion to Women and Gender in Early Modern Europe* (Farnham: Ashgate, 2013), pp. 173–93. For more on Renaissance physicians' treatises on fertility and childbirth, see note 6 in this chapter.

2 Archivio Segreto Vaticano (hereafter ASV), Archivio Boncompagni Ludovisi, (hereafter ABL) 899 (3 September 1687).

3 This study is based primarily on the letters of Eleonora Boncompagni Borghese in the Archivio Segreto Vaticano. Two specific volumes contain her epistolary outpourings to Ippolita: Archivio Boncompagni Ludovisi (henceforth ABL), busta 899 and busta 900. Busta 900 is identified as containing letters from an administrator to Ippolita Ludovisi, but it contains Eleonora's letters as well. Only busta 900 contains folio numbers.

4 For more on the Non-Naturals, see the introduction to this volume and G.B. Risse, 'In the name of Hygieia and Hippocrates: a quest for the preservation of health and virtue', in G.B. Risse (ed.), *New Medical Challenges during the Scottish Enlightenment* (Amsterdam, New York: Brill, 2005), pp. 135–69. See especially pp. 159–60 for the key bibliography on the Non-Naturals in the medical theory of ancient authors.

5 For further insights on gender differences in healthy eating and living, see S. Cavallo and T. Storey, *Healthy Living in Late Renaissance Italy* (Oxford: Oxford University Press, 2013), pp. 209, 218, 239. In contrast to Eleonora's focus, R. Bell's summary of vernacular Renaissance manuals on pregnancy and women's health notes their close attention to women's diet. See *How to Do It: Guides to Good Living for Renaissance Italians* (Chicago: Chicago University Press 1999), pp. 89–92.

6 For a summary of this early modern literature on women's health, see Bell, *How to Do It*, esp. pp. 17–123. On noblewomen as the dedicatees and possible readership for this literature, see Cavallo and Storey, *Healthy Living*, pp. 33–4.
7 On her wishes for Ippolita, see ASV, ABL, 899 (12 September 1687).
8 *Ibid.* (23 May 1686).
9 V.A. Fildes, *Breasts, Bottles, and Babies: A History of Infant Feeding* (Edinburgh: Edinburgh University Press, 1986), pp. 12, 179–81.
10 M. D'Amelia, 'Becoming a mother in the seventeenth century: the experience of a Roman noblewoman', in A.J. Schutte, T. Kuehn and S. Seidel Menchi (eds), *Time, Space, and Women's Lives in Early Modern Europe* (Kirksville: Truman State University Press, 2001), pp. 223–44.
11 For more on the demands and the difficulties for aristocratic women in providing wet nurses for their numerous offspring and tending to their care, see C. Castiglione, 'Peasants at the palace: wet nurses and aristocratic mothers in early modern Rome', in J. Sperling (ed.), *Medieval and Renaissance Lactations –Images, Rhetorics, Practices* (Burlington: Ashgate, 2013), pp. 79–99.
12 ASV, ABL, 899 (undated letter, likely early summer 1685 [miscatalogued in packet of letters, marked '1687–1689']).
13 She claimed to have had a tumour the side of a bread loaf, though she went on to conceive afterwards. See *ibid.* (3 May 1685). Since she does not identify the tumour's location, one can only assume it was a uterine tumour or cyst.
14 *Ibid.* (31 November 1685 [*sic*]).
15 *Ibid.* (12 September 1687).
16 *Ibid.* (28 November 1685). See a similar comment in D'Amelia, 'Becoming a mother in the seventeenth century', p. 232.
17 *Ibid.* (2 August 1686). On this midwife's presence at her daughter's delivery, see *ibid.* (14 June 1686).
18 *Ibid.* (1 September 1685; 3 November 1685; 19 April 1686; 22 July 1687).
19 *Ibid.* (15 March 1686). She was similarly worried when her daughter was about to give birth. See *ibid.* (14 June 1686).
20 For the significance of the epistolary circulation of medical knowledge in another Roman family, see Cavallo and Storey, *Healthy Living*, pp. 55–61.
21 ASV, ABL, 899 (28 July 1684). For more on the familial and the medical in early modern Europe, see the recent issue of *Renaissance Studies*, 28:4 (2014), pp. 496–638. See especially, A. Rankin, 'Exotic materials and treasured knowledge: the valuable legacy of noblewomen's remedies in Early Modern Germany', pp. 533–55, and J. Stevens Crawshaw, 'Families, medical secrets and public health in Early Modern Venice', pp. 597–618.

On the medical marketplace concept and the notion of patients as consumers, see M.S.R. Jenner and P. Wallis, 'The medical marketplace' in their edited volume, *Medicine and the Market in England and its Colonies, c. 1450–1850* (Basingstoke: Palgrave, 2007), pp. 1–23.

22 ASV, ABL, 900, 85v (27 November 1688).

23 ASV, ABL, 787, fascicolo 1 (26 January 1709). On the importance of walking to Ippolita, see ASV, ABL, 787, fascicolo 1 (20 March 1709; 10 August 1709; 16 November 1709). See the place of walking discussed in A. Arcangeli, *Recreation in the Renaissance: Attitudes toward Leisure and Pastimes in European Culture, c. 1425–1675* (Basingstoke: Palgrave, 2003), pp. 18–45. Concerns over the impact to health of the Lenten diet were widespread. See Cavallo and Storey, *Healthy Living*, pp. 210, 215–18, 271.

24 ASV, Archivio Borghese, 122.

25 ASV, ABL, 899 (6 April 1685 [miscatalogued in packet of letters, marked '1687–1689']).

26 *Ibid.* (7 September 1686); ASV, ABL, 900, 76r (12 September 1688).

27 Cavallo and Storey, *Healthy Living*, p. 57. For an analysis of another Roman matron, Maria Spada, who was a 'medically informed aristocratic lady', see *ibid.*, pp. 59–61.

28 ASV, ABL, 900, 76r (12 September 1688). On 'trifles' ('*bagatelle*'), see ASV, ABL, 899 (23 March 1685; 19 August 1686; 21 August 1686; 1 November 1686).

29 D. Gentilcore, 'The organisation of medical practice in Malpighi's Italy', in D. Bertoloni Meli (ed.), *Marcello Malpighi: Anatomist and Physician* (Florence: Olschki, 1997), pp. 75–110, esp. pp. 107–8. On midwives, see also N.M. Filippini, 'The Church, the State and childbirth: the midwife in Italy during the eighteenth century', in H. Marland (ed.), *The Art of Midwifery: Early Modern Midwives in Europe* (London: Routledge, 1993), pp. 152–75. While R.M. Bell and G. Pomata have posited a more positive view of menstruation as a salubrious form of bloodletting among some medical authorities, the notion of menstrual blood as impure had deep European roots. On the latter, see O. Niccoli, '"Menstruum quasi monstruum": monstrous births and menstrual taboo in the sixteenth century', in E. Muir and G. Ruggiero (eds), *Sex and Gender in Historical Perspective* (Baltimore: Johns Hopkins University Press, 1990), pp. 1–25, esp. pp. 2, 9. For a summary of the more positive views of menstrual blood in early modern medical treatises, see Bell, *How to Do It*, pp. 66–8. Pomata's more nuanced view of menstrual blood is articulated in 'Menstruating men: similarity and difference of the sexes in Early Modern medicine', in V. Finucci and K. Brownlee (eds), *Generation and Degeneration: Tropes of Reproduction in Literature and History from Antiquity through Early Modern Europe* (Durham,

NC: Duke University Press, 2001), pp. 109–52, esp. pp. 123–4, 130, 133–4, 141–4, 152.

30 ASV, ABL, 899 (3 January 1686).

31 In these issues, Eleonora resembles the opinions of an eighteenth-century Scottish physician analysed by Risse, 'In the name of Hygieia and Hippocrates'.

32 On all things in their 'just measure', see ASV, ABL 899 (3 January 1686; 1 March 1686; 7 September 1686; 26 September 1686 [a letter from Eleonora to her brother]). For further insights on the relevance of '*buona regola*' and the problems of its omission, see *ibid.* (24 March 1685 [mis-catalogued in packet of letters '1687–1689']; 1 June 1685; 3 January 1686; 7 September 1686; 10 October 1686; ASV, ABL, 900, 64r (22 June 1685); 141r (20 January 1688).

33 On the benefits of breast milk over medicine see ASV, ABL, 899 (26 October 1685). On the problems of overmedicating infants, see *ibid.* (9 June 1685); and ASV, ABL, 900, 58r (28 June 1685). For more on both issues, see C. Castiglione, *Accounting for Affection: Mothering and Politics in Early Modern Rome* (Basingstoke: Palgrave, 2015), pp. 114–17.

34 ASV, ABL, 899 (23 June 1684; 7 March 1687).

35 *Ibid.* (19 September 1685; 3 September 1687; 14 March 1687; 6 May 1687; 24 April 1687; 30 April 1687; 21 March 1687; 21 March 1687). On melancholy, see A. Groppi, 'La sindrome malinconica di Lucrezia Barberini D'Este', *Quaderni Storici*, 129:3 (2008), pp. 725–49; *idem*, 'La Malinconia di Lucrezia Barberini D'Este', in F. Cantù (ed.), *I Linguaggi del Potere nell'Età Barocca*, vol. 2, *Donne e Sfera Pubblica* (Rome: Viella, 2009), pp. 197–227.

36 ASV, ABL, 899 (2 June 1687; 12 July 1687; 22 July 1687).

37 *Ibid.* (22 July 1687; 1 September 1685; 3 November 1685; 24 August 1685; 1 September 1685; 21 November 1687; 4 April 1687; 21 March 1687; 6 May 1687; 12 June 1687; 24 August 1685).

38 On walking in pregnancy as essential, see *ibid.* (5 January 1686; 4 February 1686); on walking just before the birth, see *ibid.* (23 February 1686). For more on women's exercise in the vernacular medical manuals, see Cavallo and Storey, *Healthy Living*, pp. 152–4.

39 ASV, ABL, 787, fascicolo 1 (20 March 1709; 10 August 1709; 16 November 1709; 30 September 1713).

40 The combination of male and female efforts to the family was first elaborated by R. Ago, 'Giochi di squadra: uomini e donne nelle famiglie nobili del XVII secolo', in M.A. Visceglia (ed.), *Signori, Patrizi, Cavalieri in Italia Centro-Meridionale nell'Età Moderna* (Rome: Laterza, 1992), pp. 256–64 (esp. pp. 260–3). For an overview of this argument in English see her

'Ecclesiastical careers and the destiny of cadets', *Continuity and Change* 7 (1992), pp. 271–82. B. Borello has underscored the necessity of continuing such activities, even during pregnancy. See *Trame Sovrapposte: La Socialità Aristocratica e le Reti di Relazioni Femminili a Roma (XVII–XVIII Secolo)* (Naples: Edizioni Scientifiche Italiane, 2003), pp. 31–2. For more on women as *mater litigans* or judicial and familial advocate, see Castiglione, *Accounting for Affection*, pp. 11–19.

41 For the contradictory implications of these varied activities for Roman aristocratic mothers, see Castiglione, *Accounting for Affection*, esp. pp. 93–128.

42 ASV, ABL, 899 (5 October 1686).

43 *Ibid.* (6 February 1686; 11 September 1687; 27 September 1687; 15 March 1686; 7 September 1686; 26 September 1686 [in letter to Gregorio]).

44 *Ibid.* (19 April 1686).

45 On the mechanical demands of writing, see D. Goodman, 'Designing an education for young ladies', in her *Becoming a Woman in the Republic of Letters* (Ithaca: Cornell University Press, 2009), pp. 63–160.

46 ASV, ABL, 899 (10 October 1687).

47 All of these dire warnings come from a letter written about three weeks after the birth of Ippolita's third child, Costanza. *Ibid.* (27 September 1687).

48 *Ibid.* (27 September 1687; 11 September 1687; 23 March 1686; 9 May 1686; 23 March 1686).

49 *Ibid.* (an undated letter, likely early summer 1685 [miscatalogued in packet of letters, marked '1687–1689']).

50 *Ibid.* (12 September 1687).

51 *Ibid.* (an undated letter, likely early summer 1685 [miscatalogued in packet of letters, marked '1687–1689']).

52 *Ibid.* (12 July 1687); ASV, ABL, 900, 122v (5 May 1688). On the concept of complexion, see S. Cavallo, 'Health, hygiene and beauty', in M. Ajmar-Wollheim and F. Dennis (eds), *At Home in Renaissance Italy* (London: V&A Publications, 2006), pp. 174–87, esp. p. 178. For a summary of the early modern discourse on complexion, and the decline in its significance over time, see Cavallo and Storey, *Healthy Living*, p. 32.

53 ASV, ABL, 900, 48v (5 March 1689); 46r (12 March 1689); 55v (2 April 1689). B. Borello's interdisciplinary approach to family resemblances in early modern Italy underscores that epistolary records rarely mention shared family resemblances except as an issue of inherited responses to disease, or 'complexion' (as in note 70 in this chapter) and temperament. See 'I segni del corpo: fratelli, sorelle e somiglianze nelle famiglie italiane (XVII–XVIII secolo)', *Quaderni storici*, 145:1 (2014), pp. 9–40, esp. 25–31.

54 ASV, ABL, 899 (6 April 1685 [miscatalogued in packet of letters, marked '1687–1689']).
55 *Ibid.* (23 May 1687; 16 May 1687; 28 July 1684; 9 June 1685; 13 December 1687).
56 ASV, ABL, 900, 79r (18 October 1688).
57 *Ibid.*, 95v–96r (7 September 1688).
58 *Ibid.*, 95v (7 September 1688); 54v (2 April 1689).
59 *Ibid.*, 81v (27 September 1688).
60 ASV, ABL, 899 (23 June 1684).
61 *Ibid.* (11 August 1684).
62 *Ibid.* (11 August 1684; 28 July 1684).
63 *Ibid.* (3 August 1684): 'ne vengo avvisata dal Duca che state bene e che vi è venuto bene il tempo vostro ne stimo gran fatto sia ritardato se il Capo parto vi venne stentato'.
64 ASV, ABL, 900, 79r (18 October 1688): 'sento che havete doppo [*sic*] l'acqua havuto bene il vostro tempo ma scolorito'.
65 *Ibid.* Bell notes the concern in vernacular medical treatises with variations in menstrual blood (too red or yellowish) as a sign of problems with the temperature of the uterus: *How to Do It*, pp. 58–9.
66 ASV, ABL, 899 (9 September 1684).
67 *Ibid.* (21 July 1685; 19 April 1686; 26 April 1686; 28 July 1684; 24 August 1685; 28 July 1684; 3 August 1684; 29 November 1687).
68 *Ibid.* (24 March 1685 [miscatalogued in packet of letters '1687–1689']).
69 *Ibid.* (24 December 1687; 7 September 1684; 11 August 1685; 16 May 1687; 25 January 1687).
70 Eleonora referenced the complexion of Ippolita's children as an explanation for their character. Ippolita's daughter Constanza, for instance, was spirited due to her humoral balance. ASV, ABL, 900, 82r (27 September 1688).
71 ASV, ABL, 899 (27 September 1687).
72 *Ibid.* (22 December 1686; 10 January 1687; 18 January 1687).
73 On the harm to the unborn child, see *ibid.* (27 September 1685; 19 October 1685; 26 October 1685; 31 November 1685 [*sic*]; 30 March 1686; 13 August 1686; 10 January 1687; 18 January 1687; 25 January 1687; 1 March 1687; 16 May 1687).
74 *Ibid.* (7 February 1687).
75 *Ibid.* (22 December 1687; 10 January 1687).
76 *Ibid.* (27 September 1687).
77 *Ibid.* (24 March 1685 [miscatalogued in packet of letters, marked '1687–1689']).

78 For more on Eleonora's devotion to quietism, and that movement's connection to her world view, see Castiglione, *Accounting for Affection*, pp. 124–8.
79 ASV, ABL, 899 (5 October 1686; 10 October 1686).
80 *Ibid.* (17 August 1685; 6 February 1686; 8 July 1684; 7 February 1687; 10 January 1687; 7 February 1687; 6 October 1684; 19 March 1686; 23 March 1686).
81 Eleonora faults her mother by failing to mention her among those who loved her and by implying that she made Eleonora's life an unhappy one. See *ibid.* (26 April 1686; 11 May 1686).
82 *Ibid.* (18 December 1685).
83 *Ibid.* (7 September 1684). Eleonora's sympathetic praise was accompanied by the precaution against allowing their co-sleeping to make Ugo 'an enemy of the cradle'. She expressed no concern about co-sleeping as a possible moment for suffocation, as did some medical authorities. See Fildes, *Breasts, Bottles, and Babies*, pp. 195–7.
84 Castiglione, *Accounting for Affection*, esp. pp. 123–8.
85 Eleonora's dismay over the poor health habits of men pervades her correspondence. Examples include her concern over Ippolita's uncle: ASV, ABL, 899 (23 June 1684; 21 March 1687; 23 March 1687). She similarly complained about the 'extravagances of her brother'; *ibid.* (19 September 1684).

3

'Ordering the infant': caring for newborns in early modern England

Leah Astbury

In 1985 in his groundbreaking article, 'The patient's view: doing history from below', Roy Porter demanded historians re-evaluate their methodological approach to doing medical history and consider patient experience. In his five 'broad guidelines for future investigations', Porter complained that historians were overly concerned with diagnosis and cure. Instead, he suggested scholars turn their attention to the everyday acts of health care; the preventative measures individuals took to ward against disease. Porter opined, 'We commit gross historical distortions if we fail to give due weight and attention to traditional medical interest in the weather, in diet, in exercise, in sleep – or, in other words, in the whole field of "non-naturals".'[1] Roy Porter's work became field-defining, but while the patient-centred approach has become dominant, few have taken to Porter's other recommendation. Until recently there has been little concerted attempt to redress the relative historical silence on the role of the Non-Naturals in early modern regimes of care, or to properly integrate practices aimed at promoting longevity into extant histories of the way bodies were experienced.[2]

The ebb and flow of humours were central to the way early modern people understood the body and the way it functioned.[3] Health was dependent on the air one breathed, how one slept, the movements the body made, what one ate and drank, the regularity of excretion and the passions of the soul. Within this framework each person had their own particular complexion, which meant that individualised regimes were considered to be more favourable for the maintenance of health than universal ones. Lifestyle and social standing played a role in this: for example, scholars did not have the same health needs as labourers. Complexion was also gendered and age-related.[4] Adult females were cold and wet, men hot and dry. At birth, bodies were at their hottest and wettest whilst ageing meant losing radical moisture and heat.

Scholars have long noted the importance of considering how age determined complexion in early modern European medicine, but with the exception of Hannah Newton, who has examined the health of children, this has also remained an area of relative scholarly silence.[5] Here, I hope to speak to two neglected areas of research: preventative medicine and the health of infants.

There have been several important studies about the bodily experience of pregnancy in early modern Europe.[6] However, the infant – its body and health – have been entirely absent. This chapter will address these absences by showing how babies were medically unique, demanded their own specific care, and how this changed over time after birth. Understanding the ways in which the infant body was readied for later life, and the role that Non-Naturals played in preventative health care, is important not just to the study of childbirth and parturition, but also to deciphering the ways early modern people thought about well-being.

The chief source for this study is childbearing manuals printed in England in the seventeenth century. The late sixteenth and seventeenth centuries witnessed a particular explosion in the publication of vernacular medical texts. Elizabeth Lane Furdell has uncovered 200 printers and sellers who handled medical books in London between 1475 and 1700.[7] Similarly, Mary E. Fissell has stated that by 1700 there was one vernacular medical work in circulation in England for every four families.[8] Of particular currency were guides directed to midwives and women in 'child-bed', providing advice on the whole process of parturition. Richard Jonas' 1540 and Thomas Raynalde's 1545 English translations of Eucharius Rösslin's *Der Rosengarten* were the first of many such guides.[9] Childbearing guides were, like many early modern vernacular medical books, composite texts that combined passages from ancient sources and often reprinted swathes of material from each other, verbatim.

Essentially, childbearing manuals, which were generally written by physicians, served to reinforce the authority of the ancients while popularising knowledge so that 'breeding' women and their midwives might be better informed about the correct way to manage generation. They were structured chronologically: they provided advice on how to conceive; what to expect during pregnancy; how to prepare for birth; what positions to adopt in labour; how to recover from childbirth; and finally, how to care for an infant in the first months of life. This latter stage was often termed 'ordering the infant', and such chapters set out the various acts of care designed to ensure infant survival. The Non-Naturals were a dominant theme in this literature. The hot and wet constitution of infants drove the care they received. Excretion of moisture was important in facilitating the gradual maturation of the infant. This was achieved through hygiene, promoting crying and through creating friction on the infant's body by rubbing and stroking. A prominent theme in regimens was also ensuring babies were contented and their passions were not roused: distress could cause illness or death.

In addition to vernacular medical texts, this chapter also draws on a group of sources which have been termed 'life-writing' – that is, family correspondence, diaries and journals – which allow the historian to access the ways in which prescription and practice interacted. This is a difficult task. The very nature of the time immediately after birth, in which the mother was confined to bed and the household played host to visitors, means that in-depth written descriptions of care are hard to come by. Letters informing family members about births were generally not sent until a week or two later, and often these are frustratingly brief. What is present in family correspondence, however, are expressions of concern that the mother-to-be was adequately prepared for impending labour and had all the necessary people and things on hand so that both mother and child could survive the birth and the precarious first few days. This of course, applied to the newly delivered woman as much as to the infant, but it nevertheless indicates that there was an acceptance that babies would need care, and often professional help, after birth.

In 1699, for example, Penelope Mordaunt, who was heavily pregnant, wrote to her husband expressing her worries that she was poorly prepared if she were to go into labour prematurely:

> I grow very uneasie now a days as well as nights w[hi]ch has made mee this day send to Mrs Barns for blankets and things for the child, Lest I

> should be caute [caught]; and if I be Pen must be norse [nurse] for I have none yett; the woman I write to you about has not given me her answar yet.[10]

Pen was her youngest daughter, and was ill-equipped to play nurse. In early modern England, nurses were often hired in addition to a midwife to attend to the newborn child, thus we can assume Pen would probably have been caring for her sibling rather than her mother.[11] By representing only the female experience in childbirth we have obscured the important processes of care that were enacted on the infant body after birth, for which a nurse was often acquired. A considerable proportion of the scholarly discussion of early modern English childbirth has been devoted to the idea that premodern women were gripped by an overwhelming fear of birth.[12] The emphasis on how women understood and perceived maternal mortality has meant that the period after birth has invariably been represented as one of social relief and celebration. Laura Gowing, thus, has argued that after birth, 'the focus of the social ritual which surrounded new mothers shifted from pain and fear to thanksgiving and celebration', although she notes that the infant was 'carefully watched'.[13] Whereas watching the infant has previously been represented as a passive activity, I argue that the processes of care enacted on the newborn body after birth demanded considerable effort and investment. Although it was often a nurse or midwife who 'ordered the infant', mothers were not excluded from this process of care – but helped to direct it, and as their own health improved, took over the regimen of bathing, clothing and feeding. In this way, the bodily work of labouring for the infant's well-being did not end with birth, but rather when the infant was perceived as healthy.

Crying and changing colour

Immediately after birth, the first task of the nurse or midwife was to encourage the baby to cry. Crying played a prominent role in ensuring the regulation of several of the Non-Naturals in the early days of an infant's life. The Welsh medical writer John Jones observed as early as 1579 that if an infant 'weepe a little', at birth 'then (as sayth Avicen) it shal not be unwholesome, nor to many fathers irksome, but rather joyfull news'.[14] When Anne, Countess of Arundel, looked after her daughter's newborn son in 1689, she wrote to a family member, observing that although she was worried that the child had not been able to feed, the fact it was 'a most ernest crier' was a promising sign of future health, despite it sometimes holding its breath until 'he look black'.[15] Weeping signified that an infant was able to cope with life and function independently of the maternal body. It was only once an infant cried that medical authors suggested that the midwife or nurse should cut the navel cord.

One reason medical writers interpreted crying as an important sign of viability was because it was seen as an impulse that was unbidden and uncontrollable that expressed the baby's needs for future care. Jacques Guillemeau, in the English translation of the French manual, explained that infants were unable to cry in the womb, but 'as soone as he is born, and sees the light', out of 'necessity, and his owne feeling doe force and as it were wring from him cries and moanes'. Through these noises, newborns demanded and craved 'the succor of … [their] owne Mother'.[16] Pregnancy meant women had little active choice in whether or not they nourished and cared for their infants, but after birth, medical texts stressed that women had to choose to look after their infants, and crying was a plea for comfort and warmth that demanded a response.

Perhaps the most medically important reason crying was paramount to infant survival immediately after birth was because it allowed the baby to expel the moisture that had clogged its throat, brain and stomach during pregnancy. The midwife Jane Sharp argued that, at birth, infants ought to cry clear and loud 'for it is better for the brain and lungs, that are thus opened and discharged of superfluous humours'.[17] Mucus was thought to be particularly dangerous to the brain, something which crying shed.[18] Timothy Bright, the author of *Treatise on Melancholy,* explained that tears were the 'excrementitious humidity of the brayne, not contained in the vaynes'.[19] As tears formed, the brain compressed and forced moisture out of the tear ducts.[20] For this reason crying was more suitable for certain bodies than others. Women, for example, had 'loose, soft and tender' flesh and were more moist, and this was why women seemed to weep more often than men.[21] Importantly, babies had an even greater need to cry because they were both naturally more moist *and* they had been surrounded by fluid in the womb for nine months. Hence, Nicholas Culpeper described how the brain of infants was 'very moist, and hath many excrements which Nature cannot send out its proper passages'.[22] Crying thus marked the first act of excretion which continued steadily over the first days and weeks of the infants' life. By raising the temperature of the body, weeping was additionally a form of exercise.

Moderate exercise was understood as an important part of a healthy regimen. However, for infants, even the exercise involved in excessive crying was seen as dangerous to their bones which were excessively flexible. Medical authors were anxious to ensure that crying was occasional and that sobs did not wrack the body. Vigorous crying could distort an infant's wax-like bones and cause strains and ruptures. Authors warned of the possibility of 'broken belly' in infants, a condition that could cause the navel cord to bleed.[23] Indeed, crying was such a concern for medical authors that Robert Barret the author of *A Companion for Midwives* argued that 'Above all' other concerns, the nurse or mother should be 'very careful not to suffer the Child to cry too much'. By 'turning it clean and dry, and removing what may fright or grieve it', he proposed that infants could be soothed and placated.[24] Domestic recipe books also contain a large number of remedies for convulsions and swellings, and often identify these cures as specifically for infants. The recipe book of Elizabeth Okeover, for example, compiled between *c.*1675 and 1725, lists five remedies for convulsive fits, three for troubled or fretful young children and two for rupture in the belly.[25]

As well as facilitating breathing, expelling harmful moisture and representing potentially dangerous movement of the body, crying was related to another Non-Natural: the passions of the soul, or the emotions. Passions acted on the spirits and humours; they were influenced by, and a product of, humoral balance. Hence Barret's recommendations point to another underlying assumption in vernacular medical literature: that babies, like adults, cried because they were provoked emotionally.[26] Crying in contemporary society is seen as the occupation of a young child. Babies are thought to cry for all manner of reasons that might not be cause for concern. For seventeenth-century medical writers, however, after the first cry, successive episodes of weeping indicated to the carer that all was not well. Over the seventeenth century weeping was increasingly connected to overflowing passions, and medical writers explained that babies often cried because they had a desire for physical affection or comfort.[27] John Pechey, for example, noted 'most commonly Children do not cry without a cause, but are provoked by something that disturbs them'. Driving home a distinctly moral message he noted that a 'Prudent Mother or Nurse, will endeavour to find out what is the cause that being removed, the Child may be quiet'.[28] An affectionate relationship between carer and child could ward against emotional distress, and its dangerous consequences. In this way, the quality of care – how attentive and affectionate the mother or nurse was in tending to the infant – determined its well-being and health.

Watching newborns carefully formed the basis for the next important stage in vernacular childbearing guides: observing the colour of the baby's skin as a barometer of health. Medical writers argued that if a baby was born pink, the prognosis for survival at least into childhood was good, whilst infants born pale or black were perceived as dead, dying or unwell. However, more crucial than being pink was that in the days after delivery its visage slowly changed. Sharp commented that children that 'look white and pale when they are born, are weak and sickly, and seldome live long'. If, on the other hand, the infant was a 'reddish colour all over the body, when it is first born, and this colour change by degrees to a Rose colour, there is no doubt of the child but it may do well'.[29] Similarly, Pechey stated that 'you must mind what is the colour of the new-born infant', stating that ideally it should be 'reddish all over the body, for that by degrees turns daily florid'. This change had to be gradual or progressive, since babies that were 'at first Florid or White', Pechey explained, would not live long, or would otherwise mature to be of 'an ill temperament, Cold, Dull'.[30] The change ought to be gradual and 'daily', something Sharp and Pechey both called 'turning'.

Bodily development after birth, guided by the care administered by a mother or nurse, would give indications not just of how likely it was for a baby to survive into childhood and adulthood but it could reveal future personality. Pechey's observation that infants born florid or white would grow up to be 'cold' and 'dull' adults suggests that an individual's complexion or humoral make-up was in some way present at birth. This early period of care was about discovering the nature of the baby; a process in which the Non-Naturals played an important role. Crying and the changing colour of a baby's skin were external manifestations of internal transition and maturation that had to be steady and gradual. Although the Galenic-Hippocratic tradition saw the young as invariably hot and moist, newborns were not homogenous and varied in complexion. Between womb and cradle, newborns occupied a somewhat problematic state. Not only was the child an unstable figure in the family structure and its religious state undefined prior to baptism, but bodily it was in a way becoming itself.

Searching the body and enabling excretion

After the baby had cried and its skin seemed increasingly pink, medical writers stressed that it was important to search the body of the infant so as to identify any bodily impediments. Ensuring and enabling excretion was central to this searching process. Hygiene in early modern medicine did not just refer to the removal of external 'dirt', but rather incorporated various processes of care that aimed to facilitate the body's expulsion of harmful impurities and residues.[31] Similarly the removal of excrement did not just refer to faeces and urine, but sweat, oil and other waste from the body. For infants, there was an urgent need to manage the excretion of moisture owing to their period in the womb. Crying, as I have shown, was an important preliminary act in emptying the brain and passages of problematic moisture and mucus, but it only freed the lungs and passages of excrement, and did little to contribute to the general drying of the body.

In order to facilitate this process of maturation, any blockages had to be removed. First, the midwife or nurse was instructed to insert her fingers into the baby's mouth to clear any phlegm. Raynalde described in 1545 how 'with youre fynger (the nayle beynge pared) open the chyldes nosetrelles, and purge them of flythynesse'. With a tented cloth, the midwife should clear the ears. Similarly, by rubbing the belly, carers could encourage the baby to void its bowels. Raynalde told nurses to 'handle so the chyldes syttnge [sitting] place that it maye be prouoked to purge the belly'.[32] The 1656 edition of the *Complete Midwifes Practice* suggested offering newborns wine because it 'cuts the flegm which the Child has in its throat'. This had the triple benefit of promoting defecation, clearing the throat and allowed 'the spirit' to rise up to the head, which 'comforts and strengthens it', preventing epilepsy later in life.[33]

The need to ascertain whether the infant was capable of opening its bowels led to some toe-curling interventions. 'Slipping' of the fundament (anus), or prolapse, was thought to be a particularly common condition in infants, caused by excessive crying or straining, something that could obstruct defecation. Similarly, medical writers worried that some newborns were born entirely lacking fundaments. The East Riding gentlewoman Lady Margaret Hoby who famously attended to her neighbours in their many ailments, cared for an infant born without a fundament in 1601. An incision was made in order to ensure that the infant was able to defecate, a measure that was unsuccessful. The baby died not long after.[34]

The broader need to discover bodily abnormalities triggered a process of searching the whole body, which was intrinsic to after-birth care regimes. Vernacular medical guides instructed carers to 'search whether any thing be amiss in any part that it may be rectified as much as may be'.[35] In this, the arms and legs were extended to observe movement, and the mouth was probed to ensure the infant was not tongue-tied. This was not simply about knowing what was wrong with a newborn, but also marked the beginning of a process of potentially remedying such ailments, so the infant could go on to lead a healthy life. Although moisture was something that needed to be managed, it also meant the bodies of newborns were malleable. Medical texts were optimistic that this flexibility could be harnessed to straighten crooked limbs, and lengthen parts that appeared stunted. This was primarily achieved through the process of swaddling. This phase of identifying parts that were 'amiss' in Pechey's words, points to an underlying belief in vernacular medicine that this early period of life was bodily unique and could be capitalised upon for future health.[36]

We can find this same process of searching and identifying what might be 'amiss' in life-writing sources. In 1686, Dorothy Osborne wrote to her daughter-in-law Bridget Osborne passing on advice about Bridget's newborn son. She instructed Bridget to 'take care he [the infant] does not use exercise to[o] soon and pray good advice about it that you may be sure there is nothing out'. She stressed, 'I don't Doubt your care' but could not resist communicating her anxieties 'because I fear my nephew Herberts lamness was first occasioned by a fall w[hich] was not known or thought dangerous'.[37] Understanding whether there was anything amiss with an infant, or in Dorothy's terms, 'nothing out', meant that these problems could be potentially fixed. By not recognising the severity of her nephew's fall, Dorothy feared she had failed to capitalise on a period of bodily flexibility, a mistake she was not willing to make again.

Similarly, the Yorkshire gentlewoman, Alice Thornton, described in her spiritual meditations the birth of her second child, Naly, in 1653, and catalogued the newborn's appearance including all that was amiss. Naly became stuck during the long labour 'staing one full hoeur in the birth at neck & shoulders'. When delivered, Naly was 'well nigh choaked with Pleagme and the nauill string ... twice about her necke, & Arms' so that 'she was without any breathing or appearance of life'. Thornton's reflections belie a preoccupation with the problematic presence of mucus and moisture in newborns shared by medical authors, as well as the systematic way in which newborn bodies were searched to account for and classify their health. Despite these initial troubling signs – we can assume that Naly did not cry immediately after birth – Thornton stressed that Naly was not small, weak or imperfect. Rather, she was 'sweet & beautiful, comlie'.[38] Indeed, Naly went on to recover and survived into adulthood. There are many striking echoes of the medical literature in this reflection: the emphasis on breathing as a tool for discovering infant health. Thornton's account also encapsulates the optimism of seventeenth-century medical authors that impediments in infants could easily be overcome owing to their excessive moisture: they could simply be reshaped back into health.

Pamphlets and court cases detailing instances of infanticide are also a useful source in thinking about the ways in which individuals might define an infant as healthy or unhealthy, and also normative expectations of after-birth care, something infanticidal mothers obviously failed to meet. Women accused of infanticide often argued that they had suffered a miscarriage.[39] According to a 1624 law if an unmarried woman concealed a pregnancy and the body of an infant was discovered she was automatically guilty.[40] Courts were, however, willing to consider strong evidence that an infant had been born before it was full-term or had obvious impediments which made stillbirth a more likely explanation. In such cases, the infant body became a central site of evidence and the 'evidence' mostly about newborn health or lack thereof.

This is clearly seen in the 1651 pamphlet describing the charges brought against Anne Greene, a 22-year-old maid from Oxfordshire, who was accused of delivering her infant into the 'house of office' (lavatory) and abandoning it. The infant upon inspection was judged to be 'very unperfect'. In the first place it was 'not above a span in length, and the sexe hardly to be distinguished: so that it rather seemed a lump of flesh, then a well and duly formed Infant'; it lacked hair on its head.[41] The midwives employed by the court to inspect the infant's body determined that it had never lived. Anne herself described how the baby had fallen from 'her unawares' and that the delivery was quick and painless.[42] The same process of inspecting bodily proportions which is present in vernacular medical literature is rehearsed in this pamphlet – the limbs and length of the child were noted and its relative state of bodily perfection – adding to Anne's case that she had miscarried rather than murdered her child.

In this way, the poor and unhealthy appearance of the body of a newborn might be used to acquit women accused of infanticide. Conversely, however, if the infant was shown to be healthy and viable, as in the 1610 pamphlet, *The Bloudy Mother*, which describes the crimes of Jane Hattersley, searching the body could expose a mother's double sin: murder *and* duplicity. Jane's baby was a 'prety infant' despite originating from 'her polluted womb, into this world'.[43] The word 'prety' was often used interchangeably with 'comlie' and 'lusty' to refer to infants that were without impediment and cheerful. In this pamphlet, the author contrasted the viability of the infant, with the questionable morals of its mother. There is no way that Jane's baby could have been confused for a stillborn child: it cried, struggled and was well-coloured before its demise. When Jane concealed the baby to smuggle it out of the house and end its life away from prying eyes, it made a 'pitful [pitiful] shreeke' to 'tell his preseruers [preservers], that she told a wicked and villainous untruth'.[44] As an inversion of the ideal normative caring processes enacted by mothers or nurses in medical literature, Jane 'most carelessly wrapt [the baby] up in her apron, intending … in some impious and excreable sort to haue it made away'.[45] It was only when she was confronted by her landlords, demanding to inspect the bundle of clothes, that the infant declared its health and vitality by crying. Eventually, despite attempted interventions, Jane succeeded in murdering her infant. Once again, colour, breath, the lack of obstruction in its throat, and the face of the infant featured prominently as signs of health or increasing lack of it in the authors' description; 'the babe by his mother breathlesse, with the mouth of it soyld with some, that rose by her violent wringing'. The contrast between the promising bodily character of the baby after birth and its later poor health, made Jane's decision to murder it all the more evil. 'Good-wife', the wife of Jane's landlord, insisted that 'She knew she left the child perfectly well, and to see it so suddainly dead' only magnified and dramatised the crime.[46] Watching infant bodies for external clues of well-being features in infanticide pamphlets as a way of supplying evidence in a legal sense. This suggests, however, that there was a certain shared lexicon about how a healthy newborn body should behave which had a wider social practice than the middling- and upper-sort world that women like Alice Thornton inhabited. Furthermore, print culture of this kind drew on a notion of transgressive motherhood – where women not only failed to provide proper care for their infants but actively destroyed them. In this way, we can see that the regulation of Non-Naturals was seen as an intrinsic part of the role of an assiduous and attentive mother in early modern England.

Rectifying imperfections through hygiene

Surveying the baby's body for fault was useless without recourse to care that remedied these imperfections. After this process of searching and watching the infant had been conducted, carers were instructed to bathe the baby in warm water before drying and binding in swaddling bands designed to strengthen and straighten limbs. François Mauriceau explained that the 'assistance' mothers and nurses gave to infants in bathing and clothing was ultimately driven by a desire to remedy 'such many Infirmities, to which the weakness of his Age and tenderness of his Body renders him subject'.[47] The regulation of hygiene was an important way in which the infant body was heated, cleansed and made more malleable, so that swaddling bands might perform their proper function: to straighten and strengthen the limbs.

Medical writers promoted two separate acts of hygiene for babies: shifting and bathing. In 'shifting', the infant's swaddling bands were removed, and the anus and genitals wiped with a sponge to remove faeces and urine four or five times a day. Bathing was a more drawn out affair, generally performed once a day in which the baby was immersed in warm water, its head supported by a bolster or wadge of fabric.

As well as making the child 'clean and dry', however, shifting was couched in terms which suggest that the touching involved in this act was also as important to infant health as the removal of waste. Sharp, for example, stated that when changing infants, parents or carers should 'rub the belly down with butter as often as it is undressed'.[48] The friction involved in stroking and rubbing the baby was thought to function in many ways as a substitute for exercise, in distributing nourishment and promoting concoction. By touching babies, carers also settled infants. John Pechey recommended that before laying a child down to rest the nurse should 'see whither the Linnen be foul'd for Children love to be clean, and will not sleep quietly till filth close are removed from them'. If babies were 'swaithed too hard' or 'pinched by the wrinkling of the Linnen, or pricked by a pin', such distress could have a very damaging impact on the emotions and infant health more generally.[49] When shifting babies, the room had to be warm and free of draughts. Great care was taken to make sure the temperature and light in the room was suitable for the changing process, as well as that the child was held properly. Thomas Raynalde provided detailed instructions of how to 'shift' an infant:

> the nource [nurse] must geue all dilygence and hede that she bynd euery part ryght and in his due place and order, and that will all tendernesse (& gentell entreatyng, and not crokedly and confusely, the which also must be done often-tymes in the day … yf it be crokedly handled, it wyll growe lykewyse.[50]

It was important during this process that 'it must be defended from ouer much cold, or ouermuch heate'.[51] Wadges of material may have been inserted near the baby's genitals to absorb excrement, termed 'clouts'. Daniel Sennert, for example, described in his 1664 *Practical Physick* a particular rash that occurred on babies' hips 'when the clouts are not changed often'.[52] The word 'clout' referred to a small cloth, particularly those used in washing dishes and removing dirt.[53] Sara Read has recently suggested that the inclusion of 'clouts' in women's inventories, indicates that these pieces of fabric were used more broadly for hygiene purposes, chiefly as menstrual rags, but also for removing faeces in adults.[54] Clouts may have been an early form of cloth nappy, and shifting therefore aimed at removing specific kinds of excrement. Bathing served related but slightly different purposes.

Bathing babies was an important and relatively frequent part of after-birth regimes of care. Raynalde recommended washing babies 'two or thre times in the daye' in a warm bath, hotter in winter, until the 'body begyn to ware red for hete'.[55] After the first weeks, medical writers recommended decreasing the regularity of bathing. Jane Sharp proposed that in the early months carers should 'wash the body of it twice a week with warm water', but that once 'it be weaned' babies should be bathed as irregularly as adults.[56] Bathing was no doubt a crucial and medically important act of care in early modern English medical texts, and certainly babies were washed more regularly than adults.[57] The reason for this was not that infants were perceived as particularly filthy, but rather that through bathing, they lost some of the excessive moisture that was considered to be detrimental to health.[58]

What appears to be crucial to the rationale for bathing babies was both the temperature of the water (warm) and, as in shifting, the fact that the infant was touched, rubbed and contented. Bathing represented a mixed experience for medieval and early modern people because of the belief it interacted with the 'cooking' process of digestion, and could lead to a loss of radical moisture and heat in the body, prematurely ageing it.[59] Babies' bodies were wax-like, and easily distorted, and thus excessive movement was thought to cause deformity and illness. In this way, bathing provided an important and safe substitute for movement in encouraging digestion. The heat and frictions which accompanied bathing, John Pechey explained, helped 'Concoction, and the distribution of nourishment, and serve instead of exercise and motion.'[60]

What went into the baby's bath along with warm water was of the utmost concern for authors. Early modern medical writers departed from the ancients in their prescriptions of how to cleanse babies perhaps more so than in any other aspect of the after-birth regimen. John Jones stated, 'we differ from our elders, for we neyther sprinkle them with salte … nor spred on them Mirtle leaues'. He recommended ten parts warm water to one part milk.[61] It is unclear whether this was cow, goat or human breast milk. Marylynn Salmon has shown that breast milk was a relatively common ingredient in seventeenth-century English and American recipes to cure inflammation and to help restore strength after illness.[62] For Jones, milk was a more appropriate addition to water than salt because it comforted and soothed. Salt was an astringent, and in this way could disrupt the process of excretion. Pechey explained that 'it is to be feared that the salt biteing quality was soon left off, and instead of it they washed the new-born Children with Wine'.[63] Wine increased natural heat, making the body even more malleable. The cleansing routine Pechey recommended 'upon its coming into the World' was to 'rub [the infant] all over with hot Canary or White-wine and fresh Butter, or Lard, and dry the Child with a hot Flannel'.[64] The heat, friction and comforting properties of these hygiene regimens secured newborn development by facilitating excretion.

Early modern English medical writers expressed considerable anxiety about the potentially damaging effects of cold water on the infant body. Cold bathing not only hardened the body, but it also could be a sudden and abrupt change from what newborns were used to in the womb: it was at odds with the predominantly hot bodies of infants, and disrupted this gradual and incremental process of 'turning'. In the late sixteenth century, John Jones recorded in his treatise the tragic mistake made by some priests who typically plunged newborn infants too vigorously to the 'bottome of the font, not knowing ... that all sodayne mutations could be most daungerous'. He explained that 'if the naturall heate within, shoulde be ouwercome of the outward colde, the liuing creature must needs perishe, when as of immoderate vse of Elements death ensueth'.[65] One hundred years later, John Pechey warned of the dangerous consequences of cold bathing. The 'barbarous people' of Germany, he explained, 'dip the warm Infant from the Womb in the next Brook, that thereby it may be rendred more strong and lusty, and to try the strength of their Children, whom they chiefly design for the Wars; for without doubt none but strong Children would survive such a dipping'.[66] Sudden changes from the environment that the infant had become accustomed to – the womb – were dangerous to infant well-being. Warm bathing facilitated the transition from womb to cradle by allowing the body to adapt to the outside world: it heated and dried the body slowly and safely.

Soothing and sleeping

After these acts of hygiene and the baby had been shifted and swaddled, vernacular medical authors instructed carers to set the baby down to sleep. 'A Child new born sleeps more than he wakes, because his brain is very moist, and he used to sleep in the womb', the famous herbalist Nicholas Culpeper explained.[67] Sleeping aided consumption of the excessive heat and moisture in the infant body, but also crucially was understood as the natural state for babies freshly out of the womb. For this reason authors recommended allowing newborns to sleep without restriction. After this early period, however, mothers and nurses should be prudent not to let their charges sleep for too long lest they become sluggish and slow, which would stunt their development.

Vernacular medical texts reveal an assumption that it was only when a baby was relaxed, happy and soothed would it sleep. Strategies centred on touching and comforting the baby; writers recommended that mothers or nurses ought to set the baby down to sleep once it had been bathed and clothed. In this way, laying a child to rest was part of the process of shifting, bathing and clothing which involved touching, rubbing and stroking the infant. Guillemeau explained newborns could be pacified by 'rocking', 'by singing to them' and after the first sleep by 'giuing them the breast', all acts of affection and care.[68] Parents could additionally offer their child pleasant sights, objects that pleased them or to carry 'them abroad', a phrase that appears to have encompassed carrying the infant around the home, or venturing outside for short distances. Such practices reveal the centrality of managing the passions of the soul to securing health after birth.[69]

Rocking was particularly prominent in the strategies writers listed to induce sleep in babies. François Mauriceau instructed the carer to 'rock him gently with equal motion, without too great shaking'. Rocking too vigorously could 'hinder ... the digestion of the Milk in his Stomach, provoke him to vomit it up'.[70] The soothing motion of rocking could work in harmony with the nurse or mother's singing. Singing could foster affectionate ties, but it also settled the child and allowed the carer to shake off their own troubles. A distressed or frustrated nurse could adversely affect the health of the baby she held. Robert Barret in his instructions for choosing a suitable nurse, informed parents that although some nurses 'are huffing and bounding about, and do not mind the poor Child', good nurses would 'sing with a soft voice to lull it to sleep, rocking gently all the while'.[71] John Jones described how 'lullies' (lullabies) served a dual purpose. First, 'children disquieted may be brought to reste', but second, 'light affections [that] may happen to annoy' the nurse could be uttered and tension alleviated through singing.[72] This, he argued, would cool the passions and excitements of both nurse and child. It meant that animosity towards the child dissipated and did not contaminate milk, if the rocker was the same individual who fed the child.[73] Intense emotions such as anger or resentment in a breastfeeding mother or nurse could cause the milk to corrupt or dissipate.

Medical writers universally condemned allowing newborns to sleep in the bed with parents or nurses.[74] Mauriceau stated that the infant should be kept away from sleeping nurses 'lest unawares she overlay it', but rather 'let her lay it in a Cradle close by the Bed-side, and put a Mantle over the head of the Cradle to prevent the falling of dust on its Face, and that the Day-light, Sunshine, Candle, or Fire in the Chamber, may not offend it.[75] Likewise, Guillemeau stated that an infant must 'be laid in his cradle: fitted with a little mattresse'.[76] This should be 'laid deepe to the bottome, that the sides of the cradle may be a great deale aboue the mattress' so the infant would not 'feare least he fall out of it'. He recommended tying strings around the infant so that if rocked, it would not fall out.[77] Cradles appear to have been common accoutrement in even middling-sort families, so much so that Alice Thornton recorded that both her one-year-old and newborn had separate cradles, laid next to each other in their mother's bedroom, until the illness of her elder child necessitated shifting the cradle to the 'Blew Parlor, a great way off from me, least I hearing her sad scriks should renue my sorrowes'.[78]

The ideal sleeping position of infants was much debated in childbearing guides. Most writers recommended laying infants on their back, with the head 'sumewhat hyer than the rest of the bodye', to help the excrements of the brain flow through the body.[79] Additionally, mothers and nurses were instructed to continually shift the child from the left to right side of the bed so as to ensure asymmetry did not develop. Lighting was particularly important. If the light source was consistently on one side of the room in which the cradle was placed, the infant could develop a squint. Sleeping was the final step in the regime of care nurses and those tasked with caring for the child had to accomplish after birth. It was only once excretion, movement and passions of the soul had been regulated that a baby could be allowed to indulge in sleep.

Conclusion

The six Non-Naturals played a prominent role in securing infant survival in the minutes, hours and days after birth. They were tools in the carers' arsenal to ready the baby for life outside the womb, and they facilitated the gradual transition from womb to cradle. Sudden 'mutations' in John Jones's terms were potentially fatal; babies were vulnerable and impressionable. While this could be problematic – infants that moved excessively could rupture their bellies or break and bend bones – it also meant their bodies were malleable, something that the practices of hygiene and swaddling made use of. Breathing was the prerequisite for life and it was only once the baby had voiced its vitality and viability that carers were instructed to embark on any of the above acts of care. The moisture that had sustained the infant during pregnancy, became life-threatening after birth and had to be excreted. As exercise was dangerous for young bodies, seventeenth-century childbearing manuals offered ways in which this Non-Natural could be managed through touch. Friction aided concoction and digestion, but it also settled infants and prevented the rousing of the passions of the soul. Through these tactile practices of care, the body could be shaped and moulded.

Here, I have discussed the stages of care and caregiving that have largely excluded food and drink. This is because medical writers were adamant that these acts should be carried out before the infant suckled. John Jones stated that if the 'youngly ... be ordered as you haue harde [heard], it shall be time to giue it sucke', stemming from the belief that greedy unborn children did little else but eat during pregnancy.[80] Babies were born gluttons, but their ability to digest and excrete was limited and needed to be carefully managed. The author of *Paidon nosemata* explained, 'by reason of the tendernesse and softnesse of [their] Palat ... they being unaccustomed to meat being newly born' had insatiable appetites and could suck 'more than they can digest'.[81] Nurses or mothers were instructed to wait until both the infant appeared well and the mother's milk was thin and white to begin breastfeeding. This advice appears to have been upheld within upper-sort seventeenth-century English families.[82] The parliamentarian Simonds D'Ewes recorded in his diary that when his first son, Clopton D'Ewes, was born, doctors advised that the 'child should not sucke any other till her [his wife's] breasts were drawn, and made fit for it'. D'Ewes attributed the 'cursed ignorance of such as were employed about my wife during her lying-in' for his child's premature death. Having delayed breastfeeding 'it was so weakened as afterwards proved the cause of its ruin'.[83] Excretion had to be established before the infant took on sustenance, and thus the practices of care discussed in this chapter were very much about preparing infants for their first feed. Previous accounts of early modern infant feeding practices have focused on social and cultural attitudes to breast milk and wet nursing.[84] More work is needed on what these measures reveal about concepts of infant health.

I have shown here that newborns were seen as bodily distinct from adults and children. This was inscribed in the formulaic regimen of care set out in childbearing manuals, of which the Non-Naturals were central in guiding the infant slowly to bodily independence.

Notes

1 R. Porter, 'The patients' view: doing medical history from below', *Theory and Society*, 14:2 (1985), pp. 175–98, on p. 193.

2 S. Cavallo and T. Storey have been the first to make Non-Naturals the centre of a historical study: *Healthy Living in Late Renaissance Italy* (Oxford: Oxford University Press, 2013).

3 B. Duden, *Woman Beneath the Skin: A Doctor's Patients in Eighteenth-Century Germany* (Cambridge MA: Harvard University Press, 1991); U. Rublack and P. Selwyn, 'Fluxes: the early modern body and the emotions', *History Workshop Journal*, 53 (2002), pp. 1–16.

4 Duden, *Woman Beneath the Skin*; L. Wynne Smith, 'Reassessing the role of the family: women's medical care in eighteenth-century England', *Social History of Medicine*, 16:3 (2003), pp. 327–42; 'The relative duties of a man: domestic medicine and France, ca. 1670–1740', *Journal of Family History*, 31:1 (2006), pp. 237–56; 'The body embarrassed? Rethinking the leaky male body in eighteenth-century England and France', *Gender & History*, 23:1 (2011), pp. 26–46; O. Weisser, 'Grieved and disordered: gender and emotion in early modern patient narratives', *Journal of Medieval and Early Modern Studies*, 43:2 (2013), pp. 247–74.

5 H. Newton, *The Sick Child in Early Modern England, 1580–1720* (Oxford: Oxford University Press, 2012).

6 V.A. Fildes (ed.), *Women as Mothers in Pre-Industrial England* (London: Routledge, 1990); U. Rublack, 'Pregnancy, childbirth and the female body in early modern Germany', *Past & Present*, 150:1 (1996), pp. 84–110; L.A. Pollock, 'Childbearing and female bonding in Early Modern England', *Social History*, 22 (1997), pp. 286–306; D. Cressy, *Birth, Marriage, and Death: Ritual, Religion, and the Life-Cycle in Tudor and Stuart England* (Oxford: Oxford University Press, 1999); A. Wilson, *The Making of Man-Midwifery: Childbirth in England, 1660–1770* (London: UCL Press, 1995),

and *Ritual and Conflict: The Social Relations of Childbirth in Early Modern England* (Farnham: Ashgate, 2013); L. Gowing, *Common Bodies: Women, Touch and Power in Seventeenth-Century England* (New Haven and London: Yale University Press, 2003).

7 E. Lane Furdell, *Publishing and Medicine in Early Modern England* (Rochester, NY: University of Rochester Press, 2002), p. 49.

8 M.E. Fissell, 'The marketplace of print', in M.S.R. Jenner and P. Wallis (eds), *Medicine and the Market in England and its Colonies c. 1450–c.1850* (Basingstoke: Palgrave Macmillan, 2007), p. 114.

9 R. Jonas, *The Byrth of Mankynde* (London: Tho. Ray, 1540) and T. Raynalde, *The Byrth of Mankynde, otherwise named the Womans Booke* (London: Tho. Ray, 1545).

10 Penelope Mordaunt to Sir John Mordaunt, 12 October 1699, Warwickshire Record Office, CR1368, vol. 1, f. 21.

11 M.E. Fissell has shown that 'wet-nursing, sick-nursing, rearing older children, or "doing for" men who lacked female relatives to provide such labour' were all called 'nursing' in early modern England: 'Women, health, and healing in Early Modern Europe', *Bulletin of the History of Medicine*, 82:1 (2008), pp. 1–17, 12–15. M. Pelling has similarly commented on the ambiguity of the role 'nurse': 'Nurses and nursekeepers: problems of identification in the Early Modern Period', in M. Pelling (ed.), *The Common Lot: Sickness, Medical Occupations and the Urban Poor in Early Modern England* (London: Longman, 1998), pp. 179–202.

12 A. Wilson terms this the 'fear thesis' in 'The perils of Early Modern procreation: childbirth with or without fear?' *British Journal of Eighteenth Century Studies*, 16 (1993), pp. 1–19, on p. 2. See also: R. Schofield, 'Did mothers really die? Three centuries of maternal mortality', in L. Bonfield et al., *The World We Have Gained. Histories of Population and Social Structure* (Oxford: Basil Blackwell, 1986), pp. 230–60; H. Roodenburg, 'The maternal imagination. The fears of pregnant women in seventeenth-century Holland', *Journal of Social History*, 21:4 (1988), pp. 701–16, and S. Howard, 'Imagining the pain and peril of seventeenth-century childbirth: travail and deliverance in the making of an Early Modern world', *Social History of Medicine*, 16:3 (2003), pp. 367–82.

13 Gowing, *Common Bodies*, p. 172.

14 J. Jones, *The Arte and Science of preseruing Bodie and Soule in Healthe* (London: Henrie Bynneman, 1579), p. 32.

15 Anne, Countess of Arundle to Mary Talbot, 21 August 1689, Lambeth Palace Library (henceforth L.P.L), MS 3205, f. 143.

16 J. Guillemeau, *Child-birth or, The happy deliuerie of women* (London: A. Hatfield, 1612), sig. Kk3v.

17 J. Sharp, *The Midwives book, or, The whole art of midwifery discovered* (London: Simon Miller, 1671), p. 374.
18 Cavallo and Storey, *Healthy Living*, pp. 240–70.
19 N. Culpeper, *Culpeper's Directory for Midwives: or, A guide for women* (London: Peter Cole, 1662), p. 144.
20 F.W. Stahnisch, 'The Tertium Compartionis of the Elementa Physiologiae – Johann Gotfried von Herder's conception of "tears" as mediators between the sublime and the actual bodily physiology', in M. Horstmanshoff, H. King and C. Zittel (eds), *Blood, Sweat and Tears: The Changing Concepts of Physiology from Antiquity into Early Modern Europe* (Leiden: Brill, 2012), pp. 595–629.
21 L. Lemnius, *The Secret Miracles of Nature* (London: Jo. Streater 1658), p. 274.
22 Culpeper, *Culpeper's directory*, pp. 246–7.
23 J.S., *Paidon Nosemata. Or, Childrens Diseases* (London: W.G, 1664), p. 31.
24 R. Barret, *A Companion for Midwives, child-bearing women, and nurses* (London: Tho. Ax., 1699), pp. 80–1.
25 Wellcome Library, London, MS3712, Elizabeth Okeover, pp. 119, 203, 210, 212, 213; 142, 142 and 157; 91 and 198. This recipe book has been discussed in more detail: Richard Aspin, 'Illustrations from the Wellcome Library: who was Elizabeth Okeover?' *Medical History*, 44 (2003), pp. 531–40.
26 Hannah Newton argues that medical writers understood children to experience emotions more powerfully than adults. See *The Sick Child in Early Modern England*, pp. 41–5.
27 R. Anselment, 'Mary Rich, Countess of Warwick, and the Gift of Tears', *The Seventeenth Century*, 22:1 (2007), pp. 336–57.
28 J. Pechey, *A general treatise of the diseases of infants and children* (London: R. Wellington, 1697), p. 7.
29 Sharp, *The midwives book*, p. 372.
30 Pechey, *A general treatise*, p. 1.
31 Cavallo and Storey, *Healthy Living*, p. 241.
32 Raynalde, *The byrth of mankynde otherwyse named the womans booke*, f. 110r.
33 Although formally attributed to Thomas Chamberlayne, Doreen Evenden has claimed that it was in fact written by female midwives. *The Compleat Midwifes Practice* (London: Nathaniel Brooke, 1656), p. 98. See: D. Evenden, *The Midwives of Seventeenth Century London* (Cambridge: Cambridge University Press, 2000).
34 M. Hoby, *Diary of Lady Margaret Hoby 1599–1605*, ed. D.M. Meads (London: Routledge, 1930), p. 184. For discussion of Lady Margaret Hoby's medical role see L. McCray Beier, *Sufferers and Healers: The Experience of Illness in Seventeenth-Century England* (London: Routledge, 1987),

esp. chapter 2; E. Botonaki, 'Dissecting bodies and selves in the Early Modern period', in Z. Detsi-Diamanti, K. Kitsi-Mitaka and E. Yiannopoulou (eds), *Flesh Made Text Made Flesh: Cultural and Theoretical Returns to the Body* (New York: Peter Lang, 2007), pp. 75–86.

35 Pechey, *A general treatise*, p. 2.

36 *Ibid.*

37 D. Osborne to B. Osborne, *c.*December 1686, British Library (henceforth B.L.), MS Add 28050, f. 63r.

38 A. Thornton, B.L., Add MS 88897/1, p. 135.

39 K. Wrightson, 'Infanticide in earlier seventeenth-century England', *Local Population Studies*, 15 (1975), pp. 10–22, and L. Gowing, 'Secret births and infanticide in seventeenth-century England', *Past & Present*, 156:1 (1997), pp. 87–115.

40 21 James I c. 27 (1624). For a discussion of the law see C. Damme, 'Infanticide: the worth of an infant under law', *Medical History*, 22 (1978), pp. 1–24.

41 R. Watkins, *Newes from the Dead. Or A True and Exact Narration of the miraculous deliverance of Anne Greene* (Oxford: Leonard Lichfield, 1651), pp. 6–7. Anne Greene is a particularly famous case because she miraculously revived after execution for infanticide and was then acquitted. See, S. Mandelbrote, 'William Petty and Anne Greene: medical and political reform in Commonwealth Oxford', in M. Pelling and S. Mandelbrote (eds), *The Practice of Reform in Health, Medicine and Science, 1500–2000* (Aldershot: Ashgate, 2005), pp. 125–51.

42 L. Gowing has argued that 'It was established knowledge that poor women, and in particular the mothers of bastards, bore their children quickly and more easily than those full prepared for a lying-in', and that such labours were 'shamefully easy'. 'Secret births and infanticide in seventeenth-century England', *Past & Present*, 156:1 (1997), pp. 87–115, on p. 99.

43 T.B., *The bloudy mother, or, The most inhumane murthers, committed by Jane Hattersley vpon diuers infants* (London: John Busbie, 1610), sig. A3v.

44 T.B., *The bloudy mother*, sig. A3v.

45 *Ibid.*

46 *Ibid*, sig. B1v.

47 F. Mauriceau, *The accomplish't Midwife* (London: John Darby, 1673), p. 353.

48 Sharp, *Midwives Book*, pp. 378–9.

49 Pechey, *A general treatise*, p. 7.

50 Raynalde, *The byrth of mankynde*, f. 110v.

51 *Ibid*, f. 110r.

52 Sennert, *Practical Physick*, Chap. 31, p. 267.

53 *OED*.
54 S. Read, '"Thy righteousness is but a menstrual clout": sanitary practices and prejudice in Early Modern England', *Early Modern Women: An Interdisciplinary Journal*, 3 (2008), pp. 1–25.
55 Raynalde, *The byrthe of mankynde*, f. 111r.
56 Sharp, *Midwives Book*, p. 375.
57 K. Thomas, 'Cleanliness and godliness in Early Modern England', in A. Fletcher and P. Roberts (eds), *Religion, Culture and Society in Early Modern Britain: Essays in Honour of Patrick Collinson* (Cambridge: Cambridge University Press, 1994), p. 58; V.S. Smith, 'Cleanliness: idea and practice in Britain, 1770–1850', unpublished PhD thesis, University of London, 1985, and *Clean: A History of Personal Hygiene and Purity* (Oxford: Oxford University Press, 2008).
58 Mary Douglas has argued that 'Dirt … is in the eye of the beholder'; *Purity and Danger: An Analysis of Concepts of Pollution and Taboo* (London: Routledge, 2001), p. 2.
59 F.van Dam, 'Permeable boundaries: bodies, bathing and fluxes: 1135–1333', in *Medicine and Space: Body, Surroundings and Borders in Antiquity and the Middle Ages* (Leiden: Brill, 2007), pp. 117–49.
60 Pechey, *A general treatise*, p. 6.
61 Jones, *The Arte*, p. 32.
62 M. Salmon, 'The cultural significance of breastfeeding and infant care in Early Modern England and America', *Journal of Social History*, 28:2 (1994), pp. 247–69.
63 Pechey, *A general treatise*, p. 3.
64 *Ibid.*
65 Jones, *The Arte*, p. 36.
66 Pechey, *A general treatise*, 4. Confusingly this same practice was attributed to Scottish women by John Locke in *Some Thoughts Concerning Education* (London: Churchill, 1693), p. 13. See also: M.R.S. Jenner, 'Bathing and baptism: Sir John Floyer and the politics of cold bathing', in K. Sharpe and S. Zwicker (eds), *Refiguring Revolutions: Aesthetics and the Politics of Cold Bathing* (Berkeley: University of California Press, 1998), pp. 197–216.
67 Culpeper, *A Directory for Midwives*, p. 144.
68 Guillemeau, *Child-birth*, sig. Nn3v.
69 *Ibid.*
70 Mauriceau, *The Accomplish't Midwife*, p. 368.
71 Barret, *A Companion for Mid-wives*, p. 91.
72 Jones, *The Arte*, pp. 13, 14.
73 For the modest body of scholarship on the history of lullabies see Leslie Daiken, *The Lullaby Book* (London: Edmund Ward, 1959), and

N. Tucker, 'Mothers, babies and lullabies', *History Today*, 34:9 (1984), pp. 40–6.

74 See recent work on changing sleeping patterns and arrangements as a result of social obligations: S. Handley, 'Sociable sleeping in Early Modern England, 1660–1760', *History*, 98:39 (2013), pp. 79–104.

75 Mauriceau, *The Accomplish't Midwife*, p. 368.

76 Guillemeau, *Child-birth*, sig. Mm3v–Mm4r.

77 Mauriceau, *The Accomplish't Midwife*, p. 369.

78 A. Thornton, B.L. Add MS 88897/1, pp. 134; 135.

79 Raynalde, *The byrth of mankynde*, f. 11r.

80 J. Jones, *The Arte*, p. 39.

81 J.S., *Paidon Nosemata*, p. 123.

82 See: V.A. Fildes, *Breasts, Bottles and Babies: A History of Infant Feeding* (Edinburgh: Edinburgh University Press, 1986).

83 S. D'Ewes, *The Autobiography and Correspondence of Sir Simonds D'Ewes: During the Reign of James I and Charles I*, ed. J.O. (London: R. Bentley, 1845), p. 44.

84 Fildes, *Breasts, Bottles and Babies*; 'The English wet-nurse and her role in infant care 1538–1800', *Medical History*, 32:2 (1988), pp. 142–73; D. McLaren, 'Marital fertility and lactation 1570–1720', in M. Prior (ed.), *Women in English Society 1500–1800* (London: Methuen, 1985), pp. 22–53; Salmon, 'Cultural significance of breastfeeding'; V. Sparey, 'Identity-formation and the breastfeeding mother in Renaissance generative discourses and Shakespeare's "Coriolanus"', *Social History of Medicine*, 25:4 (2012), pp. 777–94.

4

'She sleeps well and eats an egg': convalescent care in early modern England

Hannah Newton

Early modern diaries and letters are replete with complaints about the state of the body after illness. 'A long sicknes … has much drained mee … and indeed … my feeble hands … can scarce write', remarked Rev. Thomas Lowgh from Cumbria in 1654.[1] A few years later, the London gentlewoman Ann Fanshawe recorded in her memoirs, 'a very ill kind of fever … brought me so low that I was like an anatomy'.[2] In 1697, Elizabeth Freke from Norfolk lamented, 'God raised me up againe a miserable spectt[ac]le … hardly able to goe or stand'.[3] Serious physical illness thus left the body weak and lean, full of the 'footsteps of disease', to use the early modern term. It was not until full strength and flesh had returned that the patient was pronounced back to health. This chapter asks how doctors and laypeople measured the patient's growing strength after illness, and analyses the physiological processes through which this restitution was thought to occur. It shows that both the measures and the mechanisms for the restoration of strength were intimately connected to the 'six Non-Natural things': excretion, sleep, food, passions, air and exercise. Patients' sleeping patterns, appetites for foods, and emotions, along with other inclinations and behaviours that related to the Non-Naturals, were used to track their progression on 'the road to health'. Medical practitioners and the patient's family sought to regulate each Non-Natural in order to promote the body's restoration, and guard against possible relapse. I argue that this regulation, together with the assiduous monitoring of the patient's growing strength, constitute a concept of convalescent care.

The subject of convalescence has rarely been addressed in the historiography of early modern medicine. This is probably because scholars have assumed that the concept was a later, Victorian invention. Indeed, the word 'convalescence' conjures up images of Victorian gentlefolk at the seaside or in the mountains, an impression enhanced by the proliferation of convalescent homes and paintings of recuperating patients from the 1840s.[4] While convalescence may have attained unprecedented cultural resonance in the nineteenth century, it was *not* a new concept. The word was used throughout the early modern period: for example, a dictionary from 1657 by the London barrister Thomas Blount defines 'convalesce', as 'to wax strong, to recover health'.[5] Convalescence thus denoted the gradual restoration of strength after illness; it was understood to be the second part of recovery – the first part was the removal of disease.[6] Nonetheless, the word convalescence had yet to acquire a monopoly over this health state, since it was used interchangeably with such terms as 'the recoverer', 'the patient after illness' and 'the weak party'. By demonstrating that convalescence did exist conceptually in the early modern period, the chapter seeks to expand our knowledge of the scope of therapeutics at this time, and the role of the Non-Naturals within it.[7] It shows that the treatment of the convalescent was distinctive, differing from both the care of the sick and the healthy. A unique advantage of this subject is its potential to shed light on the vital medical concepts of disease and health: this is possible because convalescence was conceived as a liminal state, 'floating betwixt' these other two bodily conditions. As such, an analysis of the signs that were used to measure the patient's transition from illness to health yields insights into the defining characteristics of these other conditions. The discussions also reveal the little explored role of the body's life force and internal agent, 'Nature', in physiological processes. While there is a rich historiography on the wider concept of the natural world – also known by this term – the bodily agent of Nature has not received much attention.[8]

One exception to the lack of work on convalescence is a chapter by the food historian Ken Albala. Focusing on the single Non-Natural of diet, Albala avers that convalescent cookery was based on 'common sense intuition rather than theory'. From an analysis of European cookbooks and medical texts, he asserts that 'Despite major theoretical shifts in early modern nutritional theory ... the form and structure of convalescent cookery remained remarkably constant throughout the era and to a large extent even down to the present.'[9] Whilst agreeing that there was little change over time in the fundamentals of convalescent care, I argue that the treatment of recovering patients was based not on 'common sense', but on historically specific ideas about how the body regained strength. Through examining the roles of all six Non-Naturals, including diet, my chapter hopes to provide a more holistic view of convalescent care.

This study draws on a range of sources. To access medical opinions, vernacular medical texts of various genres have been used, including regimens of health, collections of remedies, and general medical treatises on all diseases 'from the head to the foot'. Most of the authors claimed to be physicians from early modern Britain or Europe, but it is not always possible to date the information contained within the texts, nor to attribute it to particular individuals. This is due to the tendency of writers to plagiarise earlier and contemporary texts, or to distort original wording in translations, new editions and posthumous publications. In view of these issues, the ideas conveyed in medical literature must be regarded as representative not so much of individual authors, but of a patchwork of viewpoints from before and beyond the lifespans of those physicians named on the title pages. The intended audiences of these texts were wide, encompassing laypeople as well as doctors. *Praxis medicinae, or, the physicians practice* (1632), by the German physician Walter Bruele, was 'published for the good, not onely of Physicians, Chirurgions, and Apothecaries, but very meete and profitable for all such which are solicitious of their health'.[10] Nevertheless, we cannot know for sure whether lay readers agreed with, or acted upon, the advice of the medical authors. Thus, in order to explore lay beliefs, it is necessary to use sources penned by laypeople themselves, such as letters between family and friends, spiritual diaries and autobiographies, and a selection of culinary and medicinal recipe books. Since convalescent care took place mainly at home, it makes sense to use sources which provide insights into domestic affairs.

While the above sources – medical and lay – are diverse in their purposes and characteristics, they exhibit certain commonalities, which makes their juxtaposition in this study appropriate. Namely, the authors embrace a humoral model of the human body, and come from the same echelons of society – the middling and upper classes. In the case of clergymen diarists and physician authors, there was degree of occupational sympathy: the care of the body and soul were connected, and ministers were often well versed in medical theory.[11] Alexandra Walsham and Alec Ryrie have shown that the religious outlook of puritan clergymen differed from those of other individuals in 'temperature' (that is, fervency) rather than substance, and therefore to use spiritual and medical sources in conjunction is reasonable.[12]

An important factor to bear in mind when analysing the above sources, highlighted by Olivia Weisser, is that the 'conventions and intentions of texts determined the kinds of stories recorded'.[13] In the case of domestic correspondence, for instance, one of its functions was to congratulate the recipient on recovery from illness, and provide kindly advice about how to promote the full restoration of strength. This is evident from letter-writing manuals, such as *The Enimie of Idlness*, by the merchant tailor William Fulwood (d. 1593). Fulwood instructs readers 'How to write Letters for our frends' upon their 'safe returne' to health, and even includes appropriate phrases for how to 'declare the joy that we have had of his mending'.[14] While these conventions do not necessarily undermine the sincerity of authors' words, they do remind us that sources should not be viewed as 'transparent window[s] onto lived experience'.[15] Another methodological challenge to consider is the over-representation of the wealthy in society: most of the authors were landowners, engaged in legal, clerical, medical or parliamentary careers. It is probable that the length of time allowed for convalescence, as well as any special foods, rest and medicines prescribed to patients were heavily dependent on finances. Nonetheless, a reasonable number of the authors came from more modest backgrounds, such as the Yorkshire diarist Joseph Lister (1627–1709), who worked as a clothier and servant.[16]

The first section of the chapter asks why the body was weak after illness; the next part categorises the convalescent within early modern schemes of bodily states; the rest of the chapter is structured around the milestones or signs of increasing strength, each of which is associated with a particular Non-Natural.

The cause of weakness

To understand why the body was weak after illness, it is necessary to go back a step, and see how contemporaries explained the removal of disease. As I have shown elsewhere, three agents were thought to be involved, and they formed a clear hierarchy: God, Nature, and the physician.[17] God's instrument for removing disease was Nature, the 'intrinsic agent' and life force of the body.[18] The word 'nature' held many meanings in this period, but in the context of galenic physiology it denoted a divinely endowed power in the body.[19] Since the body was conceived as a microcosm of the world, the Nature in the body was seen as a miniature version of the wider Nature that maintained the order of the universe.[20] Personified as a benevolent housewife, Nature was responsible for all basic physiological functions, including growth, nutrition, and most importantly here, the removal of disease.[21] Nature's vehicles for performing her functions were the 'natural spirits', highly rarefied, 'subtile and Arey' vapours, 'raised from the purer blood', and carried around the body in the veins.[22] So strong was the connection between the spirits and Nature, the two were often regarded as synonymous.[23] At the bottom of the hierarchy of healers was the physician: he was described as 'an assistant and helper of nature in time of neede'.[24] As an inferior agent, he was expected to defer to Nature when treating the sick by imitating her methods. This tripartite model was espoused by practitioners across the early modern period.[25]

Upon God's command, Nature removed disease by rectifying the bad humours that had caused it. She did this through processes known as concoction and expulsion. Concoction was a form of internal cooking, through which means the malignant quality of the humours was erased; it was similar to the complex process of digestion, which was also known as 'concoction'.[26] Expulsion was the removal of superfluous humours through the 'crisis of the disease', the sudden, spontaneous evacuation of body fluids at the height of illness, in the form of sweating, vomiting, diarrhoea or other emissions. When Nature was struggling to produce these evacuations, the physician stepped in, and administered evacuative treatments, such as emetics and purges.

Once these processes were complete, the disease was gone, but the patient was not yet pronounced back to health: the body was weak and lean. Weakness was defined as the 'slowness' or 'imbecility' of the faculties of the body, caused by the 'dissipation' or 'decay' of the natural, animal, and vital spirits.[27] As stated above, the natural spirits were Nature's vehicles for carrying out the body's basic functions. The other two types – the animal and vital spirits – drove the higher faculties of the body and mind: muscular movement, the senses and rational powers (animal faculties); and breathing, the pulse and the emotions (vital faculties).[28] In turn, all three types of spirit were responsible for distributing what were known as 'radical moisture' (an oily substance) and 'innate heat' (a glowing warmth) around the body: these were the elements in which 'life consisteth', which gradually depleted with age.[29] Crucially, the processes of removing disease consumed these several substances: the heat of concoction dried out the radical moisture, and the critical evacuations removed all three types of spirits along with the bad humours.[30] The result was multiple forms of weakness, each connected to the particular spirits that had been evacuated: the dissipation of the animal spirits caused 'feebleness of motion', memory loss and dim eyesight; the consumption of the natural spirits caused poor digestion, leanness, pale complexion and vulnerability to relapse; and the loss of vital spirits resulted in faintness and anxiety.[31] In what follows, we will see that the restoration of strength was achieved chiefly by the replenishment of the spirits, innate heat and radical moisture.

Categorising the convalescent

Where did convalescence fit in early modern categories of health states, and were the aims of convalescent care distinctive? Medical writers usually envisaged three main bodily states: healthful, neutral and unhealthful (or sick).[32] Healthful was defined as the balance of the 'primary qualities' (heat, cold, dry and wet), together with the strong functioning of the faculties (animal, natural and vital). Unhealthy was the opposite: individuals suffered the 'perceptible impairment' of the faculties, and the imbalance of the four qualities – it included diseases and wounds.[33] Suspended between these two categories was the 'neutral body', otherwise known as the 'crazie' or 'valetudinarie body'.[34] Defined by Galen as 'an exquisite medium between healthful and unhealthful Bodies', it was a melting pot for all those individuals deemed 'neither perfectly whole, nor thoroughly sicke', such as those who were falling ill but not yet sick, the 'decrepit elderly', lying-in mothers, and most crucially, convalescents.[35] The neutral body has attracted only limited attention from historians, perhaps because it is no longer recognised in modern medicine.[36]

Each category of bodily state was subject to a different therapeutic aim: the care of the healthy sought to preserve the current state; the treatment of the sick aimed at the removal of the disease or wound; and the care of the neutral centred on restoration.[37] Within the neutral category, further distinctions were drawn between subgroups of patients. The Polish physician Johannes Johnstonus (1603–75), who had trained at Cambridge and Leiden, stated that whereas those who were falling sick required measures that would prevent the illness from taking hold, 'persons ... recovering' require 'two things': '1) That they fal not back again into their sicknesses. / 2) That they may soon recover their perfect health.'[38] Thus, the aims of convalescent care were the prevention of relapse, and the restoration of strength. The term used to denote this special branch of physic was 'analeptics', which meant 'to cherish and renew the strength.'[39] In the rest of this chapter, we will see how these aims were fulfilled.

The final purge

The first component of convalescent care relates to the Non-Natural excretion. Throughout the early modern period, physicians worried that after illness the body might contain residues of malignant humours that had been 'left over' from the crisis of the disease.[40] The concern was that these remaining humours would lead to relapse; practitioners therefore sought to prevent this eventuality by giving a 'final gentle purge' to 'carry off' the remnant humour. The Scottish physician John Macollo (1576–1622) warned in his posthumously published medical canons, 'if the Cris[is]e have been imperfect, it is the duty of the Physitian to purge [the] rest of the vicious humours, fearing lest by process of time, putrifying within the body, they renew the sickness.'[41] Colourful metaphors were used to explain the need for this treatment: the remaining humour was like a dead dog in a house, or a 'brood of bees', which, if not 'quickly throw[n] out', would 'soon make you weary of your Habitation.'[42] This tendency to depict the humours and other body parts as animals is a recurring theme in early modern medical writings.[43]

Laypeople as well as medical authors were aware of the necessity of the final purge after illness, as is evident in recipe collections, which provide instructions for making a 'very good purge for a weak constitution after feavour' or some other disease.[44] In hindsight, patients and their relatives attributed relapse or further illnesses to the failure to purge the body. The Lancashire-born Presbyterian clergyman Adam Martindale (1623–86) reminisced in his autobiography that after suffering smallpox as a child in the early 1630s, he 'should have been soundly purged, but was not; which as I verily believe, caused a vehement fermentation in my bodie, which, after two or three yeares' space, [came] out in an ugly dry scurfe'.[45] As well as revealing that the bad humours were imagined to remain in the body for years, this extract indicates that the final purge was sometimes neglected. Besides the cost, this may have been because patients were tired of taking physic, and wanted to give it up at the earliest opportunity.[46]

In theory, the convalescent's final purge differed from the purges administered to the sick and healthy. Those who were still ill required stronger, and more frequent, evacuations, because their bodies contained larger quantities of bad humours. Conversely, 'those persons that be perfectlie in health ought not to take a[ny] *Purgation* since they doe not abound with corrupt humours', wrote the anonymous author of a late sixteenth-century medical manual for the poor.[47] The reason doctors were reluctant to purge the healthy was that they believed the purging medicines, finding 'no excrements' in the body, would set upon 'solid and sound parts', and 'make a colliquation of good flesh'.[48] Of course, in practice many healthy people *did* take purges, because it was believed that those bodies which were 'inclined to fall' into sickness might also contain some noxious matter.[49] Nonetheless, the term 'final gentle purge' was reserved for convalescents, which indicates that it was distinctive to this group of patients in its timing and mildness.

Sleeping through the night

The next milestone relates to the Non-Natural sleep, a function defined as 'the rest of the whole body, and the cessation of the Animal faculty'.[50] Sleep occurred when the stomach sent a 'certain vaporous, sweet, and delightsome humidity' to the brain, which blocked the nerves, the routes through which the animal spirits travelled; the result was the temporary suspension of the powers of the animal faculty – movement, sensation and understanding.[51] During serious illness, the special vapour evaporated or became 'infected' by the bad humours; the result was 'unquiet' or interrupted sleep. Upon recovery, however, sleep came more easily: the abatement of pain 'allured' the animal spirits to 'quiet rest', and the rectification of the humours restored the sleep-inducing vapour to its proper quality.[52] Throughout the period, uninterrupted sleep was interpreted as a 'good signe' of recovery. George Davenport from Leicestershire, aged 31, told his former Cambridge tutor in 1662, 'I am like to do well … if I may ghess … by … [my] most profound sleep. I never waked in the night.'[53] The fact that continuous sleep was taken as a sign of growing health has important implications for the historian Roger Ekirch's notion of 'segmented sleep'. Ekirch argued that 'Western Europeans on most evenings experienced two major intervals of sleep bridged by up to an hour or more of quiet wakefulness'.[54] If unbroken sleep was a token of growing health – the norm to which most people aspired – it could be an indication that segmentation was in fact less widespread than has been acknowledged.

As well as signifying that the patient was on the mend, sleep played a crucial restorative role. The sixteenth-century Dutch physician Levinus Lemnius stated in his posthumously translated treatise, *The secret miracles of nature*, that he who 'hath already discussed the disease … yet … is weak, feeble, [and] exhausted … may be restored by sleep'.[55] Imagery of plant irrigation was used to describe the mechanism through which strength was restored – the body was 'besprinkled' with a '*mild and pleasant vapour*' during sleep, whereby the 'whole man' was furnished with new radical moisture.[56] The spirits also benefitted from sleep – exhausted from the disease, they were 'refreshed' and 'recruited' by 'soft Slumbers'.[57] Such descriptions suggest that the spirits were inseparable from the patient's own feelings. Sleep also performed a nutritional function: digestion was at its best during sleep, since Nature was undistracted by other tasks, and could concentrate solely on building up the body.[58] Sasha Handley's contribution to this volume has found that the physical and spiritual benefits of sound sleep received unprecedented emphasis after 1660, in response to rising medical interest in the brain and nerves, together with the intensification of household religious practices. Although the restorative virtues of sleep for convalescents were well known before the mid-seventeenth century, there does seem to have been an upturn in the level of detail devoted to this subject in the later medical texts.

Medical authors prescribed different sleep routines for each bodily state. The puritan Northampton physician James Hart (d. 1639) wrote in his regimen, *Diet for the diseased*, that the sick should be 'suffer[ed] to sleep when[ever] they can', including the daytime, because it was 'often out [of] our power to accommodate it … to the right and proper time'.[59] By contrast, for the healthy 'the night should bee more convenient for sleepe than the day' because the sunlight of daytime would draw the body's innate heat in the wrong direction – outwards.[60] Convalescents fell in-between: ideally, they should remain awake in the morning, but they were permitted to nap in the afternoon.[61] Over the course of recovery, however, convalescents were instructed to let daytime sleep be 'lost by litle and litle', until at last they had acquired the 'accustomed order' of the healthy.[62]

Feeling hungry

Sleep was rarely mentioned without reference to appetite, and together the two served as a litmus test for the state of the body. The first sign of approaching sickness was 'tast[e] … insipid; … the appetite … dull'; once illness arrived in full, it was commonly observed that 'sick men loathe nothing so much as meate'.[63] The reason for these changes was that Nature, the agent of appetite and nutrition, was not proficient at multitasking: during illness she was wholly occupied with the concoction and expulsion of the bad humours, and could not be easily 'diverted from her office and work' by the task of digestion.[64] Once the bad humours had been rectified, however, this agent had time once more to carry out the digestion of food. The result was the return of appetite, a universal sign of growing strength. 'I praise God I am now in the way of recovery: I am able to … eate my meat with reasonable stomacke', wrote the Essex gentleman Henry Cromwell to his sister in 1630.[65]

Although everybody required sustenance to stay alive, dietary priorities differed in sickness, health and convalescence. In sickness, the main purpose of eating was to help Nature remove the disease by correcting the humours. To this end, the patient was supposed to be given an 'allopathic diet', which meant consuming foods and drinks of the opposite qualities to the malignant humours.[66] The healthy, by contrast, were entreated to preserve their humoral constitution by following a 'sympathetic' diet.[67] However, in convalescence, the majority of the humours had already been rectified, and therefore the aim of eating was less explicitly related to the humours, and more to do with the restoration of lost strength and flesh. How were these goals achieved? There were many guidelines and precautions to bear in mind. The first was timing: Macollo warned, 'When the body is not clear, the more it is nourish'd the more it is hurt.'[68] It was believed that if nourishing foods were eaten before the final purge, they would be greedily 'licked up' by the residual humours, resulting in relapse. There was also concern about the form of the food. The Sussex physician Thomas Twyne (1543–1613) wrote in his regimen that for the first two or three days of convalescence the 'Recoverer [should] … retain the same diet' that he had taken during illness, consuming only liquid foods. The reason was that 'it is not good to chaunge suddenly from that wherto a man is accustomed … because of custome.'[69] Twyne was referring to the Hippocratic proverb 'custom is a second Nature', which dictated that habit was almost as vital to bodily functioning as Nature herself. Liquid foods were advantageous because they were more quickly distributed around the body than solid foods; the best forms were jellies, possets, broths and soups.[70]

Another important consideration was the patient's personal food preferences. At the beginning of convalescence, it was vital to indulge the patient's dietary predilections. The Manchester physician Thomas Cogan provided the justification in his regimen for students: '[L]iking causeth good concoction [i.e., digestion]. For what the stomacke liketh, it greedily desireth: and having received it, closely incloseth it about untill it bee duly concocted … wherein wee have great delight … it doth us more good.'[71] Personified as a fussy creature, the weak stomach of the convalescent could more effectively digest foods which it desired. It was Nature who produced these cravings – she 'calls for that which is good for it self': the practitioner's role was simply to supply her with what she wanted.[72]

The next priority was nourishment: it was essential to build up the lean body by giving highly nourishing foods. The most nutritious foods were thought to be substances which resembled the human body; this was because nutrition was understood to be a process of assimilation, whereby the ingested matter was transformed into the substance of the body.[73] Consequently, meat was thought to be more nutritious than vegetables, because its 'fat and gluttonous substance has neerest affinity with mans radicall moisture.'[74] Likewise, flesh was considered to be superior to fish, since humans bore a closer resemblance to the former.[75]

Amongst non-aquatic creatures, further distinctions were drawn: animals that could fly would 'afford the body a ... subtill nourishment' because 'the wings of such fowles ... are in perpetuall motion', wrote Hart.[76] By contrast, 'four-footed beasts' that lived on the ground provided less wholesome nourishment. The favouring of flying creatures probably stems from natural philosophical notions of the 'Chain of Being', the hierarchy of living things. Allen Grieco has shown that fowl and birds were thought to be 'nobler' than quadrupeds and fish, because they were associated with the superior element of the air, whereas land- or ocean-bound creatures were analogous of the lower elements of earth and water.[77] The sky was closer to the heavens and to God, while the earth held connotations of death and damnation.[78] Given this cultural backdrop, it is unsurprising that the most nutritious creatures were judged to be those which could fly.

As well as being nutritious, the convalescent's food had to be 'easie of digestion'.[79] Easily digested foods were aliments that did not require much alteration from their present state, such as eggs and milk. Speaking of eggs, the Wiltshire MP and physician Thomas Moffet (1553–1604) wrote, 'They nourish quickly, because they are nothing but liquid flesh.'[80] The clue was the colour: white foods, like chicken and partridges, were the easiest to digest as a pale tone signified that the texture was light, and therefore could be broken down with minimum effort. Conversely, dark-coloured animals, such as beef and venison, 'may not be allowed' because they were too heavy and dense.[81] These colour preferences may have been informed by religious ideas: Christianity celebrated light, and equated darkness with evil.[82] One way to make foods more digestible was to cook them; the preferred method throughout the period was boiling, because it was most similar to Nature's own form of digestion in the stomach.[83] The easy digestibility of the food is one quality which overlaps with the diet of the diseased, since sick people's stomachs were thought to be even weaker than those of convalescents. However, healthy individuals required the opposite, as revealed in the text *Regimen Sanitatis Salerni*, allegedly written by the twelfth-century Italian physician Johannes de Mediolano:

> For they that be strong and lusty, and exercise great labour must be dyeted with grosser meat because in them the way of digestion is strong, and so they ought not to use slender meats, as Chickens, Capons ... or Kid, For those fleshes in them will burn, or be digested oversoon.[84]

The stomach of the healthy person was depicted as a fiery furnace, which would burn up slender food in a moment. These individuals therefore required much tougher meats, which would provide more sustained, slow-burning nourishment.

Turning from the quality of food to the quantity, throughout the early modern period convalescents were advised to 'be temperate in eating and drinking ... tak[ing] a little and often.'[85] Although moderation was important in all states of health, it was thought to be critical in convalescence, due to the residual weakness of the digestive faculty.[86] This advice sounds simple enough, but judging by doctors' reports, it was notoriously difficult to follow: medical texts and casebooks are full of cautionary tales of patients who overindulged, with devastating consequences.[87] Physicians warned that the appetite is 'sharp' after acute illness, which makes self-restraint a great challenge, whilst the social celebrations that were commonly arranged to mark the person's recovery added to the danger, since they provided opportunities for overeating, along with other excesses. Hence Lemnius complained,

> [W]hen men recover of their disease many witty merry companions come to see them, and they invite them to rejoyce, and make merry ... Hence they eat, and drink healths ... and commonly ... they sing bawdy songs ... To this I add the delicate and voluptuous meats, which the humours being augmented by, do stimulate and prick the obscene parts ... and cause erection ... [thus they] return to ... gluttony, and profuse lusts.[88]

In this context, medical and religious concerns coalesce: gluttony for food and other sensual appetites would lead to the double relapse of body and soul, since God used the natural consequences of immoderate eating to renew disease and punish the sinner.[89] Lemnius later became a priest, so it is possible that his emphasis on the spiritual implications of the convalescent's behaviour was especially pronounced.[90] Besides, we should be wary about how we interpret doctors' reports of patients' excesses – the authors may have been highlighting these instances as a way to divert the blame for relapse from themselves onto their patients. After all, one of the purposes of medical texts was to promote the doctor's professional reputation.

Growing cheerful

The next Non-Natural to consider is 'the passions of the soul', or to use modern terminology, the emotions, a subject of rising historical interest in recent years.[91] Medical historians have paid considerable attention to the perceived impact of the passions on the body, but much less has been said about the influence of the body on the passions.[92] The following paragraphs illuminate both sides of the relationship, thereby providing a more complete picture of the body–soul connection in early modern perceptions.

The passions provided clues into a person's state of health. The 'Messenger or forerunner' of illness was a creeping feeling of anxiety, whilst at the height of illness, 'a horror … invades the sick' wrote the popular medical writer and astrologer Nicholas Culpeper (1616–54). This claim is supported by patients' frequent expressions of fear and grief during illness.[93] Upon recovery, however, they began to grow cheerful, as testified by the Suffolk conformist clergyman Isaac Archer (1641–1700), who stated in 1679, 'My mind is more cheerly, and I get strength.'[94] Laughter and cheerfulness were taken as clear signs of growing health. Medical texts drew on Aristotelian philosophy to explain these emotional responses. Hart stated that '[A]lthough the substance of the soule and body differ much, God hath … tyed and united them so fast …, that there is no small … sympathy betwixt them: insomuch that either of them being affected, the other suffereth also.'[95] Thus, the body and soul were so bonded that they shared one another's sorrows and joys. As Erin Sullivan has recently commented, this reciprocal influence seems to have been understood 'less as cause and effect and more as simultaneous happening'.[96]

Cheerfulness was cherished during convalescence, not just because it was pleasant in itself, but because it was thought to be a means for restoring strength to the body. *The sickmans rare jewel* (1674), by B.A., states that it 'recreates and quickens all the Faculties, … helps concoction, makes the Body to be better in liking, and fattens it'.[97] Sandra Cavallo and Tessa Storey have observed that *allegrezza* (cheerfulness) was understood to be a 'calm, tranquil happiness' which gently lifts and expands the spirits, 'thereby increasing the overall body heat and vitality'.[98] Since the strength of the body was synonymous with the quantity and liveliness of the spirits, the augmentation of these substances automatically invigorated all the faculties of the body. Cheerfulness also helped the body to put on weight, since the newly enlivened natural spirits propelled the digested aliment from the interior organs to the rest of the body, thereby facilitating the process of nutrition.[99] These ideas were expressed throughout the period.[100]

Unfortunately, the cheery feelings of convalescents were not universal – some patients suffered from 'low spirits' or 'faint-heartedness'.[101] Common causes included the traumatic memory of pain, and the fear of relapse.[102] What made these emotions all the more distressing for patients and their loved ones was the belief that they could precipitate the return of disease.[103] The Essex puritan clergyman Ralph Josselin attributed the renewed illness of his 8-year-old daughter Jane in 1653 to her 'feare and griefe [at] see[ing] her mother ... tormented ... with a felon [boil] on her finger'.[104] Physicians explained these effects by reference to the spirits: anxiety made these special vapours shrink and dissipate, and recoil to the heart.[105] Since the spirits were the chief instruments through which Nature concocted and expelled bad humours, their sudden reduction in volume impeded this agent's defence against returning disease. Anxiety also hindered nutrition: the centripetal direction of the spirits from the surface of the body to the heart starved the outer parts of nourishment – the result was the continuation of bodily wasting.[106]

In view of the divergent effects of positive and negative emotions, convalescent care sought to promote the former and guard against the latter. Expressions of love and kindness, together with 'merry company', were regarded as the 'best cordials'.[107] Families strived to protect recovering relatives from sorrow by concealing bad news. The Somerset gentlewoman Ursula Venner warned her brother in 1675 that, although 'the danger is over', their father 'is soe extreamly we[e]ping at all kind of buisnesse that I would desire you to send him as little of ill news as possible'.[108] Of course, these forms of emotional support were unlikely to have been universal: it was not always possible to conceal bad news, nor did all convalescents enjoy such loving family relationships. Furthermore, domestic correspondence may provide a skewed picture of the lengths to which relatives went to promote the convalescent's happiness, since a function of this genre was to bestow consolation and advice.[109]

Unlike some of the other components of convalescent care, cheerfulness was beneficial in all bodily states. Doctors agreed that 'nothing is more necessary for the Preservation of Health, than to live merrily'.[110] In sickness, cheerfulness was thought to 'rouse up and unite' the body's spirits, so that they were able to more 'effectively co-operate with Nature, and strengthen her in the performance of the … expulsion of the noxious humours', wrote the medical writer and minister John Harris.[111] Nonetheless, in practice it was difficult to provoke cheerfulness during sickness: the pain of illness, together with the 'true sorrow for sinne' sparked by thoughts of death, conspired against their intentions.[112] Likewise, it was impractical to always promote cheerfulness in the healthy, since sorrow was an inevitable companion of life.[113] As such, the emotion of cheerfulness assumed a special status during convalescence – it was both a sign and a catalyst of growing strength.

Sitting up to going abroad

The final Non-Naturals to consider are exercise and air. Convalescence was basically a process of increasing physical exertion and exposure to the air. In acute sickness, the patient was usually confined to a bedchamber, breathing in warm air.[114] Once the illness was gone, however, the patient could begin to return to normal life, a trajectory that was measured by a number of key spatial movements. In 1666, 14-year-old Samuel Jeake from Rye in Sussex described his recovery from smallpox as follows:

> 21st July: I lay upon the bed all day.
> 22nd: Something better; but kept my bed till 27th then I rose.
> 28th: I went into my Study.
> 29th Downstairs.
> 30th into the garden.[115]

Each action signified a certain level of strength, and therefore they were useful for tracking a person's progress towards health. The final action – going outside or 'abroad' – was shorthand for complete recovery.[116] Some of the actions were gender or age specific: when men 'went abroad', it was usually to their former employment, whereas a recovered woman would be described as being 'able to doe [her] business in the house'.[117] Children were accorded their own special milestone, play.[118] The significance of the patient's location as a measure of health has not been sufficiently recognised in the historiography.[119]

The exercise and exposure to air that accompanied the above actions was thought to contribute to the restoration of strength after illness. Hart stated, 'exercise ... increase[s] the natural heat, [causes] a more speedy ... distribution of the spirits ... and addition of strength to all the members therof'.[120] Pure, temperate air 'engenders both Vital and Animal Spirits', and 'opens the pores' of the skin, thereby enabling any remnant humours to escape, and preventing relapse.[121] Since the spirits shared the 'arey' consistence of the air, breathing was the most direct way to replenish these substances. Laypeople concurred about the strengthening effects of exercise and air, although they were less likely to describe the precise physiological processes involved.[122] The best air for the convalescent was mountain or country air, a preference which endured throughout the early modern period.[123]

Nonetheless, these Non-Naturals were not without danger: namely, the patient's premature activity or exposure to the outdoor air could lead to relapse. Upon recovery from fever in 1657, the Bradford servant Joseph Lister confessed that he had 'longed to go into the garden ... and did so for a few minutes, but soon repented my folly, for next morning I was confined to my bed, and much worse than before'.[124] Even apparently minor actions, such as sitting up, could have severe consequences.[125] This was because it was believed that immediately after illness, when the body lacked strength and flesh, Nature's priority was nourishment; to force the body to exercise would therefore 'stop the Work of Nature so luckily begun' and delay the restoration of strength.[126] Exposure to cold air caused relapse by shutting the pores of the skin, thereby blocking the exits for the body's remnant humours.[127]

The intentions behind convalescent care were to prevent these potential dangers by carefully 'ordering' the patient's progression through the actions. Friends and family sent letters to recovering patients advising them to refrain from going abroad until they were quite ready 'to bear those journeys'.[128] Convalescents were also told to 'try their strength', and attempt everything gradually. The dean of the Faculty of Medicine in Reims, Nicholas Abraham de La Framboisière (1560–1636), advised, 'such [as] are newly recover'd from Sickness ...

must by degrees ... accustom themselves to a more free and plentiful Air.'[129] The reason for these incremental changes was once the notion that 'Nature abhors all sudden change', an aphorism which linked to the idea expressed earlier that custom was 'a second nature'. Temperature was also important: the convalescent was instructed to 'only stir abroad on warm days, and with very warm clothes to keep out the cold.'[130] Such measures would ensure that the pores of the skin remained open, thus providing a convenient exit for remnant humours. Finally, when possible patients and their families put in place special arrangements that would help limit the dangers posed by exercise and air, such as travelling by carriage rather than on horseback, and delegating strenuous work to friends or colleagues.[131] These arrangements were dependent on the good will of others, as well as the financial position of the individual.

Once again, the convalescent was subject to a different regime to those in sickness and health. Hart stated that in acute illness, patients should not 'use any exercise at all': such diseases were 'so violent and fierce' that Nature could not afford to divert her spirits from the vital tasks of concocting and expelling the humours.[132] Likewise, exposure to outdoor air was to be avoided in acute illness, on the grounds that it would hinder the critical evacuation of the noxious humours, instead sending them inwards towards the 'noble organs'.[133] The advice for the healthy was rather different: fresh air and 'vehement exercise' were 'so necessarie to the preservation of health' that without them 'no man may be long without sicknes', wrote the humanist and lawyer Thomas Elyot (*c.*1490–1546) in his widely published regimen.[134] These Non-Naturals maintained the strength of the healthy body by stirring up the spirits and promoting the perspiration of superfluous humours. The convalescent's regimen was a transition between these two extremes.

Conclusion

The Non-Naturals played two vital functions during convalescence in early modern England. The first was prognostic: the manifestation of each Non-Natural acted as a measure of the patient's growing strength. Miss Kemey 'sleeps well and eats an egg and sits up for two or three hours', wrote the Bishop of Bath and Wells, Thomas Ken, in 1686, which he took as a sign she was 'past danger'.[135] Cheerful passions, an appetite for food and the ability to 'walk abroad' signified that the patient was 'on the mending hand'. The second role was therapeutic: the manipulation of the Non-Naturals was the chief means through which strength and flesh were restored. Pleasant, nutritious food, pure and temperate air, and cheerful emotions served to refresh and expand the spirits, thereby enlivening and fattening the 'whole man'. Personified to a high degree, the spirits seem to have been synonymous with the patient's own strength and well-being. Ultimately, it was the body's internal agent, Nature, under the command of God, who was in charge of these processes: it was she who made the patient feel sleepy after illness, and hungry for certain foods. The practitioner was supposed to act 'in subserviency to her designs', simply promoting what Nature was already doing. Through emphasising the agency of Nature, this chapter has sought to deepen our understandings of the perceived role of this agent in bodily processes, a topic which has received little attention. These discussions have also shed fresh light on the meanings of health and disease, states traditionally defined as balance and imbalance: other crucial components were function and location – sickness was being in bed, unable to do anything; health was being able to sleep, eat, walk and go abroad. Little evidence has been found to show change over time in the care or perception of the convalescent, as the footsteps of disease – weakness, emaciation and vulnerability to relapse – were reported consistently across the period. Likewise, the methods that were used to restore strength, such as nutritious and easily digestible food, and plenty of sleep, went uncontested into the eighteenth century. Such continuity does not mean that convalescent care was based on 'common sense', or was somehow divorced from medical theory. Rather, it reflects the endurance of the belief in the role of the spirits in the restoration of strength.[136]

Whilst much work has been conducted on the gendering of bodies, far less has been written about bodily categorisations based on states of health.[137] We have seen that the convalescent was placed into the 'neutral' category of bodies, alongside other individuals who were deemed 'neither sick nor sound'. By resurrecting this forgotten category, this chapter has sought to widen our knowledge of early modern bodily classifications, and encourage comparative studies of groups within the neutral category. My prediction is that there was considerable semblance between the therapeutic priorities directed at the various neutral groups: those on the cusp of illness, the elderly, and newly delivered mothers all required strengthening.[138] The interpretive value of the neutral category is substantial, as it brings us to a closer understanding of how early modern people judged ambiguous states of health. This is nicely illustrated by an observation made by the physician Levinus Lemnius, who was of the opinion that daily experience teaches that most people 'ought not to be placed amongst the sick or sound; but partaking in both ... [:] the neutrall condition'. His evidence was that if we ask 'our friends ... what health he is in', he will almost certainly reply, 'So so, indifferent ... doubtfully, inclining, flo[a]ting between both, instable ... not as we could wish.'[139] Thus, the neutral category was indispensable because it captured the everyday reality of imperfect health.

An underlying question in the discussions has been to what extent the care of the convalescent differed from the treatment of the other categories of body. It has been shown that the therapeutic intentions clearly differed: whereas practitioners sought to remove disease from the sick, and preserve health in the sound, convalescent care or 'analeptics' was devoted to the restoration of strength and the prevention of relapse. However, we have seen that there was some overlap between the three schemes, since convalescence was a liminal state: over the course of recovery, the patient's regimen became increasingly similar to that of the healthy person.

Notes

1 [Fleming], *The Flemings in Oxford*, ed. J.R. Magrath, Oxford Historical Society, vol. 44 (Oxford, 1904), vol. 1, p. 69.
2 A. Fanshawe, *Memoirs of Lady Fanshawe*, ed. R. Fanshawe (London: Henry Colburn, 1829), p. 125.
3 E. Freke, *The Remembrances of Elizabeth Freke*, ed. R. Anselment, Camden Fifth Series, vol. 18 (Cambridge: Cambridge University Press, 2001), p. 235.
4 See the blog by the Johns Hopkins PhD student, E. Anders: http://remedianetwork.net/2014/11/07/locating-convalescence-in-victorian-england/ (accessed 20 February 2015).
5 T. Blount, *Glossographia, or, a Dictionary* (London: Thomas Newcomb, 1656), image 82.

6 On the removal of disease, see my article, ' "Nature concocts & expels": the agents and processes of recovery from disease in Early Modern England', *Social History of Medicine*, 28:3 (2015), pp. 445–64.

7 This draws on research from my book, *Misery to Mirth: Recovery from Illness in Early Modern England* (Oxford: Oxford University Press, forthcoming); I would like to thank the Wellcome Trust for generously funding this research; award reference: 095760/Z/11/Z.

8 The literature on the wider concept of nature is extensive. Here are just a few examples: R.G. Collingwood, *The Idea of Nature* (Oxford: Oxford University Press, 1945); C. Merchant, *The Death of Nature: Women, Ecology, and the Scientific Revolution* (London: Harper & Row, 1980); J. Torrance (ed.), *The Concept of Nature* (Oxford: Clarendon Press, 1992); L. Daston and K. Park, *Wonders of the Order of Nature, 1150–1750* (New York: Zone Books, 2001); L. Daston and G. Pomata (eds), *The Faces of Nature in Enlightenment Europe* (Berlin: BWV-Berliner Wissenschafts-Verlag, 2003); L. Daston and M. Stolleis (eds), *Natural Law and Laws of Nature in Early Modern Europe: Jurisprudence, Theology, Moral, and Natural Philosophy* (Aldershot: Ashgate, 2008). Much less has been written on nature in the body – see my article, 'Nature concocts & expels', for a discussion of the historiographical exceptions, most notably, M. Neuburger, *The Doctrine of the Healing Power of Nature throughout the Course of Time* (New York: privately printed, 1932; originally published in German in 1926). See also the literature on learned medicine and its relationship to natural philosophy, such as I. Maclean, *Logic, Signs, and Nature in the Renaissance: The Case of Learned Medicine* (Cambridge: Cambridge University Press, 2002); P.J. Van der Eijk, *Medicine and Philosophy in Classical Antiquity: Doctors and Philosophers on Nature, Soul, Health, and Disease* (Cambridge: Cambridge University Press, 2005); J. Bono, *Word of God and the Languages of Man: Interpreting Nature in Early Modern Science and Medicine* (Wisconsin: University of Wisconsin Press, 1995).

9 K. Albala, 'Food for healing: convalescent cookery in the Early Modern Era', *Studies in History and Philosophy of Science Part C: Studies in History and Philosophy of Biological and Biomedical Sciences*, 43:2 (2012), pp. 323–28, at p. 325.

10 G. Bruele, *Praxis Medicinae, or, the Physicians Practice* (London: John Norton, 1632).

11 D. Harley, 'The theology of affliction and the experience of sickness in the godly family, 1650–1714: the Henrys and the Newcomes', in O.P. Grell and A. Cunningham (eds), *Religio Medici: Medicine and Religion in Seventeenth-Century England* (Aldershot: Scholar Press, 1996), pp.

273–92; A. Wear, 'Puritan perceptions of illness in seventeenth century England', in R. Porter (ed.), *Patients and Practitioners: Lay Perceptions of Medicine in Pre-Industrial Society* (Cambridge: Cambridge University Press, 2002, first publ. 1985), pp. 55–99.

12 A. Walsham, *Providence in Early Modern England* (Oxford: Oxford University Press, 2003, first publ. 1999); A. Ryrie, *Being Protestant in Reformation Britain* (Oxford: Oxford University Press, 2013).

13 O. Weisser, *Ill Composed: Sickness, Gender, and Belief in Early Modern England* (New Haven: Yale University Press, 2015), p. 4.

14 W. Fulwood, *The Enimie of Idlenesse Teaching the Maner and Stile how to Endite, Compose and Write all sorts of Epistles and Letters* (London: H. Bynneman, 1568), p. 52. On epistolary etiquette, see J. Daybell, *The Material Letter in Early Modern England: Manuscript Letters and the Culture and Practices of Letter-Writing, 1512–1635* (Basingstoke: Palgrave, 2012).

15 Weisser, *Ill Composed*, p. 5.

16 J. Lister, *The Autobiography of Joseph Lister of Bradford, 1627–1709*, ed. T. Wright (Bradford: J.R. Smith, 1842).

17 For a full discussion of the role of Nature in recovery, and the relationship between this agent, God and the physician, see my 'Nature concocts & expels'.

18 For more definitions of Nature, see M. Neuburger, *The Doctrine of the Healing Power of Nature*.

19 The *OED* online lists fourteen categories of definitions, and a total of thirty-four meanings.

20 The introduction to L. Daston and F. Vidal's edited book, *The Moral Authority of Nature* (Chicago: University of Chicago Press, 2004), pp. 1–20, esp. 4–7, 11–12, draws attention to the diverse meanings of 'nature', and the idea that it could both refer to the body's internal agent and to the wider physical world.

21 On the female personification of nature, see K. Park, 'Nature in person: medieval and Renaissance allegories and emblems', in Daston and Vidal (eds), *The Moral Authority of Nature*, pp. 50–73.

22 A. Paré, *The Workes of that Famous Chirurgion Ambrose Parey* (London: T. Cotes, 1634), p. 25. On the spirits, see Carrera (ed.), *Emotions and Health, 1200–1700* (Leiden: Brill, 2013); and S. Cavallo and T. Storey, *Healthy Living in Late Renaissance Italy* (Oxford: Oxford University Press, 2013).

23 For example, J. Harris, *The Divine Physician* (London: H.B., 1676), pp. 163–4.

24 J. Hart, *Klinike, or the Diet of the Diseased* (London: J. Beale, 1633), p. 358.

25 See Newton, 'Nature concocts & expels' for examples.

26 On the concoction of food, see M. Schoenfeldt, *Bodies and Selves in Early Modern England: Physiology and Inwardness in Spenser, Shakespeare, Herbert, and Milton* (Cambridge: Cambridge University Press, 1999), pp. 25–33; K. Albala, *Eating Right in the Renaissance* (Berkeley: University of California Press, 2002), pp. 54–62.

27 L. Lemnius, *The Secret Miracles of Nature* (London: Jo Streater, 1658, first publ. 1559), p. 43; Hart, *Klinike*, p. 241; J. Macollo, *XCIX Canons, or Rules Learnedly Describing an Excellent Method for Practitioners in Physic* (London: J. Grismond, 1659), p. 44.

28 F. Platter, *Platerus Golden Practice of Physick* (London: Peter Cole, 1664), p. 148; Paré, *The Workes*, pp. 25–6.

29 *Ibid.*, p. 26; Hart, *Klinike*, p. 299.

30 Bruele, *Praxis Medicinae*, p. 223. See also Platter, *Platerus Golden Practice*, p. 149.

31 On feebleness of motion, dim eyesight and hearing, and paleness, see Platter, *Platerus Golden Practice*, pp. 58, 84, 92. On memory loss and poor digestion, Bruele, *Praxis Medicinae*, pp. 79, 247, 514. On relapse, see the section on 'The final purge' in this chapter. These various weaknesses are mentioned frequently in laypeople's personal documents.

32 T. Joutsivuo states that this scheme is derived from Galen's *Ars Medica* – see an early modern vernacular edition, *Galens Art of Physic* (London: Peter Cole, 1652), pp. 5, 8–10. T. Joutsivuo, *Scholastic Tradition and Humanist Innovation. The Concept of Neutrum in Renaissance Medicine* (Helsinki: The Finnish Academy of Science and Medicine, 1999), p. 1. A more detailed discussion of the neutral body will be provided in my book *Misery to Mirth*, ch. 2.

33 *Galens Art of Physic*, pp. 13, 18, 105. This definition is cited in most medical texts across the period.

34 Hart, *Klinike*, p. 270.

35 *Galens Art of Physick*, p. 9. See also, G. Grataroli, *A Direction for the Health of Magistrates and Students* (London: William How, 1574, first publ. Latin 1555), preface; Lemnius, *The Secret Miracles*, 245.

36 Exceptions include: M. van der Lugt, 'Neither ill nor healthy: the intermediate state between health and disease in medieval medicine', *Quaderni Storici*, 136:1 (2011), pp. 13–46; Joutsivuo, *Scholastic Tradition*. These scholars discuss the philosophical controversies surrounding the neutral body, particularly between Aristotle and Galen.

37 F. Glisson, G. Bate and A. Regemorter, *A Treatise of the Rickets* (London: Peter Cole, 1651), pp. 277–8.

38 J. Johnstonus, *The Idea of Practical Physick* (London: Peter Cole, 1657), p. 26.

39 S. Blankaart, *A Physical Dictionary* (London: J.D., 1684). See also Joutsivuo, *Scholastic Tradition*, pp. 102, 191–2.
40 Examples from either ends of the timeframe are: P. Barrough, *The Methode of Phisicke* (London: Thomas Vautroullier, 1583, first publ. 1508), p. 19; F. Mauriceau, *The Diseases of Women with Child* (London: Andrew Bell, 1710), pp. 358–9.
41 Macollo, *XCIX Canons*, p. 111.
42 W. Walwyn, *Physick for Families* (London: J. Winter, 1669), pp. 53–4. Walwyn himself contested this practice: in keeping with his Helmontian sympathies, he regarded disease not as a humoral state, but as an idea or 'seminal principle'. On Helmontian ideas about recovery, see my article, 'Nature concocts & expels'.
43 On the use of animal imagery, see A. Skuse, 'Wombs, worms and wolves: constructing cancer in Early Modern England', *Social History of Medicine*, 27:4 (2014), pp. 632–48.
44 MS 1320, 96v ('A book of physick', made in 1710), Wellcome Library, London. See also Additional MS 45196, fols 44v, 70v (Brockman Papers, 'Ann Glyd Her Book 1656'), British Library.
45 A. Martindale, *The Life of Adam Martindale*, ed. Richard Parkinson, Chetham Society, vol. 4 (Manchester, 1845), p. 20.
46 This was the case for Brilliana Harley's son Ned in 1641: in B. Harley, *Letters of The Lady Brilliana Harley*, ed. Thomas Taylor Lewis, Camden Society (London, 1853), p. 128.
47 A.T., *A Rich Store-House or Treasury for the Diseased* (London: Thomas Purfoot, 1596), 'divers & sundrye Good instructions & Rules' (n.p.).
48 *The Aphorismes of Hippocrates* (London: Humphrey Moseley, 1655), pp. 35, 68; Hart, *Klinike*, p. 269.
49 *Ibid.*, p. 270.
50 Paré, *The Workes*, p. 24. On sleep, see K. Dannenfeldt, 'Sleep: theory and practice in the late Renaissance', *Journal of the History of Medicine and Allied Sciences*, 41:4 (1986), pp. 415–41.
51 Paré, *The Workes*. See B. Maclehose, 'Fear, fantasy and sleep in medieval medicine', in Carrera (ed.), *Emotions and Health*, pp. 67–94, at p. 83.
52 J. Kettlewell, *Death Made Comfortable* (London: R. Kettlewell, 1695), p. 212.
53 G. Davenport, *The Letters of George Davenport 1651–1677*, ed. Brenda M. Pask, Surtees Society, vol. 215 (Woodbridge, 2011), p. 89.
54 R. Ekirch, *At Day's Close: A History of Nighttime* (London: Phoenix, 2005), pp. 300–10.
55 Lemnius, *The Secret Miracles*, p. 244.
56 Hart, *Klinike*, p. 332.

57 Kettlewell, *Death Made Comfortable*, p. 212.
58 Hart, *Klinike*, p. 332. On the nutritional purposes of sleep, see Maclehose, 'Fear, fantasy and sleep', pp. 78–9.
59 *Ibid.*, p. 333.
60 T. Cogan, *The Haven of Health* (London: Anne Griffin, 1636; first publ. 1588), p. 271. See also Cavallo and Storey's discussion of daytime sleep: *Healthy Living*, pp. 119–26.
61 Afternoon naps for the convalescent are mentioned in *ibid.*, pp. 122–3, 125.
62 J. Banister, *A Needefull, New, and Necessarie Treatise of Chyrurgerie* (London: Thomas Marshe, 1575), p. 91.
63 J. Donne, *Devotions upon Emergent Occasions and Severall Steps in my Sicknes* (London: A.M, 1624), p. 26 (this text is an autobiographical meditation on Donne's illness); T. Wright, *The Passions of the Minde* (London: Miles Flesher, 1630; first published 1601), p. 13.
64 Barrough, *The Methode of Phisicke*, p. 184. See also Macollo, *XCIX Canons*, p. 94.
65 *Barrington Family Letters, 1628–1632*, ed. A. Searle (London: Royal Historical Society, 1983), p. 126.
66 Hart, *Klinike*, p. 168.
67 T. Cock, *Kitchin-physick: or, Advice for the Poor* (London: J.B., 1676), pp. 31–2.
68 Macollo, *XCIX Canons*, p. 96.
69 T. Twyne, *The Schoolmaster, or Teacher of Table Phylosophie* (London: Richard Johnes, 1583, first publ. 1576), sig. B2.
70 Lemnius, *The Secret Miracles*, p. 118; Albala, 'Food for Healing', p. 327.
71 Cogan, *Haven*, p. 201. See also Lemnius, *The Secret Miracles*, p. 17.
72 R. North, *Notes of Me: The Autobiography of Roger North*, ed. P. Millard (Toronto: University of Toronto Press, 2000), p. 80; N. Biggs, *Mataeotechnia Medicinae Praxeos, The Vanity of the Craft of Physick* (London: Edward Blackmore, 1651), p. 200.
73 See Albala, *Eating Right*, ch. 2.
74 Hart, *Klinike*, p. 173.
75 *Ibid.*, p. 182.
76 *Ibid.*, p. 174.
77 A. Grieco, 'Food and social classes in late medieval and Renaissance Italy', in J.L. Flandrin and M. Montanari (eds), *Food: A Culinary History* (New York: Columbia University Press, 1999), pp. 302–12.
78 Ryrie, *Being Protestant*, p. 162.
79 Hart, *Klinike*, p. 168.
80 T. Moffett, *Healths Improvement* (London: T. Newcomb, 1655), p. 135. See also Hart, *Klinike*, p. 79; Platter, *Platerus Golden Practice*, p. 151. Eggs

were also recommended by laypeople: typically, recipes for restorative broths contain between 12 and 30 egg yolks.

81 Moffett, *Healths Improvement*, pp. 32–3; Hart, *Klinike*, pp. 79, 77–8, 173–4; Bruele, *Praxis Medicinae*, p. 249. Albala has also pointed this out: 'Food for healing', pp. 324–6, 328.

82 John 8:12. Albala highlights the preference for white meats: 'Food for healing', p. 326.

83 Hart, *Klinike*, p. 178.

84 J. de Mediolano, *Regimen Sanitatis Salerni: or, the Schoole of Salernes Regiment of Health* (London: B. Alsop, 1650; first transl. from Latin 1541), p. 125. See also Moffett, *Healths Improvement*, p. 94

85 Platter, *Platerus Golden Practice*, 159.

86 Lemnius, *The Secret Miracles*, 244.

87 For example, I. Spon, *Observations on Fevers and Febriguges* (London: Mark Pardoe, 1682), pp. 91–2.

88 Lemnius, *The Secret Miracles*, p. 135.

89 On the natural and divine causes of relapse, see Harris, *The Divine Physician*; Lemnius, *The Secret Miracles*, pp. 135–6.

90 Spon, *Observations on Fevers*, pp. 91–2.

91 For a recent review, see E. Sullivan, 'Emotions in history: a review essay', Cultural History, 2:1 (2013), pp. 93–102.

92 For example, M. MacDonald, *Mystical Bedlam: Madness, Anxiety and Healing in Seventeenth-Century England* (Cambridge: Cambridge University Press, 1981), pp. 84, 72–3; A. Wear, 'Fear, anxiety and the plague in Early Modern England: religious and medical responses', in J.R. Hinnells and R. Porter (eds), *Religion, Health, and Suffering* (London: Kegan Paul International, 1999), pp. 339–63.

93 N. Culpeper, *Semeiotica Uranica: or, An Astrological Judgement of Diseases* (London: Nathaniel Brookes, 1651), pp. 28–9. For children's emotional responses to pain, see H. Newton, *The Sick Child in Early Modern England, 1580–1720* (Oxford: Oxford University Press, 2012), ch. 6.

94 I. Archer, *Two East Anglian Diaries 1641–1729*, ed. M.J. Storey, Suffolk Record Society, vol. 36 (Woodbridge, 1994), p. 162.

95 Hart, *Klinke*, p. 398. See also T. Walkington, *Optick Glasse of Humors* (London: John Dawson, 1639, first publ. 1607), p. 8.

96 E. Sullivan, 'A disease unto death: sadness in the time of Shakespeare', in Carrera (ed.), *Emotions and Health*, pp. 159–81, at p. 164.

97 B.A., *The Sick-Mans Rare Jewel* (London: T.R., 1674), p. 30.

98 Cavallo and Storey, *Healthy Living*, p. 184.

99 *Ibid.*, p. 185.

100 For examples at either end of the timeframe, see Barrough, *The Methode of Phisicke*, p. 6; J. Pechey, *A Plain Introduction to the Art of Physic* (London: Henry Bonwick, 1697), p. 94.
101 J. Clegg, *The Diary of James Clegg of Chapel-en-Frith 1708–1755*, ed. Vanessa S. Doe, 5 vols (Matlock: Derbyshire Record Society, 1978), vol. 1 (1708–36), p. 116.
102 T. Rogers, *Practical Discourses on Sickness & Recovery* (London: Thomas Parkhurst, 1691), p. 98.
103 Sullivan, 'A Disease unto death'.
104 R. Josselin, *The Diary of Ralph Josselin 1616–1683*, ed. A. Macfarlane (Oxford: Oxford University Press, 1991), p. 297.
105 N. Coeffeteau, *A Table of Humane Passions* (London: Nicholas Okes, 1621), p. 332.
106 Hart, *Klinike*, p. 393. See Cavallo and Storey, *Healthy Living*, p. 183.
107 For example, Additional MS 36452, fol. 76r (Private letters of the Aston family, 1613–1703), British Library, London.
108 Cited by A. Stobart, 'The making of domestic medicine: gender, self-help and therapeutic determination in household healthcare in south-west England in the late seventeenth century', unpublished PhD thesis, Middlesex University, 2008, p. 72. Now published as a book.
109 On the functions of domestic correspondence, see J. Daybell, *Women Letter-Writers in Tudor England* (Oxford: Oxford University Press, 2006), ch. 6.
110 Pechey, *A Plain Introduction*, p. 95. On the pernicious effects of negative emotions see Sullivan, 'A Disease unto Death'; Cavallo and Storey, *Healthy Living*, p. 189.
111 Harris, *The Divine Physician*, p. 151. O. Weisser has found that sudden joy could bring instant healing: the sympathy between soul and body was so great that the happiness of the soul might automatically bring health to the body: 'Grieved and disordered: gender and emotion in Early Modern patient narratives', *Journal of Medieval and Early Modern Studies*, 43:2 (2013), pp. 247–73. Chapter 3 of her book, *Ill Composed*, discusses how emotions could also cause disease.
112 Hart, *Klinike*, p. 395.
113 Statements about the inevitability of affliction are ubiquitous in lay personal documents. This theme is elaborated in *Heraclitus Christianus, or the Man of Sorrow* (London: A.M., 1677).
114 Culpeper, *Semeiotica Uranica*, p. 28.
115 S. Jeake, *An Astrological Diary of the Seventeenth Century: Samuel Jeake of Rye*, ed. M. Hunter (Oxford: Clarendon, 1988), pp. 89–90.
116 For example, W. Fitzwilliam, *The Correspondence of Lord Fitzwilliam of Milton and Francis Guybon, His Steward 1697–1709*, ed. D.R.

Hainsworth and C. Walker, Northampton Record Society, vol. 36 (1990), p. 271.

117 O. Heywood, *The Rev. Oliver Heywood, B.A: His Autobiography, Diaries, Anecdote and Event Books*, ed. Horsfall Turner, 4 vols (London: Brighouse for A.B. Baynes, 1883), vol. 4, p. 168.

118 [Hatton], *Correspondence of the Family of Hatton being Chiefly Addressed to Christopher, First Viscount Hatton, 1601–1704*, ed. E.M. Thompson, Camden Society, vols 22–3 (London, 1878), vol. 2, p. 212.

119 Notable exceptions include Stobart, 'The making of domestic medicine', pp. 80, 82; A. Withey, *Physick and the Family: Health, Medicine and Care in Wales, 1600–1750* (Manchester: Manchester University Press, 2011), p. 127.

120 Hart, *Klinike*, p. 211.

121 Galen, *Galens art of physic*, p. 91.

122 J. Buxton, *John Buxton, Norfolk Gentleman and Architect: Letters to his Son, 1719–1729*, ed. A. Mackley, Norfolk Record Society, vol. 69 (Norwich, 2005), pp. 99, 103.

123 For examples at either end of the timeframe, in 1598, the Countess of Shrewsbury, Elizabeth Talbot, advised her son-in-law and step-daughter to 'come into the cuntrye[,] [because] this eayre is better for you both than London, and especially … after your ague': Cecil Project, Lambeth Palace Library, MS 3205 f75. A century later, Lady Russell gave her niece and nephew identical advice: R. Russell, *Letters of Rachel, Lady Russell* (London, 1853), vol. 2, p. 4.

124 Lister, *The Autobiography*, pp. 43–4.

125 J. Hervey, *Letter-Books of John Hervey, First Earl of Bristol, vol. 1, 1651–1715* (Wells: Ernest Jackson, 1894), p. 145.

126 Y. van Diemerbroeck, *The Anatomy of Human Bodies* (London: W. Whitwood, 1694), p. 81.

127 J. Symcotts, *A Seventeenth Century Doctor and his Patients: John Symcotts, 1592?–1662*, ed. F.N.L. Poynter and W.J. Bishop, Bedfordshire Historical Record Society, vol. 31 (Streatley, 1951), p. 45.

128 Hervey, *Letter-Books*, p. 335.

129 N.A. de La Framboisière, *The art of physick made plain & easie* (London: Newman, 1684), p. 72.

130 Fitzwilliam, *The Correspondence*, p. 156.

131 *Ibid.*, pp. 125–6, 155; Mary Cowper, *Diary of Mary, Countess Cowper*, ed. John Murray (London, Privately printed, 1864), p. 23.

132 Hart, *Klinike*, p. 220.

133 Van Diemerbroek, *The anatomy of human bodies*, p. 26.

134 T. Elyot, *The Castel of Health* (London: Company of Stationers, 1610, first publ. 1534), p. 72.

135 A. Bryant (ed.), *Postman's Horn: An Anthology of the Letters of Latter Seventeenth Century England* (New York: privately printed, 1946), p. 191.
136 On the endurance of the belief in the spirits between 1200 and 1700, see Carrera, *Emotions and Health*, pp. 5, 99, 221, 224, 237–8.
137 See the introduction to W. Churchill, *Female Patients in Early Modern Britain: Gender, Diagnosis, and Treatment* (Farnham: Ashgate, 2012), for a summary of this literature.
138 Albala, 'Food for Healing', p. 324; Joutsivuo, *Scholastic Tradition*, pp. 104, 161, 191–3.
139 Lemnius, *The Secret Miracles*, p. 244.

III

Airs and places

5

Neapolitan airs: health advice and medical culture on the edge of a volcano

Maria Conforti

In January and February 1645 John Evelyn visited the Kingdom of Naples and its capital.[1] He enjoyed the food, both because it was plentiful and inexpensive: as he says, 'Provisions are wonderfully cheap.' He visited and admired the churches, even if, in the presence of St Januarius's relics, 'we obtained not the miracle of the boiling of this blood', but he was obviously mainly interested in natural phenomena. On 4 February he visited the celebrated museum of the learned apothecary Ferrante Imperato (1550–1631), 'the repository of incomparable rarities'. Over the following days he climbed up the steep path to Vesuvius, where he collected lava specimens and was duly impressed by the 'horrid barathrum', a memento of the eruption of 16 December 1631 that had caused one of the worst destructions recorded in the long history of the volcano. He then proceeded to the Phlegraean Fields, with its smaller volcanoes, mineral vapours and hot springs lost in sea waters, its ancient, imposing ruins and baths, and modern antiquarians (and forgers). Evelyn's impression of the place echoed the judgment – and the stereotypes – of many other early modern travellers: 'Summer is here eternal; caus'd by the natural & adventitious heate of the earth, so warmed through the Subterranean fires, as our guide alighting, and cutting a turfe with his knife, & delivering it to me, I was hardly able to hold it in my hands.' The warmth is the cause of the richness of the place, a land which as well as producing a wealth of fruits at all times of the year, abounded in 'silks, manna, sugar, oil, wine, rice, sulphur, and alum', and whose 'Chief Magistrates … wonderfully enrich themselves out of the miserable people's labour.' Human bodies are also influenced by the earth's heat: women are 'generally well featur'd, but excessively libidinous', and in general 'they are merry, Witty and genial; all which I much attribute to the excellent quality of the ayre'.[2] Evelyn was coming from England, where discussions on the airs were not quite as prevalent as in Italy. It is likely that visiting Naples helped him in shaping his ideas on air pollution in London and more generally in focusing on the connection between airs and disease.

The relationship between subterranean fires, waters and airs – that is between a troubling, if not downright dangerous, geology and a propitious, fertile and healthy environment – was a well-known feature of the city of Naples and even more of its immediate surroundings. Naples, as Evelyn well knew, was located in a territory whose troublesome character matched its charms. Its air and its temperate climate were celebrated and eulogised; but earthquakes, volcanic eruptions and other geological phenomena were likely to scare scholars and laypeople. This ambivalent character was considered to have been a feature of the place since antiquity. It strongly influenced the way the medicine and natural philosophy practised in the city in the Renaissance looked at disease and health, and also at phenomena concerning the earth. Indeed, the very presence of geological phenomena whose magnitude could not be ignored prompted an early interest in the connection between what happened at the surface or above the earth, and what was likely to occur in the subsoil.

One of the crucial questions for practical medicine, in Naples as elsewhere, concerned the way in which airs *change* in a given place: whether under the impact of astrological movements, winds, seasonality and climate, or as a consequence of more dramatic phenomena, such as earthquakes or eruptions. These were all crucial elements to consider both in the assessment of the origins, nature and prognostics of epidemics, and in the activity of medical counselling to individuals. On the one hand, physicians needed to be keen interpreters of the earth and of terrestrial phenomena in order to give sound advice to their patients.[3] On the other hand, they were not just concerned with individual patients but with collectivities: indeed, one of the crucial questions addressed by medical experts was the way in which the environment could cause or foster the outbreak of epidemic diseases. How was the kind of air common in Naples, rich in metallic, and thus potentially poisonous, exhalations, going to affect local people's bodies, especially in the frequent case of catastrophic events, such as earthquakes or eruptions?

In what follows, I will first deal with the paradoxical nature of perceptions about the Neapolitan environment and the way in which its airs were seen to affect human bodies and health. I will then explore the ways learned traditions such as the rich literature on *meteorae* produced at a local level by natural philosophers often intersected with medical knowledge, which accounted for the seeming paradox that dangerous, indeed threatening, phenomena such as eruptions could be seen as contributing to a healthy environment. Finally, I will trace changes in medical discourse in the late seventeenth century, a period when the airs became the object of harsh disagreement in Naples among physicians and naturalists.

Eruptions: the ambivalent influence of subterranean fires on airs

While visiting the Phlegraean Fields, Evelyn remembered a spectacular eruption, in 1538, that had caused the emergence of a totally new hill, the so-called Monte Nuovo:

> the new mountain ... which rose partly out of it [Lake Lucrinus], and partly out of the sea, and that in the space of one night and a day, [rose] to a very great altitude ... after many terrible earthquakes, which ruined divers places thereabout, when at midnight the sea retiring near 200 paces, and yawning on the sudden, it continued to vomit forth flames and fiery stones in such quantity, as produced this whole mountain by their fall, making the inhabitants of Pozzolo to leave their habitations, supposing the end of the world had come.[4]

Pedro de Toledo, the Spanish Viceroy, and governor of Naples at the time, commissioned reassuring works written by outstanding natural philosophers, such as the physician Simone Porzio (1496–1554), and built a splendid villa with gardens for himself near Pozzuoli, so as to quench this and similar opinions and encourage people to come back to the town.

Baths at Pozzuoli were still in use in the following decades, as shown by the case of one rather exceptional patient, the ailing, intellectually restless cardinal Girolamo Seripando (1493–1563), one of the protagonists of the Counter Reformation and the Council of Trent.[5] Seripando's unpublished correspondence and his recently published journal offer many interesting hints at a learned patient's experience. He was treated by two of the best physicians in Naples, whom he also befriended, Donato Antonio Altomare (1520–66) and Simone Porzio, whom we have already mentioned. Seripando was constantly on the move: writing in July 1548 to one of his best friends, Augusto Cocciano, he complained of the *aëre* in Bologna, where he was staying, and he hoped to be back in Naples soon.[6] Once there, however, physicians advised him to abandon his monastery in the humid and unhealthy centre of the city, and to move to Pozzuoli or to Torre del Greco, a village on the seashore, near Vesuvius. He preferred instead to go to Posillipo, a hill overlooking the city and the Phlegraean Fields, whose Greek name means 'suspension of suffering', at a safe distance from the dangerous fires of Pozzuoli.[7] Apparently, he was happy there, and he felt much better; he came back the following winter, and enjoyed the air as much as the conversations with Porzio, who also owned a villa there.[8]

The city of Naples was in fact, and still is, located in a territory whose geology is one of the most troubling in Europe.[9] As Iuan de Quiñones pointed out to his king, Philip IV of Spain, in 1632, Naples and Southern Italy held a place of distinction even in the lengthy catalogue of the volcanoes to be found in Spanish domains – that is, in a substantial part of the explored world.[10] Quiñones was writing after the worst geological catastrophe of the seventeenth century in this area, namely, the eruption of Vesuvius that took place on 16 December 1631, nearly a century after the emergence of Monte Nuovo in 1538. Vesuvius had been silent for centuries, and while historical memories were kept of previous destructive eruptions, especially those of late antiquity, this one took the city of Naples and the villages and *casali* scattered around the fertile mount Somma and along the coast by complete surprise. It is difficult to assess how many people were killed: prudent modern estimates evaluate the casualties at *c.*5000, while contemporary publications hint at a much larger figure of about 10,000. The eruption threatened the city itself – only to be stopped by divine intervention, it was commonly held – and left a lasting memory, which represented a turning point in the very image and iconography of the city. Comparisons were immediately drawn with the events of 1538, but this eruption changed everything, even more than the Monte Nuovo one had. Destruction was on a far larger scale and it struck nearer to the centre of the city. Its ashes were projected as far as the Montenegro (Bocche di Cattaro), it was accompanied by frightening earthquakes, and was followed by a peculiar and by all (textual) standards inexplicable event, a violent inundation, today known as *lahors*, coming from the mouth of the volcano, which partially covered with water the land already destroyed by fire.[11]

Despite the prominence of these events and the great number of narratives they produced, the inhabitants of the place and natural philosophers all around Europe knew very well that Vesuvius and the Monte Nuovo were only two of the many volcanoes, or geological phenomena, to be observed in the Campania region. A journey to Naples was considered incomplete without a visit to the area of Pozzuoli and to Solfatara, an active volcano, less threatening, more easily accessible and perhaps even more fascinating than Vesuvius itself. The place was constantly used for experiments on animals and humans, intended to assess the role of poisonous exhalations on respiration and life. For example, not far from Solfatara was the Grotta del Cane in Agnano, where miasmatic exhalations could 'kill' a small animal in a few minutes, only for it to be revived in the waters of the lake of Agnano by tourist guides. Rather sinister and more dangerous experiments were attempted by Viceroy Pedro de Toledo, who tested the effects of the poisonous *effluvia* on Turkish slaves, probably in an effort to better understand the events of 1538. Contrary to all expectations, however, these men did not recover after being immersed in water.[12] Earthquakes and what we now call bradisismic phenomena were widespread in the area and *tsunamis* and lesser tidal waves, in connection with volcanism, could affect the seashores and human activities connected with fishing and navigation.

However, and somewhat paradoxically, there was also a very positive side to the worrying geology of the city and its surroundings. Despite their violence, subterranean fires, hot springs of mineral waters, *fumarole* (exhalations of hot vapour, also called *mofete* when they stank) and active volcanoes were considered throughout the early modern age to be the direct or indirect causes of the most celebrated features of the place. The very healthiness of its airs and environment, and the richness of its soil, meant that local trees bore fruit twice a year, a level of fertility which was perceived as deriving from sulphuric and other mineral exhalations, caused by the burning of subterranean fires.

Moreover, only passing mention can be made here of the celebrated mineral and therapeutic baths of the area, which were also deemed to derive their medical qualities from the phenomena occurring in the subsoil.[13] And as we have noted, John Evelyn's description of the mild and 'merry' nature of the inhabitants, who inclined towards music, singing and playing, as well as to love and sociability, was accounted for, in true Hippocratic fashion, with recourse to the warm and temperate 'airs' of the locality. The whole area – that is, Naples itself – was celebrated for possessing one of the most 'temperate' climates in Europe: the city was in fact named '*gentile*', gentle, both in a climatic and moral sense.[14]

The volcanic Phlegraean Fields, where Monte Nuovo was born, had first acquired its reputation in antiquity, when it was the fashionable resort for upper-class Roman inhabitants. Long before the rediscovery of Herculaneum and Pompeii in the eighteenth century, an event that reversed the map of antiquarian tourism at a local and indeed European level, it was Pozzuoli, Bajae and Misenum, not the area surrounding Vesuvius, that formed a staple of the Grand Tour.[15] Starting in the middle ages a rich literature of erudite 'guides' to the area was produced and printed, which contained descriptions of the splendid locations and antique ruins of the baths and *sudatoria*. The role and activity of subterranean fires, while mentioned, was rather downplayed in this genre, which was meant for travellers, whom it would not have been wise to scare.[16] However, guides, descriptions, booklets containing instructions for touring and bathing, all mention the ambivalent character of the environment.

The air around Vesuvius was considered in such a positive light that it was thought to produce an eternal springtime, in a context in which spring was considered to be the most temperate, and therefore the healthiest season. These qualities, caused by constant communication between the surface of the earth and the processes, mainly combustions, going on within its bowels, *viscera*, were matched by the extension to the airs and indeed to the skies, of their effects, be they positive or negative for 'animal' and human health. This motif was exploited in texts written and published from the Middle Ages well into the eighteenth century.[17] It was a common belief among physicians and lay people that sulphur and bitumen, the substances that were mainly considered responsible for the ignition and maintenance of subterranean fires, might well be the cause of the flood of hot lava, or clouds of ashes, that were life-threatening in the event of eruptions or earthquakes. However, in normal conditions sulphur and bitumen helped to keep the environment balanced towards the hot and dry, and thus to preserve bodies from epidemics, especially those caused by cold and humidity. This also affected the balance of humours of individual temperaments, inclining them towards a prevalence of the same qualities; indeed, heat and dryness were so prized as to be ideally attributed in humoral medicine to adult males. The opinion of physicians is summarised by Giulio Cesare Capaccio (1550–1634), the author of a well-known guide, in his description of the Solfatara: 'One can see about two thousand little fissures breathing out a sulphurous aluminous smoke of amoniac salt and other minerals which our physicians say is very healthy for cold and humid diseases.'[18]

Attacks aiming at the 'putrid' character of the airs of the area were not uncommon, and there was certainly a degree of parochialism behind some of the reasons for the reiterated defence of the quality of airs in Pozzuoli and the Phlegraean Fields, as well as in the city of Naples.[19] But there was also the need to protect what were perceived to be important economic enterprises. These included the maintenance of baths and *sudatoria*, but also activities such as the maceration of linen in the lake of Agnano, or the 'cultivation' of sulphur in the Solfatara, a bizarre form of husbandry grounded in the idea that the soil treated in this way was more fertile: 'The peasants turn over the earth very diligently with iron tools, so that the earth gets mixed with the vapours, and from the month of January to October cultivate the earth as if they were tending to their vegetable patches.'[20] At the same time, there was genuine wonder at the contradictory properties of natural phenomena in the area. A curious example of the ambivalence associated with the mineral exhalations and their effects is to be found, for instance, in the discussion on the edibility of fish killed or thrown ashore by the thousands by volcanic eruptions or submarine exhalations. Giulio Cesare Braccini, the author of one of the richest booklets on the 1631 eruption of Vesuvius, mentions that such fish may possibly represent a damage to health, while also admitting to having eaten them himself and not having found them noxious.[21]

Despite the violent and at times dangerous character of terrestrial phenomena in the area surrounding the city of Naples, the airs in the area were made healthy, indeed salubrious, by these same phenomena. This might have been a paradox for the traditional doctrines, given the poisonous character that was commonly attributed to exhalations produced by 'winds' in subterranean caves. However, lay perceptions of the healthiness of the airs in Naples, shared by local inhabitants and by travellers, constantly underlined the benign character of skies and earth.

Interpreting meteorae: learned traditions and natural philosophy in Naples

'Airs' cannot be properly addressed without stepping over disciplinary boundaries. For the medical historian, appraising their role in pathology and therapeutics means walking a fine line between different, and often diverging, approaches, many of them with a distinct tradition of their own and extending over a *longue durée* often coming from antiquity. Early modern discourses on 'airs' followed at least two ancient medical traditions: the Hippocratic view, as set forth in *De aeris aquis et locis* and in innumerable commentaries, and the Galenic one, with what was in fact its largely post-Galenic doctrine of the Non-Naturals. However, as the case of Naples demonstrates, 'airs' were also strictly connected to the earth and to its modifications and phenomena: exhalations and earthquakes, springs and volcanic eruptions. There is thus an equally important non-medical tradition to be taken into account, the one dealing with geological phenomena and going back to Aristotle's *Meteorologica*, and to its early modern followers and critics, among them, prominently, René Descartes, who published his innovative *Meteorae* in 1637.[22] Among ancient authors writing on the subject who were much quoted by authors writing on the earth, we find Lucretius, the *De Rerum natura*, and Seneca, with his *Naturales Quaestiones*. The bricolage between the different models and explanations, ancient and modern, and their influence on medical texts, was obviously variable, depending on chronology and cultural geographies, and it produced results so diverse that a contemporary reader may even wonder at their consistency. However, to a certain extent, and from the point of view of Italian and especially Neapolitan texts, these traditions merge and they were all meaningful in shaping medical discourses which discussed the way the airs affect individual and collective bodies.

Natural philosophers active in the Kingdom and in the city of Naples were keenly interested in the question of the local airs. I will briefly mention here only two of these authors and their works, to show how the interplay between ancient theories and recent developments occurred in practice. The first is a short treatise by the Calabrian natural philosoher Bernardino Telesio (1509–88), *De his, quae in Aere fiunt; & de Terrae motibus* (1570).[23] Telesio was critical of Aristotle's natural philosophy as it was expressed in *Metereologica*, but he also knew this text well: he commented on it at length and accepted some of its conclusions. In fact, contrary to Aristotle's theories, Telesio believed that air is a body (*corpus*) in its own right, as are the earth and the sea; moreover, the air is in perpetual movement, animated by *vapores*, vapours moving in different fashions and because of different causes (mainly, heat and cold). He also thought that terrestrial phenomena have an influence on what happens in the air, and that earthquakes are caused by exhalations imprisoned in underground cavities – and in this was more or less following what Aristotle himself had said. However, Telesio underlines the role of nitre and saltpetre in causing subterranean 'explosions', and here Telesio is using practical chemical notions that he may have gathered from the rich milieu of 'chymists', active in Italy and in the Kingdom of Naples at the time.[24]

The *Historia Naturale* (1599), written in Italian by Ferrante Imperato, also dealt at length with airs, in connection with underground *miniere*, that is, mineral mines. Imperato was a remarkable medical man: an apothecary, he owned a well-known museum and his *Historia* is mainly devoted to minerals and stones ('miniere, & pietre'), to their characteristics, properties and medicinal uses. But before this, by way of introduction, Imperato deals with the elements – *earth, waters, air, fire, hot, cold* – showing a strong propensity for what he calls 'medicina filosofica', that is, 'chymistry'. This is not surprising, since chemical preparations may have been controversial at times, but in the late sixteenth century they had become almost commonplace, alongside traditional ones, among Italian *speziali*. Imperato briefly comments on the airs of Naples and especially on those of the Phlegraean fields, whose quality should theoretically have been very bad, given the abundance of noxious or downright poisonous exhalations coming from places such as the Grotta del cane, and from other *mofete*.[25] He says that the foggy (*caliginosa*) character of the air in the area makes it 'suspicious' (*sospetta*) from the point of view of health. He even mentions one of the baths in Pozzuoli (the *Ortodonico*) where the vapours, normally considered helpful for patients, become toxic when the Borea (northern) wind is blowing. At the same time, he underlines the belief that waters and airs that have been in contact with subterranean fires help to restore people to perfect health, by promoting the fluidity of humours and thus dissolving obstructions in the vessels – a crucial element in the maintenance of the humoral balance required for a healthy disposition. In his opinion, fires and heat are also extremely helpful in purifying the airs (and waters) and restoring them to a balanced, indeed healthy, state. He goes as far as to say that the air in the surroundings of Pozzuoli is to be considered 'aria medicata', that is, medicinal air – and, as with every medicinal remedy (*pharmakon*), to be prescribed following carefully assessed proportions and doses.[26] This is a common and exceptionally long-lasting theme in the works published in Naples in the early modern age, and it can be found in many different kinds of works, from learned treatises to the medical literature of *consultationes*.

The literature on baths in Pozzuoli and Ischia is so rich that it is impossible to give it but a passing reference; however, it is worth mentioning here the substantial work on mineral springs and medical baths in the island of Ischia published in 1558 by the physician Giulio Jasolino (1538–1622). He was a teacher at Naples *Studium*, an anatomist and a man with a deep interest in chemistry.[27] In his text, Jasolino attempts a complete 'anatomy' of the island, recently delivered from the danger of incursions by pirates from North Africa. He proposed that its waters could be used as an alternative to the baths in Pozzuoli, which had been badly damaged, or destroyed, by the 1538 eruption of the Monte Nuovo. What is fascinating in Jasolino's work is the way in which he analyses each spring and its surroundings, taking into account both the underlying *minera* and the effect they have on their immediate environment, on airs, and especially on human bodies. He says, for instance, that in the village of Barano women are beautiful and people are healthy because of the effects of a spring that Nature itself has heated to just the right point (*cotta dalla natura giustamente*).[28] He thus traces a complete map of the island, also providing a lengthy catalogue of successful treatments for each locality. Jasolino's case is also extremely interesting because his work, fastidiously listing the localities and features of a not very large area, shows the extent and the scale to which the discourse on airs, like the one on waters and places, could be *local*. Springs have obviously different mineral properties, but they (or better, the soil they are coming from) determine different 'ecologies' that can be known and observed only by gathering news and information – and by experimenting, as Jasolino does, with distillations – about a very circumscribed and limited space. The specificity of localities is obviously already to be found in Hippocrates' texts, but the presence of fires and minerals, and their action on waters and airs, subtly changes the approach and promotes a sort of 'microgeography' of the territory.

The puzzling contradictions between observed phenomena and textual explanations or prescriptions were likely to show to what extent, and on which occasions, traditional scientific or medical knowledge became useless, or too sketchy to be helpful. Hence there was a constant struggle to accommodate these explanations to unlikely and unpredictable phenomena in local writers on natural philosophy.

Medicine and eruptions: air, disease and epidemics

The physical effect of eruptions on animal and human bodies was a cause for widespread anxiety. Already in 1538, Simone Porzio, writing at the instance of Pedro de Toledo, underlined that the only effect of the Monte Nuovo eruption might be drought, thence a shortage of food that might ultimately cause disease, and that the exhalations arguably produced by the volcanic fire would thus not cause any specific illness.[29] Was this the opinion of a particularly enlightened physician, or was it shared by other medical practitioners? In fact, with some variations due to the development of new or conflicting explanations for geological phenomena, this is also what is said in the rich literature concerning the 1631 eruption. This event, as already noted, produced an eruption of paper throughout the continent. A complete census does not exist, but a prudent estimate sets the number at about 200 works, printed in Naples and elsewhere in the kingdom, in Rome, but also in Venice, Paris, in Germany and in other European countries, prominently Spain.[30] Among them we find broadsheets, sometimes mere illustrations accompanied by short texts; a sizeable number of *relazioni* (reports) by direct witnesses (real or fictional), often written in the first person and mainly consisting of a *giornale* (diary) of the events; longer chronicles, accompanied by scientific comments, usually on the remote chronology, causes and prognosis of the event; and a small number of texts written by 'experts' – natural philosophers, many of them physicians – who explicitly say they were writing under commission and using or collecting information provided by eyewitnesses. There were also lengthy treatises, written months or years after the events, with higher scientific ambitions and goals. While stereotypical, to a certain extent, these works are by no means uniform in the description or explanation of what was observed in the dramatic days of December 1631 and January 1632; many of them addressed the question of the effects on human bodies and of the consequences of the event for public health.

Physicians were asked to, and claimed to be able to, predict the impact of eruptions on individual bodies and on public health. Fears that magical or demonic influences were causing eruptions were constantly being attributed to the *volgo* (the common, uneducated people) but undoubtedly the anxiety concerning the events, their predictability and their immediate and remote consequences, was widespread.[31] I will quote here from two texts dealing with the medical consequences of the eruption. The first is interesting because the author, the physician Francesco Porrata Spinola (1535–1639), was not a direct witness, since he lived in another Southern Italian region, the Puglie. He also had a strong interest in poetry and astrology and he styled himself as 'Medico, Filosofo et Astrologo'.[32] In fact, he claimed to have made elaborate calculations, which showed that the eruption might have been observed in astrological conjunctions; as such, the event was not isolated and it would undoubtedly be followed by other consequences, among them fevers and other pathological conditions affecting individual bodies: 'Double tertiary fevers, ardent malignant fevers … stomach symptoms and afflictions of the heart, which bring a loss of strength and death with diaphoretic sweats, vomiting and malign flux of the body (diarrhoea), some kinds of pleurisy and sore throats and catarrh in the throat.'[33] However, he too ruled out the possibility of epidemic diseases. In his opinion, these are impossible because the pestilence (*contagio*) was not apparent in the skies, and also – and mainly – because sulphur, by which volcanic exhalations are composed, protected the body from putrefaction and plague; in fact, it helped respiration:

> During earthquakes the mountain 'Somma' doesn't really give off pestilent vapours of the kind others have written about or expect to find, because where there is fire there can be no putrefaction. Furthermore, there is such an abundance of sulphur there, which is the principle

> secret against plague ... and it is unequalled as a remedy for breathing difficulties.[34]

Sensibly, he added that the inundations that have followed the eruption may indeed cause diseases, if waters are left to stagnate.

We find more or less the same opinions in one very different work, by the Roman physician Pietro Castelli (1570–1661), arguably one of the best written on the 1631 eruption.[35] Castelli's background was very different from Porrata Spinola's; he was not interested in astrology, but in chemistry. Despite the differences, the two texts closely resemble each other on the topic of diseases: Castelli goes as far as to predict an increased healthiness of the air after the eruption. The purifying action of the sulphur exhalations will help avoid pestilence, and even syphilis (*mal franzese*):

> I predict in future that the air will be healthy. Nor can one argue that plague will result from this fire: Because if these fires lead to a drier temperament in the air, dryness is a remedy for putrefaction: And as regards the plague, preventing putrefaction acts as a preservative as I have already said many times in my book on the plague.[36]

Castelli openly addresses the question of why airs that have been long closed in subterranean cavities are normally noxious or poisonous, as also happens in the Grotta del Cane, in Agnano; whilst the airs from the underground of the Vesuvius and other volcanoes are not harmful, or even healthy.[37] The answer, once again, is fire – subterranean fire that can burn noxious particles: 'If at first there had been ... any pestilential fomites, the fire has eradicated and dissipated it.'[38] Castelli has had a direct experience of its effects in Pozzuoli, where it had burnt his fingers and shoes: 'I have experienced the fire of Pozzuoli since as I was trying to gather sulphur and salt armoniac I scorched my fingers and burnt my shoes.'[39]

Generally speaking, physicians ruled out the possibility that bad airs set free by catastrophic conflagrations such as those we have described would cause disease or epidemics (*pestilenze*). This opinion on the effects of eruptions in the long run is shared by later physicians. In 1661, Giovan Battista Zupi, writing after one of the many events following the catastrophe of 1631, observes and describes its effects on his patients. Many of them suffered from inhaling the ashes, also experiencing difficult digestion and feeling as if they had a 'lead ball' in their stomach;

eyes were also affected. But on the whole, nothing really remarkable had happened to their health.[40]

Echoes of the view that airs in localities subject to eruptions were harmless, indeed even healthy, can be found more than a century and a half later, in the early eighteenth century *Consulti* by the university teacher and follower of 'modern' philosophy Nicola Cirillo (1671–1734). One of the most common remedies he offers to an impressive number of patients' complaints is moving to Pozzuoli or Ischia, to be able to breathe better air and go to the baths. The language employed by Cirillo and his 'geology' are obviously very different from those of the previous century: he believes that the medical properties of mineral waters and exhalations derive their power and strength from subterranean fermentations, which changed with the season.[41] This is only one of innumerable instances of the fact that while the airs of the area surrounding the urban centre were considered healthy by the population at large, even therapeutic, especially when nearer to the fires in the Phlegraean Fields, the city itself was by no means deemed a salubrious place. Overcrowded and poor, filthy and humid, the centre of the city was hardly a good place to stay, by early modern medical standards. Hence the two largest hospitals in the city, the Incurabili and the Annunziata, had facilities for convalescent patients in the areas near Vesuvius or in Pozzuoli.

With the exception of the advice on bathing in localities such as Pozzuoli or Ischia, and of changing air by abandoning the unhealthy urban centre, diets and *regimina* in Naples seem broadly to have followed the pattern of those we find in other Italian localities. Airs were taken into account, but this did not alter dramatically the way other Non-Naturals were dealt with. For instance, as regards diet, exercise and sleep, there is no remarkable difference between advice given in Naples by Cirillo or that coming from Tuscan, Roman, Paduan or Bolognese physicians. However, despite the shifts in the underlying scientific explanation, the therapeutic effects Cirillo and other physicians of the late seventeenth and early eighteenth centuries expected from immersion in mineral waters or from the 'medicated airs' in Pozzuoli are not dissimilar to those described by Ferrante Imperato in the late sixteenth century.

The same was true for outbursts of epidemic diseases. In 1656 a violent bubonic plague epidemic shook the city of Naples, and killed one third of its inhabitants.[42] There was, however, no question of how the disease had spread. The explanations advanced by physicians, and especially by the 'modern' or innovative ones, ruled out the possibility that the air was responsible for the epidemic, laying the blame on contagion by contact with people or objects coming from other Italian localities which had already been affected.[43] Some years after this crisis, in 1663, a new – and fortunately less threatening – fever epidemic caused heated discussions in the medical community in the city. The lake of Agnano was used to macerate linens, and some of the physicians, those who adopted a traditional, pro-Galenist position, blamed this activity, and the 'bad air' that it produced. The 'moderns', who were often adept at chemistry, and closer to the Jesuits who profited from the linen industry, chose to defend the lake and its 'innocence', claiming that the presence of *putredo* was no longer a viable explanation for epidemics, and that something else 'in' the air – namely, mineral particles or *semina* – was needed to cause disease. So the idea that fevers and diseases, and especially the plague, were not necessarily caused by 'bad' airs alone was already a common acquisition.[44]

In the seventeenth century the way the earth was envisaged changed dramatically. In 1658 the French philosopher Pierre Gassendi published the *Syntagma philosophicum*. Despite, or maybe because of, Gassendi's commitment to corpuscularism, the *Syntagma* soon became – at least in Italy – a sort of encyclopaedic text, offering a ready explanation for an array of natural phenomena, including *meteorae*.[45] The texts and explanations belonging to the tradition of early modern 'chymistry' and iatrochemistry, from Paracelsus to Jean Baptiste van Helmont, from Robert Boyle to his followers, the physicians and experimenters known as the 'Oxford physiologists', dealing with the composition and nature of air in relation with respiration and other bodily phenomena, must also be taken into account when trying to understand Italian medical discussions on airs in the seventeenth century. What happened to the Galenic and humoral doctrine of the 'Non-Naturals', and especially to its understanding of airs, in this period? While a simplistic narrative of modern developments in 'iatromechanism' or 'iatrochemistry' as radically changing – but in fact 'improving' – medical knowledge in the seventeenth century can no longer be accepted, the doctrine of the Non-Naturals had to face new challenges and adapt itself to a changing landscape in medicine and therapeutics in this period. Challenges came from innovative scientific theories and explanations of the body, its anatomy and physiology, as well as from chemistry. Chemistry, as Craig

Martin has shown, for example in the case of the Italian Jesuit Niccolò Cabeo, by no means always discarded Aristotelian theories concerning *meteorae*. On the contrary, it changed and adapted the ancient theories to include new findings and new practices.[46] In Naples, the confrontation between 'the ancients' and 'the moderns' became at times very harsh, and chemistry was one of the banners of the moderns; but even then, chemical and mechanistic explanations were used alongside ancient theories of the airs and their influence on bodies.

In the same months in which the Lago di Agnano crisis was taking place, in 1663, the well-known physician Leonardo Di Capua (1617–95) read lessons on *mofete*, stinking exhalations, at the Accademia degli Investiganti, the stronghold of free-thinkers and modern natural philosophers in the city.[47] The 1683 published version of the lessons is a puzzling text which tries to keep together different approaches, among them a literary and historical one, in order to explain the action of 'bad' airs on bodies and respiration. In fact, as many others had done before, the *accademici* had organised expeditions to Agnano to experiment on the Grotta del Cane and on other *mofete*. However, no certain conclusion could be reached as to the action of noxious exhalations from the Grotta, Di Capua prudently stated. Nevertheless, he employed one explanation that we can find in all the texts of the time, namely, that in some cases the substances underground ferment, and this process of fermentation produces noxious exhalations. Water, like air, is projected upwards by the fermentation of minerals, 'pushed upwards by some subterranean fermentation of various and diverse mineral (gases/fumes) which are constantly arguing and struggling with each other'.[48] Di Capua's opinion is based on the notion of the fermentation of bodily fluids, and especially of the blood, as the cause of fevers, a theory that became widespread in Italy at the time, following the reception of works by Robert Boyle and especially Thomas Willis. Fermentation became a catch-all explication, for life and disease in animal bodies, as well as for earthquakes and eruptions affecting the body of the earth.

The fermentation model is to be found in the text by Giovanni Alfonso Borelli on the Etna eruption that destroyed part of Catania (1669) and in many works on Vesuvius published in subsequent years by followers of Di Capua and his fellow *Investiganti* academicians, such as Giuseppe Macrini and Gaspare Paragallo.[49] Macrini believes explosions and eruptions were due to *semina ignis* present in sulphur and bitumen. And it is remarkable that after more than a century, Paragallo expresses – in a totally different scientific language – the same opinion as Imperato: fires can reduce the noxiousness of exhalations to nothing; the eruptions are not the cause of diseases – on the contrary, the air that has been in contact with subterranean fires could almost be considered as possessing therapeutic properties.[50] In the 1740s, Francesco Serao (1702–83) would once again connect the fertility of the soil, the salubrity of the airs and the presence of natural remedies such as the baths in the Kingdom of Naples to the abundance of the 'seeds' of fire diffused in its environment.

Discourses and narratives on airs and on their medical role, in the form of analyses of the environmental features of a specific place, seemingly abound in the Kingdom of Naples in the sixteenth and early seventeenth centuries; however, they are somewhat lacking in the late seventeenth century, with a sharp increase in the eighteenth century. This is an interesting, if puzzling, fact and it would be interesting to compare it with the discussions on local airs at a European level. The revival of Hippocratism in (early) Enlightenment medicine meant a renewed attention to the territory and to ecology in explaining health conditions.[51] But while 'neohippocratism' certainly is a useful label, we should perhaps give a closer look at the question of what happens to 'airs' in the late seventeenth century. The centrality of the notion of fermentation may perhaps account for the disappearance, at least in the Neapolitan context, of medical works on the salubriousness of specific localities in the late seventeenth century. In the eighteenth century the close attention to public health took yet another new turn in the city, as we gather from a text published by Giuseppe Mosca, that in spite of the traditional title (*Of the air and the diseases depending on air*), was in fact an attempt at assessing the healthiness of the different quarters of the city itself.[52] Even though he was not able to offer such a detailed map – he says his fellow practitioners failed to provide the information he required – his book paved the way for the 'medical topographies' of the nineteenth century.[53]

Conclusion

Adopting the point of view of a local culture and knowledge is likely to offer a fresh and interesting, if obviously partial, answer to how pathologies were understood and therapeutics were constructed in specific localities, and to how these ideas and practices changed over time. From this point of view, Naples is extremely interesting in that it shows how controversial and quizzical the very notion of a 'local' medicine can be. The texts examined here show a tendency to become more and more focused on 'smaller' scales, that is, on airs in specific localities, villages or quarters of a city.

Especially in the seventeenth century, therefore, when chemistry and iatrochemistry were developing in Italy and elsewhere in Europe, Naples became an exceptional case study for testing innovative theories concerning what John Evelyn calls 'subterranean Fires'. In Evelyn's terms, as in other reports by contemporary foreigners or locals, the presence of nitrous and sulphuric exhalations were the cause of the fertility of the soil and of the temperate climate; but they also posed questions to physicians regarding the way airs, enriched and/or poisoned by exhalations, could affect human and animal health and individual temperaments. In other words, the merry and witty character of Neapolitans, together with their general good health, could be explained by recourse to a corpus of knowledge that was both traditional, humoral and Galenic, as well as being new, thanks especially to the influence of iatrochemistry. In Naples, one of the Italian centres for chemical experimentation from the late sixteenth century, it was particularly evident that chemistry was likely to be useful for medicine, both as a theory and as an operative and therapeutic means, and that, more generally, the way medicine envisaged health had to take into account terrestrial phenomena. When theories of the earth slowly began to change in the late sixteenth and seventeenth centuries, so did medical theories, which also had to consider changing the advice they offered to their patients. The Neapolitan case offers therefore a particularly striking example of the strong connections that existed at the time between medicine and earth sciences, chemistry, air mechanics and medicine. Today we conceive of those disciplines as being far apart, thereby neglecting the strong connections drawn between them at the time.

Physicians in Naples put themselves forward as the main interpreters of the worrying phenomena affecting the earth, the waters and the airs. As I have shown through many examples, their expertise in these matters, while not entirely unchallenged, due to competition with other professions (e.g., with engineers or architects), was rather commonplace.

The analogy between the body of the earth and the 'animal' body was so obvious that it elicited little explicit discussion in early modern medicine; recently, moreover, it had been revived in the Paracelsian and chemical tradition.[54] The 'anatomy' of the earth, of its fires and waters, also involved a precocious and strong interest for chemistry.

Despite changes in natural philosophy, such as the emergence of chemical explanations and of models both for human and animal physiology and pathology, along with models for geological phenomena affecting the body of the earth, physicians in Naples continued to envisage airs and the environment in the area surrounding the city not just as healthy, but as likely to produce therapeutic effects, healing or improving a number of diseases. This was true both for individual bodies and illnesses as for inhabitants of the area as a whole, provided they abandoned as often as possible the damp and filthy centre of the urban area. In the opinion of the lay public, of natural philosophers and physicians active locally and abroad, Neapolitan volcanic airs helped improve health, both individual and public. This was not the least reason for the European fascination with Vesuvius and with the Phlegraean Fields, apparent as much in travellers' reports as in works of science and art.

Notes

1 J. Evelyn, *Diary*, ed., W. Bray, 2 vols. (New York and London: Dunne, 1901), vol. 1, pp. 146–60.

2 *Ibid.*, pp. 148, 149, 150, 152, 153, 160. See also J. Evelyn, *Fumifugium* (1661) (Exeter: The Rota at the University of Exeter, 1976), pp. 1–3, for a theorisation on the relationship between airs and places; M.R.S. Jenner, 'The politics of London air: John Evelyn's Fumifugium and the Restoration', *The Historical Journal*, 38:3 (1995), pp. 535–51.

3 See S. Cavallo and T. Storey, *Healthy Living in Late Renaissance Italy* (Oxford: Oxford University Press, 2013), ch. 5.

4 Evelyn, *Diary*, pp. 156–7; see also S. Porzio, *De conflagratione Agri Puteolani* (Florence: Torrentinus, 1551; first ed. 1538), and D. Castelli, 'Il De conflagratione di Simone Porzio: la collazione delle tre edizioni, un volgarizzamento e il ms. Phill.12844 dell'HRC di Austin', *Rinascimento Meridionale*, III (2012), pp. 81–104.

5 H. Jedin, *Girolamo Seripando. Sein Leben und Denken im Geisteskampf des 16. Jahrhunderts*, 2 vols (Würzburg: Rita-Verlag, 1937).

6 Biblioteca Nazionale Napoli, BNN Ms XIII AA 49 (ex 50), XXI luglio 1548, Seripando to Augusto Cocciano from Bologna, c. 24r.
7 *Ibid.*, Di Napoli alle VIII di Novembre del L a A. Cocciano Roma, 46r.
8 *Ibid.*, Di Posilypo. L'ultimo di Ottobre del LI a A. Cocciano a Roma, 69r.
9 On the geology of the area, B. De Vivo (ed.), *Volcanism in the Campania Plain. Vesuvius, Campi Flegrei and Ignimbrites* (Amsterdam: Elsevier, 2006).
10 J. Quiñones, *El Monte Vesuvio a ora la Montaña de Soma* (Madrid: Por Juan Gonçalez, 1632).7
11 S. Cocco, *Watching Vesuvius: A History of Science and Culture in Early Modern Italy* (Chicago: University of Chicago Press, 2013).
12 Evelyn, *Diary*, p. 154; see also S. Majoli, *Dies caniculares, Hoc est, Colloquia physica noua & admiranda* (Mainz: Ioannis Theobaldi Schonnvetteri, 1615, first ed. 1608), p. 693.
13 M. Conforti, 'Subterranean fires and chemical exhalations: mineral waters in the Phlegraean Fields in the Early Modern age', in D. Boisseuil, J. Coste and M. Nicoud (eds), *Le Thermalisme. Histoire d'un Phénomène Culturel et Médical* (Paris: CNRS éditions, 2015), pp. 123–36.
14 M. Rak, *Napoli Gentile: la Letteratura in Lingua Napoletana nella Cultura Barocca, 1596–1632* (Bologna: Il Mulino, 1994).
15 L. Ciancio, *Le Colonne del Tempo: il Tempio di Serapide a Pozzuoli nella Storia della Geologia, dell'Archeologia e dell'Arte (1750–1900)* (Florence: Edifir, 2009), while dealing mainly with the eighteenth and nineteenth centuries, is a wonderfully rich introduction to archeology and science in this area.
16 See e.g. G.C. Capaccio, *La Vera Antichita di Pozzuolo, Descritta … A modo d'Itinerario* (Naples: Gio. Giacomo Carlino e Costantino Vitale, 1607).
17 See e.g. C. Pellegrino, *Apparato alle Antichità di Capua o vero Discorsi della Campania Felice* (Naples: Francesco Savio, 1651), Disc. III, pp. 482ff.; cf. the much later F. Serao, *Istoria dell'Incendio del Vesuvio Accaduto nel Mese di Maggio dell'Anno 1737* (Naples: Novello de' Bonis, 1788).
18 'Si veggono intorno a due mila fossette, dalle quali esala un fumo sulfureo, aluminoso, di sale armoniaco, e di altri minerali, ch'i nostri Medici dicono che sia molto salutifero a' morbi freddi, & humidi'; Capaccio, *La vera*, p. 105.
19 See e.g. G.N. Eustachio, *Opusculum de aere, Situque Beneventanae civitatis* (Naples: Io. Baptistae Subtilis apud Scipionem Boninum, 1608), p. 100, where the author explains that Benevento is not prone to earthquakes as is Pozzuoli, where airs are putrid because of volcanism and exhalations.
20 '[I] paesani con molta diligenza detta terra col ferro rivolgono, acciò che con quella si vada mescolando il fumo, e dal mese di Gennaio infino all'Ottobre la coltivano, come sogliono coltivare gli horti'. Capaccio, *La Vera*, p. 106.

21 G.C. Braccini, *Dell'Incendio Fattosi nel Vesuvio a 16. di Dicembre M.DC. XXXI. E delle sue Cause, ed Effetti* (Naples: Secondino Roncagliolo, 1632), ch. 7.
22 C. Martin, *Renaissance Meteorology* (Baltimore: Johns Hopkins University Press, 2011). On seventeenth-century debates on the earth, W. Poole, *The World Makers: Scientists of the Restoration and the Search for the Origins of the Earth* (Oxford: P. Lang, 2010).
23 B. Telesio, *De his, quae in Aere fiunt; & de Terrae motibus, liber unicus* (Neapoli: Ios. Cacchium, 1570). See M. Mulsow, *Frühneuzeitliche Selbsterhaltung. Telesio und die Naturphilosophie der Renaissance* (Tübingen: Niemayer, 1998).
24 A. Clericuzio, 'Chemical medicine and Paracelsianism in Italy, 1550–1650', in M. Pelling and S. Mandelbrote (eds), *The Practice of Reform in Health, Medicine and Science. Essays for Charles Webster, 1500–2000* (Aldershot: Ashgate, 2005), pp. 59–79.
25 F. Imperato, *Dell'historia naturale* (Naples: Costantino Vitale, 1599), b. VIII ch. XXI.
26 *Ibid.*, pp. 265–6.
27 G. Jasolino, *De Rimedi Naturali che sono nell'Isola di Pithecusa, hoggi detta Ischia* (Naples: Gioseppe Cacchij, 1558).
28 *Ibid.*, p. 36.
29 'Quare ego, quod a me alibi disputatum est, nihil certi haec significare, praeter siccitatem, affirmo: cui frugum penuria succedere consuevit. quin & pestem multis ante saeculis accidisse accepimus', Porzio, *De conflagratione*, p. 8.
30 F. Furchheim, *Bibliografia del Vesuvio: Compilata e Corredata di Note Critiche Estratte dai più Autorevoli Scrittori Vesuviani* (Naples: F. Furchheim di Emilio Prass, 1897).
31 J.E. Everson, 'The melting pot of science and belief: studying Vesuvius in seventeenth-century Naples', *Renaissance Studies*, 26:5 (2011), pp. 691–727.
32 G.F. Porrata Spinola, *Discorso sopra l'origine de' Fuochi gettati dal Monte Vesevo, ceneri piovute, et altri successi, e Pronostico d'effetti maggiori* (Lecce: Pietro Micheli Borgognone, 1632).
33 '[T]erzane doppie, febbri ardenti maligne … sintomi di stomaco & afflittioni di cuore, d'onde nasce perdita di forze, e presta morte con sudori diaphoretici, vomiti, e flussi di corpo maligni, & alcuni mali di punture, e … mali alla gola, e discesi al collo'. *Ibid.*, p. 39.
34 '[L]a Montagna di Somma ne' terremoti non manda vapori tanto pestiferi, come altri scrive, o pensa, perché dov'è fuoco non si permette putredine, di più lo zolfo là abbondante è secreto principale contra la peste … e contra la difficoltà della respirazione non ha ugual rimedio'. *Ibid.*, p. 40.

35 P. Castelli, *Incendio del Monte Vesuvio* (Rome: Giacomo Mascardi, 1632). On Castelli, A. Clericuzio, 'Chemical medicines in Rome: Pietro Castelli and the vitriol debate, 1616–1626', in M.P. Donato and J. Kraye (eds), *Conflicting Duties: Science, Medicine and Religion in Rome, 1550–1750* (London: Warburg Institute, 2009), pp. 281–302.

36 '[P]redirò salubrità futura dell'aere. Nè si può in modo alcuno da questo incendio argumentar futura peste: perche se questi incendii inducono un temperamento secco all'aria, la siccità è rimedio della putredine: e nella peste, il prohibir la putredine è rimedio preservativo, come ho già diffusamente scritto nel mio libro della peste.' *Ibid.*, p. 64.

37 *Ibid.*, p. 68.

38 '[S]e per l'avanti vi fosse stato … qualche fomite pestifero con il fuoco l'ha cacciato, e dissipato'. *Ibid.*, p. 66.

39 '[I]l cui fuoco io ho provato havendomi scottato alcune dita, & abrugiate le scarpe, volendo raccorre del solfo, e del sale armoniaco'. *Ibid.*, pp. 7, 31.

40 '[C]ome una palla di piombo', G.B. Zupi, *Continuazione de' successi Del prossimo Incendio del Vesuvio con gli effetti della cenere, e pietre da quelli vomitate* (Naples: Gio:Francesco Paci, 1661), pp. [A6]–[A6v].

41 '[P]er le mutate sotterranee fermentazioni'. N. Cirillo, *Consulti medici* (Venice: F. Pitteri, 1741; first ed. 1738), p. 142.

42 G. Calvi, 'L'oro, il fuoco, le forche: la peste napoletana del 1656', *Archivio Storico Italiano*, 3 (1981), pp. 405–58.

43 G. Gatta, *Di una gravissima peste Che nella Passata Primavera & Estate dell'anno 1656 depopulò la Città di Napoli, suoi Borghi, e Casali, e molte altre Città, e Terre del suo Regno* (Naples: Luc'Antonio di Fusco, 1659). For a similar attitude see e.g. A. Mariani, *De peste anni MDCXXX Bononiae. Cuius generis fuit, & an ab aere* (Bologna: Clementis Ferronij, 1631)

44 M. Torrini, 'Un episodio della polemica tra "antichi" e "moderni": la disputa sulla macerazione dei lini nel Lago di Agnano', *Bollettino del Centro di Studi Vichiani*, 5:1 (1975), pp. 56–70.

45 S. Murr (ed.), *Gassendi et l'Europe (1592–1792)* (Paris: Vrin, 1997); see also F. Bernier, *Abregé de la Philosophie de Gassendi* (Lyon: Anisson, Posuel et Rigaud, 1684), v. V, b. I.

46 Martin, *Renaissance Meteorology*, ch. 5.

47 L. Di Capua, *Lezioni intorno alla natura delle mofete* (Napoli: per Salvatore Castaldo, 1683). As shown by the dedication to Christina, Queen of Sweden, by Cesare Di Capua, the lessons were printed twenty years after having been delivered.

48 '[I]n su spinta da qualche sotterranea formentazione di vari, e diversi aliti minerali, che continuo tempestano, e dibbattonsi fra esso loro'. *Ibid.*, p. 16. See also n. 46.

49 G.A. Borelli, *Historia et meteorologia incendii Aetnaei anni 1699* (Reggio di Calabria: Ferri, 1670); G. Macrini, *De Vesuvio* (Naples: Hieronymi Fasuli, 1693), pp. 68–9; G. Paragallo, *Istoria Naturale del Monte Vesuvio* (Naples: G. Raillard, 1705).

50 Serao, *Istoria*, pp. 16–17.

51 D. Cantor (ed.), *Reinventing Hippocrates* (Aldershot: Ashgate, 2002).

52 G. Mosca, *Dell'aria e de' morbi dall'aria dipendenti* (Naples: Alessio Pellecchia, 1746).

53 B. Marin, 'La topographie médicale de Naples de Filippo Baldini, médecin hygiéniste au service de la Couronne', *Melanges de l'Ecole française de Rome. Italie et Méditerranée*, 101 (1989), pp. 695–732.

54 See e.g. the comparison between the erupting Vesuvius and an animal body suffering from a violent disease in V. Alsario Croce, *Vesuvius ardens siue Exercitatio medico-physica ad rigopyreton* (Rome: Guilelmi Facciotti, 1632).

6

The afterlife of the Non-Naturals in early eighteenth-century Hippocratism: from the healthy individual to a healthy population

Maria Pia Donato

This chapter explores the afterlife of the Non-Naturals in late seventeenth- and early eighteenth-century medical culture. It is concerned with two processes that supposedly took place in this period and are normally regarded as being only loosely connected. On the one hand, the collapse of traditional health advice based on the care of the Non-Naturals (food and drink, air, motion and stillness, evacuation and retention, sleep and wakefulness, the passions of the soul); on the other hand, the emergence of an early form of environmental medicine and of medical policing, concerned with the prevention of disease and the avoidance of health hazards. What happened when the philosophy that for centuries had underpinned the doctrine of the Non-Naturals fell apart? Which aspect of the tradition in which the doctrine was embedded could be reframed and how?

In their recent book, Sandra Cavallo and Tessa Storey have illustrated the growing importance attached to the Non-Naturals in early modern culture, and how widely prophylactic concerns were disseminated through various textual genres which went well beyond the medical literature of *regimina sanitatis*.[1] They also showed, however, that by the end of the seventeenth century, this genre declined. This did not mean the end of preventative medicine altogether, of course, nor the complete disappearance of popular handbooks for the preservation of health nor even the extinction of learned medical literature on the six Non-Natural things.[2] Yet, the culture of healthy living undoubtedly underwent change, as we will see.

Around the same period, new concerns over public health and salubriousness emerged in European medicine and culture. Drawing on Hippocrates, especially on the Hippocratic texts *Airs, Waters and Places* and *Epidemics* I and III, medical writers and, to a certain extent, natural philosophers and lay authors sought to explain health and disease by looking at the role of particular agents, especially underscoring the impact of some of the old Non-Naturals, namely air and food. Such was their interest in the impact of air and climate on bodies, in the quality of water and food supply, in the nature of soil and in the dangers posed by organic or industrial waste that it gave rise to a new kind of medical climatology and geography. As James Riley noted, in the Hippocratic tradition the physician was urged to examine winds, waters, site, soil, diet, and the other characteristics of a place, but he did not think 'that environmental circumstances influencing local diseases might themselves be modified', whereas modern Hippocratism sought 'to determine what aspects of the environment might be modified to weaken or eliminate their capacity to cause disease'.[3] Accordingly, improvements to methods of sanitation were put forward while public officials took a more active role in the surveillance of community health.

The aim of this chapter is to investigate the relationships between these processes by focusing on the transformation of the notion of Non-Naturals in the eighteenth century, and the changing role assigned to them in preserving health. It mainly, though not exclusively, deals with Rome. Although Rome was part of a broader picture, focusing on one precise context brings deeper insight into the interaction between intellectual and social change. As we shall see, against the backdrop of collapsing Aristotelian and Galenic views, new philosophical ideas emerged that provided a new framework for explaining the impact of environment on the human body, and eventually resulted in a new emphasis on public health. However, the transformation of medical theories, though crucial, was not the only reason for such a shift in focus from the healthy individual to a healthy population; indeed, new theories combined with reforming trends in the social organisation of medicine were already at work. While not completely overturning the preventative paradigm based on the care of Non-Natural things, this was now reinterpreted in a more innovative fashion.

The decline of a medical tradition?

The health regimen literature had flourished in early modern Rome. A wealthy town, where social elites from all over the Catholic world lived and refined courtly and civic cultures coexisted, the city was home to a prosperous and active medical community. Notwithstanding such a well-established tradition, the genre seems to have fallen into neglect by the end of the seventeenth century and only a few new regimens were published in Rome and the vicinity in the period spanning 1670 to 1730. The new titles included *L'oro della sanità* by Barnaba Ciccolini, a prolific medical practitioner and a staunch opponent of modern mechanical medicine and natural philosophy, and *Sopra le cure preservative* by Domenico Passeri, a town physician in nearby Orvieto, north of Rome.[4]

The very profile of both authors – a traditionalist and a provincial practitioner – would seem an indictment of the decline of health regimens. In his booklet and in his later Latin tract *Aeris salubris specimen*, however, Passeri professed modern tenets.[5] Discussing the impact of earthquakes on human health, he wrote of the air as a spirituous and elastic element, 'a mass of impure sulphurs and a variety of vitriolic, aluminous and especially nitrous salts', which 'pervert the motions and compositions' of the blood, namely 'the little globules or round molecules observable through good microscopes'. Acids can indeed alter 'the site, shape and movements' of all bodily fluids. Hence, the correct management of each Non-Natural thing should seek to 'preserve and promote the natural fermentation of the blood and ... keep it in the right mixture, on which depends the right rule of its movements, both circular and fermentative'.[6] In practice, Passeri's advice was as conventional as Ciccolini's, but his rationale referred to the circulatory pathology of Frans de la Boë (Sylvius) and Thomas Willis. This theory was extremely popular in the medical culture of the time, and posited that most ailments arose from impairments in the natural circulation and fermentation of the blood due to a chemical imbalance.[7]

The *Consigli preservativi e curativi in tempo di contagio* published by the Roman state Chief Physician (*protomedicus*) Domenico Gagliardi in 1720, the year of the plague in Marseille, is another work to be mentioned.[8] Plague tracts had long been a peculiar subgenre of regimen literature, often written by the most prominent medical figures, and Gagliardi's tract follows in this tradition. His advice for the people of Rome falls into three categories: *preservativa prudenziale* (regimen and care of the house), *preservativa medica* (hygiene and preventative medicine) and curative medicine for those struck by the plague without medical assistance. A further subgenre was advice on the Lenten diet, which was the preserve of medical officials too: hence, in 1703, the *protomedicus* in office, Paolo Manfredi, published his own *Instruction* on how to follow religious precepts without prejudicing one's health.[9]

The paucity of new works arguably reveals the overall decline of health regimens, and not only in Rome. Introducing his learned and courtly *Adnotationes* on Alvise Cornaro's *Della Vita Sobria,* Bernardino Ramazzini, professor at Padua, lamented that publishers refused to print regimen anymore, as physicians 'by far prefer [to buy] books explaining how to cure diseases, rather than how to protect health.'[10] Ramazzini himself, however, had also printed a further regimen on the health of princes, and this, like the rest of his books was widely known in Rome, where he had many friends and correspondents.[11]

True, a more nuanced picture of the decline of preventive advice literature emerges if we turn our attention to new editions of older works. For instance, Cornaro's *Della vita sobria,* originally published in 1588, was reprinted in Rome in 1673 by the official printing press of the Camera Apostolica in Lessius's Latin translation, a fact that is probably connected with the peculiar moralistic stance of this work on food and sobriety, well attuned to the moral concerns of the papal curia. This same work also continued to circulate as an appendix to cheap reprints of the medieval regimen of the school of Salerno.[12]

Nonetheless, judging by the number of editions and the many copies still remaining in historical Roman libraries, by the end of the seventeenth century books of secrets and recipes seem to have enjoyed a greater success among Romans than regimens, though it is difficult to draw a clear dividing line between the two genres.[13] Francesco Domenico Auda, a friar and chief apothecary at the main city hospital of Santo Spirito, actually tried to bring them together. His *Breve compendio di maravigliosi segreti,* which went through several editions, was composed of four sections pertaining to medicinal remedies, house and beauty care, chemical secrets and medical astrology with an appended tract on 'how to maintain health'.[14] It was, however, unoriginal in style and content. Far more innovative was another book related to food and health that was popular in Rome at that time, though by a French author: the *Traité des aliments* by Louis Lémery.[15] Lémery analysed each foodstuff and drink according to its peculiar balance of acids, alkalis and other salts, and systematically adapted the traditional discourse on nutrition and well-being (the title clearly alluded to Galen) to chemical ideas.

Of course, material evidence suggests that books often remained in circulation for decades, even centuries after their first publication,[16] although older regimen were made more attractive for the market by being published together with tracts on 'modern' beverages like chocolate, tea and coffee.[17] As a matter of fact, Rome was witness to a heated debate on the beneficial effects that drinking these 'exotic' substances had on digestion, evacuation and wakefulness, involving lay authors[18] and physicians as prominent as Giorgio Baglivi, professor of *medicina theorica* at the university of Rome, and Luca Tozzi, physician to pope Innocent XII and later to the King of Naples.[19]

Altogether though, much evidence points towards the eclipse of a medical tradition. Of course, the decline of the regimen literature did not imply that Non-Naturals ceased to be resorted to in medical theory and practice all at once. First, hygiene was still part of the standard medical education in Rome just as it was throughout Europe, and the basic principles of dietetics were cursorily taught in the university course of *medicina theorica* or *institutiones medicinae*.[20] The correct management of the Non-Naturals for the preservation of health was an ordinary topic in comprehensive medical handbooks or academic orations, replete with quotations from classical authors.[21]

Second, at the turn of the seventeenth and eighteenth centuries the Non-Naturals still recurred in many practical medical works, regardless of the philosophical tenets of their authors, be they Galenists or 'neoterics'. So for instance, on the one hand, Tozzi could append a learned tract on *de recto usu non naturalium* to his commentary on Galen's *Of the art of medicine* (which had been one of the core texts on hygiene over the centuries), in which he set out to modernise Hippocratic and Galenic teachings in the light of modern natural philosophy. On the other hand, as late as 1726 an aspiring doctor in philosophy and medicine at the

Sapienza could dedicate his still strictly Galenist thesis on hygiene and on the regimen for the ill to the pope.[22]

The Non-Naturals in medical theory and practice: debating health, lifestyle and death

The debate surrounding sudden death that was sparked in 1705 by a series of mysterious casualties, which terrorised the whole of Rome, offers excellent insight into the transformation of the Non-Naturals in medical culture. Sudden death provides a very good standpoint from which to investigate the notion of health and the role assigned to the Non-Naturals over time.[23] It is not a proper disease and yet it threatens life and indeed, because with no time to confess one might die in a state of mortal sin, it also threatens the afterlife. Ever since antiquity, the misuse of the six Non-Naturals was regarded as the primary cause of sudden death, that is as the outcome of an abrupt loss of vital heat or a sudden obstruction of the ventricles of the brain responsible for the distillation of the animal spirits. These problems were caused precisely by a mismanagement of the Non-Naturals which had altered the balance of humours and had produced overabundant viscous matter. Alternatively, the Non-Naturals could kill by acting as a contrary quality (as when an excessively cold drink abruptly extinguishes vital heat), or by consuming vital and animal spirits at once, for example through excessive and untimely sexual activity. Increasingly complex justifications of why and how this occurred went hand in hand with the growing sophistication of scholastic and Renaissance medicine. At the same time, the Non-Naturals were seen as crucial for preserving health and life itself. They not only formed an essential part of medical treatment (together with surgery and pharmacy), but were the main pillar of the measures of preventative health care adopted under the guidance of the physician, responsible for adapting general principles to individual patients and their idiosyncrasies.[24]

In the second half of the seventeenth century, the Galenic and Aristotelian principles that had underpinned such interpretations were challenged. Humours and qualities gave way to various new views of the workings of the body in terms of chemical operations and mechanical actions. Yet both laypersons and experts still somehow took the Non-Naturals into account. After the onset of the 'epidemic' of sudden deaths, the people of Rome attributed them 'to the instability of the season, first cold North winds, then the burning Sirocco'.[25] Accusing fingers were then pointed at chocolate, at the poor quality of tobacco and the abuse of liquor. The most widespread opinion, however, was that this epidemic was an outcome of the earthquakes and volcanic eruptions over the previous years, which produced a 'malign influence' which 'alters the air and makes it of such bad quality'.[26] The idea that earthquakes corrupted air was as ancient as Aristotle's *Meteorology* and Pliny's *Natural History*, and yet it still operated within the corpuscular paradigm of the moderns, which had gained momentum in the late seventeenth century. No less an author than Boyle had validated such an interpretation in his *General History of the Air* (1692). In the papal city itself, prominent men of science and medicine and proponents of Galilean and Cartesian philosophy like Giovanni Alfonso Borelli and Giorgio Baglivi defended similar theories. As we have seen, a provincial doctor like Passeri deemed it necessary to devise an ad hoc regimen to preserve health from the effects of earthquakes.[27]

The doctors who were involved in the debate on sudden death suspected that it was caused by air intoxicated with noxious exhalations from earthquakes and harmful winds, by rotten food and alcoholic drinks and, last but not least, intemperate lifestyles. However, they provided rather different explanations of it, some drawing heavily on an old humoral understanding of the body – which now incorporated, however, circulatory physiology – whilst others gave greater importance to mechanical ailments. For Manoel da Sylva, a Portuguese doctor practising in Rome, the air was the primary cause of the abrupt deaths savaging the city in 1706, for it contained noxious vitriolic ferments which coagulated the blood.[28] These 'vitriolic, arsenical and nitrous' exhalations, which ordinarily only cause light fevers, emanate from underground in harmful quantities during earthquakes, and make the blood unable to ferment and circulate properly, causing apoplexy or syncope.

According to Angelo Evangelista, apoplexies were caused by 'bad mixtures in the blood', when blood was corrupted by a 'very strong ferment or juice of an alien and perverse nature' from food.[29] Food produces such fermentation especially when warm and chilly periods alternate. But air might also harm the body, and especially the blood, filling it 'with nitro-sulphur that some authors call elastic'; this causes the vessels to become thicker so that they sometimes lacerate and bring about sudden death. In Antonio Bernabei's *Dissertazione delle morti improvvise* of 1708 sudden deaths were considered in a similar vein, as the outcome of a 'stomach syncope' or a 'suffocating catarrh, produced by a superabundance of serums, or lymphs or serous blood tending to stagnation', or possibly as a result of humoral plethora from excessive food and *acquavite*.[30] Otherwise, imbalances in the bodily fluids could be attributed to irritating acrid and mercurial corpuscles in the air; blood, with its very tiny 'reddish little globules', is particularly liable to contamination by such particles, which render it too dense or 'fixed' to circulate and ferment healthily. But, Bernabei added, a major threat came from suppressed evacuations too, namely from the fashion of wearing wigs that hindered the evacuation of 'excrementitial matter' through the hair.

Doctors who explained sudden death in mechanical terms did not fail to evoke the role of the Non-Naturals either. For instance, Domenico Mistichelli, physician at the hospital of Fatebenefratelli, based his explanation of apoplexy on an updated anatomical understanding of the brain and viewed it as an impairment of the brain meninges and nerves. But as for causes, Mistichelli still used the scholastic distinction between proximate and remote causes, among which he listed the abuse of food and drink, especially 'certain food and unripe fruits ... full of rigid salts', suppressed or excessive evacuations, excessive study, and first and foremost, the air.[31] He considered air both as a physical agent, which by virtue of its elasticity rarefies and condenses the humours in the body (as proven by Torricelli's and Boyle's experiments) and as a chemical agent: 'urinary spirits, or ammoniac vapours' can coagulate the spirits' nitrous part, which is indispensable for the motion of the blood and the distillation of animal spirits, and thence of life.

The most accomplished mechanical explanation of sudden death was that of Giovanni M. Lancisi, papal physician and professor of theoretical medicine at the Roman university. His *De subitaneis mortibus* was printed in 1707 as a report of the official medical investigation into the 'epidemic' ordered by Pope Clement XI.[32] In Lancisi's authoritative view, sudden death only results from the impairment of the 'flux and reflux' of the three major bodily fluids, that is, air, blood and nervous fluid, or of the main organs responsible for life, that is, lungs, heart and brain. In most cases, it is the outcome of the rupture of major blood vessels, as shown by dissection. Lancisi nevertheless also pointed to the role of noxious particles in the air, and to air pressure and swift temperature changes which alter the mechanical and chemical behaviour of the body's fluids, drying up its tissues and making them more likely to tear and ulcerate. The papal physician also reminded readers of the role of food and lifestyle: thus, the poorest part of the population fell victim to rotten food and to improper medication sold by charlatans, whereas the rich indulged in excessively rich food and were prey to sudden death too.[33]

Moreover, regardless of their tenets in physiology and pathology, all authors put some emphasis on the Non-Naturals as the best, and possibly the only, means to prevent sudden death. No one was out of danger unless he followed 'the exact and regulate life' prescribed by the doctor, and to support this statement da Sylva quoted no lesser authority than Avicenna and the Salernitan *Regimen Sanitatis*. For Evangelista there was not, in fact, any real treatment, only prevention. Therefore, the doctor should adapt a few good universal rules to individual patients, both when they are sick and when they are in (apparently) good health. Both authors emphasised that it was of utter importance to avoid affliction and sadness, recalling the standard precepts of earlier writers on this point. But since noxious ferments originated mainly from food, diet was the key to healthy living. After all, warned da Sylva, 'gluttony kills more than the sword'.[34] Most physicians, for example, recommended light wine as a solvent for thick blood; since light wine was the most common early modern drink, the preventative use of wine was already a commonplace in all regimen literature. Now, however, the advice was reframed into circulatory pathology and referred to contemporary theories on the blood fermentation.

A tenet especially dear to Bernabei was that any regimen should be individual. And yet he provided 'some details of almost generic method' on each of the canonical Non-Naturals in order to remove 'from the bodies the bad dispositions they may have and remove those humours that can bring a man to the edge of the precipice'. Hence people should live in the mountains where air is purer, burn juniper to improve it through its perfumed fumes, make use of tobacco that stirs 'the dormant spirits in the brain wonderfully', drink coffee, tea or chocolate and eat sorbets as much as 'one's temperament wishes or requires, and as much as the physician deems it good, just remembering that only excess makes them dangerous'. Last but not least, one ought to 'live happily', since fear is the enemy of health. In a word, 'keep away from any extreme in everything', as he wrote in a perfectly classical mode.[35]

A few physicians maintained the distinction between 'dietary' and 'preservative' treatment which combined Non-Naturals with a few medical or surgical remedies, be it the customary spring bloodletting and purge or light cordials. According to Mistichelli, the former consisted in 'not abusing the six Non-Natural things' while the latter amounted to 'a certain way of life consisting on the one hand of a perfect diet, and on the other of the use of appropriate remedies'.[36] Among these he listed 'spirituous cephalics', 'volatile liquors, nearly pure spirits' and the anti-apoplectic waters of chemical classics like Donzelli, Crollius, Rivière and Quarcetanus. His colleague Bernabei recommended the 'morsel called cephalic': clearly a well-established preparation, as he gave no further details.[37]

As a proponent of modern natural philosophy, Lancisi was more reluctant than his colleagues to mention the Non-Naturals openly, as they were arguably too reminiscent of the humoralism that mechanical medicine opposed, at least in principle. Also, his tract was of wider scope than those of other practitioners, who wrote for an audience of potential patients. Yet, Lancisi did not omit to write on how to safeguard 'bodies that appear to be healthy' and resorted to traditional rules of hygiene, especially on food, reinterpreting them in the light of mechanism. Accordingly, he recommended fasting and bloodletting as these reduce the blood mass, pressure and fat, as well as moderate exercise and light frictions to invigorate the tissues of the body, whose healthy movements are necessary for life. As for 'sick bodies', everything depended on the type of ailment they were affected with, so that only the treating physician could discern the individual mix of diet and medicines. However, Lancisi added, 'there are times when all medical precautions deceive us, but one ... has never failed: namely, a sober regimen of life, and a tranquil and undisturbed mind, in good health or ill'.[38]

Non-Natural things made real

Hence, at the beginning of the eighteenth century, the Non-Naturals still represented a key notion for medical practitioners in a city like

Rome when explaining health and disease. The overlapping of chemical and mechanical words and concepts with older humoral ideas in their writings arguably reinforces continuity. Notably, in this regard, Roman physicians were not alone. Writing on apoplexy in the same period, Pierre Dionis, royal surgeon in Paris, blamed sophisticated *ragouts* and delicacies that engross the blood and cause deadly *coups de sang*; and in his tract on the health of princes, Ramazzini accepted the view that too cold a drink could kill swiftly.[39]

The 'moral' approach to illness and health, focused on individual dispositions and conduct and on the counselling role of the physician, remained a pivot for the professional ethos of academic medicine. It was also through this that experts and the public found common ground in their effort to cope with sickness.[40] This perspective also continued to provide the conceptual and cultural framework within which hygiene could be adapted to contemporary medical and philosophical ideas and modern urban lifestyles.

Under this veil of continuity, however, shifts cannot pass unnoticed. First and most obvious, the emphasis on prevention was now laid mainly on air, eating and drinking. None of this was new,[41] yet these aspects of everyday life were given even greater importance, whereas the complex of Non-Naturals worked holistically in the Galenic medical tradition. Air especially stands out, which, considering the amount of research and speculation over air in seventeenth-century science, is hardly surprising.[42] Second, both air and food are clearly no longer thought of as entities defined by their qualities, but as composite bodies or material aggregates acting either through chemical reactions or through physical properties. This is true in later regimens as well as in practical medical literature. Winds, for instance, were key preoccupations in traditional preventative medicine. According to Hippocrates and Galen, winds impact on health by disturbing through their own qualities the optimal balance of qualities in the body, especially during the change of seasons and in particular on dangerously hot or cold days. In these terms, their role is underscored by older texts still circulating like Durante's *Tesoro della sanità*.[43] In contrast, at the beginning of the eighteenth century, the pathogenic action of the air was conceived differently. Winds were understood to carry particles and chemical agents that interact with the components of the body. Furthermore, many authors now discussed air as an elastic body endowed with weight and other physical properties.

Indeed, all physical realities are more or less explicitly deemed to be non-elemental: blood is made of 'reddish globules', nervous fluid is made of nitro-aerial components, tissues are made of fibres, viscid matter of acrid particles, and air is made of chemical corpuscles. According to Lancisi, all the fluids and solids of the human body and of Nature at large are composed of discrete entities, which have both chemical and mechanical properties. His approach is similar to that of prominent natural philosophers and physicians like Boyle, Borelli and the great anatomist Marcello Malpighi.[44] Although these and the lesser Roman authors writing on health or debating sudden death did not agree on the actual composition of corporeal realities or the ultimate nature of their smallest components, they shared a corpuscular understanding of physical bodies. As Mistichelli put it, whether

> the blood [is] composed either according to the galenists by the four humours ... or according to chemists by salt, sulphur, mercury, water and earth, or even, according to democritics and platonicists, by a single substance or matter, variably modified in site, number, shape and size ... it will still be true that the different ways in which the continuous motion of fermentation, agitation and circulation can mix these visible and sensible components ... can pervert vital and animal economy and bring about grave and serious illnesses.[45]

What is more, they all agree on the corporeality of Non-Natural things, especially air, in line with the overall materialisation of the natural world and of the human body in late seventeenth- and early eighteenth-century natural philosophy and medicine. Whereas the canonical Non-Naturals were actions and principles of qualitative balance in the *crasis* of humours and faculties, in modern medicine their materiality seems to take over. And whereas in the Galenic tradition hygiene was more a matter of behaviour in general rather than of single potentially harmful substances, this seems to be no longer true.

The corpuscular view coupled with circulatory physiology can explain why the emphasis was put mainly on food and air. In actual fact, through the corpuscular paradigm, the vulnerability of bodily fluids and tissues (themselves corpuscular in nature) to these external agents was perfectly understandable. Conversely, other Non-Naturals were now perceived to exert a less direct action upon the body and received less attention, though mechanical explanations of the animal economy did not exclude their impact on human health. In fact, Lancisi and others did point at fibres as being the smallest component of the solid parts of the body, and did praise motion and friction as part of healthy living. In the same years in Rome, Baglivi devised a whole pathology of solids which underscored the value of exercise and rest in preserving and restoring health; he also emphasised the importance of transpiration (that is, of excretion) in the wake of Santorio, whose work he edited as an early instance of mechanical medicine.[46] Yet, this early 'fibre medicine' did not really succeed in making the whole set of the canonical Non-Naturals relevant.[47]

Furthermore, an emphasis on air, food and also on water could help explain why places had different diseases and 'morbid constitutions'. According to Bernabei, for instance, Roman air was 'heavy' with 'bituminous, sulphurous, arsenic, vitriolic corpuscles and others', which 'penetrate into the red and animal fluids and dispose bodies to sudden, deadly diseases'.[48] For Mistichelli, the Roman climate had always been slightly adverse, due to southern winds and the mineral-rich soil, problems which were exacerbated by the habit of eating 'unripe' fruits and vegetables.[49]

Drawing on the Hippocratic treatise *On Airs, Waters and Places*, Lancisi argued that Rome was liable to adverse climate conditions from time to time. He thus explained the wave of sudden deaths in 1705–06 through the abrupt shifts between warm and cold periods and the predominance of south winds experienced in those times; these had arguably increased the normal dispersion of the volatile components of corporeal fluids, thereby provoking the untimely demise of so many. Hippocratic teachings could thus be understood in the light of modern physics. This made research into climate, waters and soil all the more urgent for early eighteenth-century Roman physicians, just as it had become for their colleagues in other cities and countries.

Bad air, bad water, unhealthy places?

The quality of air and waters and the impact of environment on health is precisely the subject of papal physician Lancisi's second tract *De nativis, deque adventitiis Romani coeli qualitatibus*, published in 1711, the year when he also held the post of state chief physician. Lancisi's scope in this work is manifold, and, to a certain extent contradictory. On the one hand he intended to extol the healthiness of the Roman habitat and to praise the papal government and civic authorities for their care of the city's welfare, but on the other hand he wished to account for the persistence of endemic diseases and the outburst of epidemics. Also, whilst his work bears comparison with that of his great Renaissance predecessors like Antonio Porzio, Andrea Bacci, Alessandro Petronio and Marsilio Cagnati who had written on Roman air and waters most learnedly,[50] he set out to revise old ideas in the light of modern natural philosophy and what he claimed to be a new understanding of Hippocratic methods of observation.[51]

The book is divided into three parts. In a very Hippocratic manner, the first part analyses the air, waters and weather conditions which could be expected in Rome under normal circumstances. It drew upon a variety of classical and modern sources, providing a wealth of medico-topographical and meteorological observations. Since the 'atmosphere is a liquid and compressible body', all climatic phenomena must be considered on that basis. Winds are composed of 'a mixture of particles, which either impart motion to the air, or mix with it in its motion': they are not hot, cold, salubrious or insalubrious 'unless they are accompanied by various sorts of corpuscles' that exert their forces on the living. These theoretical premises allowed him to discard the claim that Roman air was naturally unhealthy.[52] Lancisi then provided chemical analyses of the water from various Roman sources (*Acqua Vergine, Acqua Felice* etc.), an experimental procedure that had been keeping virtuosi and academies throughout Europe busy for some time.[53] The potability of water was not a new concern, as some Renaissance authors had already discussed it, but it was attracting growing interest against the backdrop of modern chemistry, which enabled a fresh understanding of water qualities and curative properties. A whole new culture of mineral waters (to drink and to bathe in) was in fact about to develop in European medicine and society.[54]

The second part of the book examines the factors that altered optimal conditions, leading to periods of 'morbid constitution'. Lancisi attributed insalubriousness to the neglect of sanitation in cities and the desertion of land, which was left uncultivated and eventually turned into marshes or wastelands. In Rome, the recurrent flooding of the Tiber was especially dangerous since stagnant water lingered in surrounding neighbourhoods. In his several capacities, whether as the pope's personal physician and trusted advisor, as a university professor, as a leading member of the Roman College of physician and as *protomedicus*, Lancisi suggested how Pope Clement XI could amend such hazards, and particularly how to sanitise the city which was still affected by the major flooding of the Tiber in 1702. He also suggested draining the Pontine marshes, a project that had had once again become a concern for the papacy at the end of the seventeenth century. Finally, the third part of the book deals with a 'rheumatic epidemic' that had raged in 1709. Lancisi writes that according to 'the testimony of thermometers' the most rigid winter in memory had followed a mild autumn. This had resulted in innumerable people suffering with coryza, angina, pleurisy and pneumonia between January and February. He argues that harmful salts in the atmosphere had mixed with bodily fluids and were not contrasted by a suitable regimen; so when the cold interrupted transpiration and the wind brought further nitrous and subacid salts, many died.[55] At the end of his tract, Lancisi detailed all the sanitation measures and improvements in food supply and medical care suggested by physicians and graciously put into practice by the pope. He also included a copy of the official edicts issued by the city's government.

In his later works, Lancisi would use the same narrative device. Both his *Dissertatio historica de bovilla peste* of 1715 on the cattle plague that was spreading across Europe and the wide-ranging study about marshland effluvia and tertiary fevers, *De noxiis paludum effluviis*, focused on public health.[56] Again, he discussed the various ways in which air was contaminated, whether by fixative chemical particles or, in the case of tertiary fevers, by micro-organisms dispersed by those insects that prospered in the marshlands like mosquitos. He then collected all expert reports, edicts and regulations adopted over time to combat epidemics and extol the pope's paternal care for his subjects. He thus urged active intervention. The scientific and the political sections of the book are clearly connected: because air was no longer considered to be an element that could be corrupted in its essence but was understood as being a vehicle for particles or for living micro-organisms which only reproduced in specific ecosystems; hence the idea that sources of contamination could be removed was reinforced. Individual regimen were not to be discarded, of course, and yet they were insufficient for protecting people's health.[57] And this was, after all, the main scope of the government and of the medical profession through its governing bodies such as the *Protomedicato*, the College of Physicians and the papal physician himself.

The political bent of Lancisi's work, therefore, introduces a further element that differentiated this new Hippocratism from older traditions of health advice, though both approaches still shared a number of assumptions. Unlike regimen literature, it cannot pass unnoticed that these 'Hippocratic' works were not intended for a lay readership and individual patients (or rather, groups of patients), but for the political elites. And unlike lesser medical practitioners, Lancisi, who held the most prestigious offices in the Roman medical establishment, acted to enhance the public role of the medical profession and to strengthen the prerogatives of its collegiate organisation through closer connections with political power. Thus, the fading importance of the older regimen genre, with its peculiar focus on the individual and the relationship between a doctor and his patients, coincided with the rise of a new environmental medicine in Rome and with renewed efforts to restore the control of the College of Physicians over all aspects of medical practice; even to expand it to new areas. Indeed, while he was writing about the healthiness of Rome, Lancisi himself carried out his duties as *protomedico* with a firm hand.[58]

Arguably, then, an emphasis on those things that could be actively managed must be seen in connection with such political developments. Whereas sleep and exercise, repletion and passions of the souls remained individual matters in the private realm, air, food and water supply could, at least to a certain extent, be the object of the medical police, that is to say, of management by medical and political authorities jointly. In other words, the collapse of Galenism, though crucial, would not appear to be the single cause for the demise of a traditional discourse on healthy living based on the individual care of the Non-Naturals. New explanations which recast the traditional understanding of the doctrine of the Non-Naturals and shifted the emphasis onto collective health should also be set against a background of reforms in the organisation of medical practice.

Conclusion: Rome in the European context

This brief excursus into the afterlife of the Non-Naturals from the standpoint of Rome would thus suggest that at the beginning of the eighteenth century, healthy living was still largely a matter of managing the six Non-Natural things correctly. New philosophical and medical theories, however, helped modernise older ideas about how the Non-Naturals preserved health or caused disease, and especially the nature and effects of air, food and water – whether considered as drinking water or as a source of effluvia. It was still a matter of devising the right regimen for each individual or group of persons with the physician's advice and of avoiding deleterious habitats or dangerous behaviours, but it was also, and increasingly, a matter of managing these things collectively and of protecting public health regardless of individual constitutions. Such an ambition was not new to eighteenth-century medicine, of course, but novel in the intensity with which it was held all over Europe. As a matter of fact, such developments were not unique to papal Rome. It is therefore useful to enlarge the picture both in space and time, especially to the rest of Italy and to Britain, given the focus of this book, in order to draw some provisional concluding remarks.

At the turn of the seventeenth and eighteenth centuries, the connections between locality, lifestyle and illness were at the core of a rising strand of environmental medicine, where references to Hippocrates, modern natural philosophy and elements of a revised doctrine of the Non-Naturals intersected. It advocated the need to conduct in-depth observations of climate and other environmental circumstances to identify seasonal and local morbidity patterns. After the 1670s, therefore, we see a common endeavour to collect systematic observations on the 'natural history' of disease, which led to the recording of weather conditions (measured with thermometers and barometers), and of outbursts of specific illnesses and their most recurrent symptoms, and the most effectual remedies reported. The information was then shared through academies such as the Royal Society and other learned and administrative networks.[59] The 'rheumatic' epidemic of 1709 studied by Lancisi notably caught the attention of all those who sought to investigate the 'morbid constitution' and unhealthy qualities of seasons and places in the wake of Sydenham, including physicians like Ramazzini, Lukas Schroek and Friedrich Hoffman.[60] These and other experts were later active in tackling the cattle plague, which marked a consistent advancement in the international coordination of quarantine.[61]

Many of these physicians occupied leading roles in the government of medicine in their towns or countries. As in Rome, various European countries, including England, were at that time undergoing some degree of reform in order to enhance the central control of medical practice. 'Hippocratic' observations on climate and disease and the collection of demographical data were generally put forward as part of these reforms.[62] In the medical writings of this epoch, air figured as the most important explanatory principle, either as vector of noxious particles or in the form of climatic conditions, and ancient aerism was therefore recast into a modern mould. According to Ramazzini, for instance, the causes of malign fevers and other common diseases should definitely be searched for in the Non-Natural things, and namely in the quality of food and water. Yet,

> because among the six Non-Natural things there is no cause which is more common than air … one must necessarily think of some kind of defect and pollution of the air that has brought such strong dispositions in the blood as to waken this malignant fever … we consider it without doubt that the air we breathe and the whole atmosphere keep within themselves various particles of different kinds, both for the superior (i.e., celestial) and the inferior (i.e., terrestrial) bodies.[63]

Italian and British authors like Wainewright, Cheyne, Burton and Arbuthnot thus made a special plea for the impact of air on the body, giving, however, what Jeremiah Wainewright termed 'a mechanical account' of the Non-Naturals which fitted into the framework of modern natural philosophy.[64]

In the course of the eighteenth century, European medical reformers also revived the genre of health advice, adapting the Non-Naturals both to modern physiological ideas and ways of living, and sometimes adding an overtone of social and political criticism. Indeed, during the Enlightenment the positive emphasis placed on Nature as opposed to the corruption of modern urban and courtly life encouraged just such a revival, which was further boosted by increasing literacy and a rapidly growing print industry. Samuel Auguste Tissot's *Avis au Peuple sur sa Santé* (1768) for example, had forty-six editions in French, twenty-nine in English, twenty-four in German and several others in Italian, Spanish, Dutch and Portuguese.[65] At the same time, air, food, water and drinks came under the supervision of an expanding medical police. Their quality was to be attained through the sanitation of sewers and stagnant waters, the regulation of industrial waste, the reform of burial practices and waste disposal, rational urban planning and building legislation, and controls on all crafts, especially those handling edible goods and drinks. All these aspects, although already subject to regulation in towns since the Black Death and even earlier, received unprecedented attention in the age of reforms. Peter Johannes Frank systematised each field of intervention in his *System einer vollständigen medicinischen Polizey*, which began to appear in 1779 and grew into several volumes while Frank was director general of public health for Austrian Lombardy.

Actually, these two strands of medical discourse on health coexisted all through the eighteenth century and beyond under the new labels of 'private' and 'public' hygiene. Further research could draw a finer picture of their interactions, and maybe bring to light a political geography of the medical discourse on health, that is the prevailing of one approach or the other in connection to specific political and social contexts.[66] However, both approaches featured the ambition to apply the same rules of healthy living to larger and larger sections, if not the totality, of a given population. Enlightenment optimism underpinned this effort to extend both health advice, which acquired an overt educational purpose, and centrally controlled medical police as far as possible. The Non-Naturals may still have been part of a medical discourse on healthy living, but this more collective stance on health eventually led to the relinquishing of the original Hippocratic concept of idiosyncrasy and the Galenic and scholastic notion of individual complexion, in which the traditional doctrine of the Non-Naturals had been embedded rather more deeply than into mere humoralism.

Notes

1 S. Cavallo and T. Storey, *Healthy Living in Early Modern Italy* (Oxford: Oxford University Press, 2013).

2 H. Mikkeli, for example, has traced the persistence of a learned medical discourse on hygiene over time. H. Mikkeli, *Hygiene in the Early Modern Medical Tradition* (Helsinki: Finnish Academy of Science and Letters, 1999).

3 J. Riley, *The Eighteenth-Century Campaign to Avoid Disease* (London: MacMillan, 1987), p. ix. On the perception of the link between places and health in early modern culture at large, see A. Wear, 'Place, health and disease: the airs, waters, places tradition in Early Modern England

and North America', *Journal of Medieval and Early Modern Studies*, 38:3 (2008), pp. 443–65.

4 B. Ciccolini, *L'oro della sanità ritrovato nel clima romano* (Rome: Vannacci, 1697); D. Passeri, *Riflessi consultivi sopra alle cure preservative da farsi in quest'anno 1703 da chi desidera conservare la sanità* (Orvieto: Tosini, 1703).

5 D. Passeri, *Aeris salubris specimen* (Todi: Pascutium & Sambuchium, 1715).

6 Passeri, *Riflessi consultivi*, pp. 5–6.

7 W.F. Bynum and V. Nutton (eds), *Theories of Fever from Antiquity to the Enlightenment* (London: Wellcome Institute for the History of Medicine, 1981); A.G. Debus, *Chemistry and Medical Debate: van Helmont to Boerhaave* (Canton, MA: Science History, 2001).

8 (Rome: S. Michele, 1720) on which see M.P. Donato, 'La peste dopo la peste. Economia di un discorso romano (1656–1720)', *Roma Moderna e Contemporanea*, 14:1 (2006), pp. 159–74.

9 P. Manfredi, *Instruzzione medica … con la quale s'insinua il modo di osservare il precetto quaresimale, anche da chi patisce qualche indispositione* (Rome: Camera Apostolica, 1703). On Lenten diet see Cavallo and Storey, *Healthy Living*, pp. 213–18.

10 B. Ramazzini, *Annotationes in librum Ludovici Cornari de vitae sobriae* (Padua: Conzatti, 1714), p. 5.

11 B. Ramazzini, *De principum valetudine tuenda* (Patavii: Conzatti, 1710), on which W.F. Kümmel, 'The morbis aulicis: on diseases found at court', in V. Nutton (ed.), *Medicine at the Courts of Europe 1500–1837* (London: Routledge, 1990), pp. 15–48.

12 The circulation of late seventeenth- or eighteenth-century editions of this tract is attested in Rome, either by possession marks or because these texts are among the holdings of Roman libraries or private collections like the Collegio Romano's (now in the Biblioteca Nazionale Centrale in Rome) or Chigi's (now in the Vatican Library).

13 Indeed, some particularly popular collections of chemical remedies, like G. Donzelli's *Teatro farmaceutico dogmatico e spagirico* (1667) or N. Lémery's *Recueil de secrets* (1692) still included non-curative secrets for the preservation of health and the care of the house.

14 D. Auda, *Breve compendio di maravgliosi segreti rationali … con un trattato … per conservarsi in sanitá* (Rome: de' Lazari, 1652).

15 Published in Paris in 1702 and translated as *Trattato degl'alimenti, e della maniera di conseruarsi lungamente in sanitá; … secondo i principij chimici, e mecchanici* (Venice: Albrizi, 1704); both the French and Italian version had several editions.

16 On this point, see Cavallo and Storey, *Healthy Living*, pp. 31–7.

17 For instance, new editions of C. Durante, *Herbario nuovo ... hora in questa novissima impressione vi si è posto in fine l'herbe thè, caffè ... e cioccolata* (Venice: Hertz, 1684 and further 1717 and 1718).

18 [D. Magri], *Virtù del Kafe bevanda introdotta nuovamente nell'Italia con alcune osservazioni per conservar la sanità nella vecchiaia* (Rome: Hercoli, 1671); [F. Nairone], *Discorso della salutifera beuanda cahue, ò vero Café* (Rome: Hercoli, 1671), also published in Latin in the same year; *Dichiaratione delle virtù della bevanda del caffé* (Rome: Bernabò, 1683).

19 G. Baglivi, *De praxi medica,* now in *Opere complete medico-pratiche ed anatomiche* (Florence: Coen, 1842), pp. 124–5; L. Tozzi's writings on this topic are included in the 1716 and later editions of Magri's *Virtù del caffé*; see above note 18.

20 For instance, Ms London, Wellcome Library, 4612–13, *Institutiones medicae* by Alessandro Pascoli and Giacomo Sinibaldi, unpaginated. On the place of hygiene in medical studies, see Mikkeli, *Hygiene,* especially pp. 98–118, according to whom, however, this was shrinking at the beginning of the eighteenth century.

21 For instance, by the famous German professor F. Hoffmann, *Dissertationes physico-medicae curiosae selectiores, ad sanitatem tuendam* (Leyden: Haak, 1708).

22 L. Tozzi, *In librum artis medicinalis Galeni paraphrastikē anakephalaiōsis. ... Huic adjectum est practicum opusculum de recto usu sex rerum nonnaturalium* (Naples: Porpora, 1710); F.A. Georio, *Flores medicinae theoricae ac fructus medicinae practicae necessarii ad diu vitam prolungandam* (Rome: S. Michaelis ad Ripam, 1726).

23 On these debates, see M.P. Donato, *Sudden Death. Medicine and Religion in Eighteenth-Century Rome* (Farnham: Ashgate, 2014), where the topic of this section is discussed in greater detail.

24 See P. Grassi, *Mortis repentinae examen ... cum brevi methodo praesagendi et praecavendi* (Modena: I. Cassianum, 1612). Grassi lists three types of rash extinction of the vital heat: *per subitam suffucationem, aut per repentinam dissolutionem, aut per improvvisam corruptionem.* It is caused by humoral plethora and unbalance of different kinds, all largely depending on the misuse of the Non-Naturals; hence, he devotes a chapter to each of them expatiating on the better conduct for each sort of people according to their age, sex and completion. On the 'pastoral' role of physicians, see H.J. Cook, 'Good advice and little medicine: the professional authority of Early Modern English physicians', *Journal of British Studies,* 33:1 (1994), pp. 1–31.

25 F. Valesio, *Diario romano,* ed. G. Scano (Milan: Longanesi, 1977), vol. 3, p. 388.

26 Ms Biblioteca Nazionae, Rome, Vittorio Emanuele 790, fol. 133.
27 G.A. Borelli, *Delle cagioni delle febbri maligne della Sicilia negli anni 1647 e 1648* (Cosenza: Rosso, 1649) and *Historia et meteorologia incendii Aetnaei anni 1699* (Reggio di Calabria: Ferri, 1670); G. Baglivi, *De terremoto romano*, in his *Opere complete medico-pratiche*, pp. 596–677. For an overview on earthquakes and meteorology see V. Jankovich, *Reading the Skies. A Cultural History of English Weather, 1650–1820* (Chicago: University of Chicago Press, 2000), and Conforti in this volume. For earlier aerist theories connected to epidemics see J. Henderson, 'The Black Death in Florence: medical and communal reactions', in S. Bassett (ed.), *Death in Towns. Urban Responses to the Dying and the Death 1000–1600* (Leicester: Leicester University Press, 1992), pp. 136–50; S.K. Cohn, *Cultures of Plague: Medical Thinking at the End of the Renaissance* (Oxford: Oxford University Press, 2010).
28 M. da Sylva, *Romanorum lachrymae subitaneis mortibus effusae exsiccantur* (Rome: Herculis, 1706), pp. 9–10.
29 A. Evangelista, *Lettera informativa intorno alle cause delle morti improvise* (Rome: Stamperia Camerale, 1706).
30 A. Bernabei, *Dissertazione delle morti improvvise nella quale si ragiona delle perucche e degli acidi* (Rome: Gonzaga, 1708), p. 10.
31 D. Mistichelli, *Trattato dell'apoplessia* (Rome: de Rossi, 1709). The idea that excessive study is bad for health is an old *topos* drawn from Ficino's *De vita triplici*.
32 G.M. Lancisi, *De subitaneis mortibus libri duo* (Rome: Buagni, 1707).
33 *Ibid.*, pp. 118–20.
34 Da Sylva, *Romanorum lachrymae*, p. 25.
35 Bernabei, *Dissertazione*, pp. 42, 45.
36 Mistichelli, *Trattato dell'apoplessia*, pp. 159, 162–3.
37 Bernabei, *Dissertazione*, p. 45.
38 Lancisi, *De subitaneis mortibus*, p. 79.
39 P. Dionis, *Dissertation sur la mort subite et sur la catalepsie* (Paris: d'Houry, 1710); Ramazzini, *De principum valetudine*, p. 69.
40 R. Jütte, 'The social construction of illness in the Early Modern period', in J. Lachmund and G. Stollberg (eds), *The Social Construction of Illness* (Stuttgart: Steiner, 1992) pp. 23–38; M. Stolberg, *Experiencing Illness and the Sick Body in Early Modern Europe* (London: Palgrave Macmillan, 2011).
41 M. Nicoud, *Les régimes de santé au Moyen Âge: naissance et diffusion d'une écriture médicale (XIIIe–XVe siècle)* (Rome: Ecole Française de Rome, 2007), pp. 285–395; K. Albala, *Eating Right in the Renaissance* (Berkeley: University of California Press, 2002).

42 S. Shapin, S. Schaffer, *Leviathan and the Air-Pump: Hobbes, Boyle, and the Experimental Life* (Princeton: Princeton University Press, 1985).
43 C. Durante, *Il tesoro della sanità* (Padova: Cezza, 1659, first ed. 1586).
44 M. Hunter (ed.), *Robert Boyle Reconsidered* (Cambridge: Cambridge University Press, 1994); A. Clericuzio, *Elements, Principles and Corpuscles: A Study of Atomism and Chemistry in the Seventeenth Century* (Dordrecht: Kluwer, 2000); D. Bertoloni Meli (ed.), *Marcello Malpighi. Anatomist and Physician* (Firenze: Olschki, 1997).
45 Mistichelli, *Trattato dell'apoplessia*, pp. 87–8.
46 S. Santorio, *De medicina statica libri octo Accedunt Georgii Baglivi* (Romae: haered. L'Hulliè, 1704). Since it could be reinterpreted in mechanical terms, Santorio's work (1614) was reprinted several times and translated into English (1676), French (1722), German (1736) and Italian (1746).
47 Hallerian physiology and, later, Brownianism would recast the issue of tonus and exercise later in the eighteenth century: H. Ishizuka, '"Fibre body": the concept of fibre in eighteenth-century medicine, c.1700–40', *Medical History*, 56:4 (2012), pp. 562–84.
48 Bernabei, *Dissertazione*, pp. 27–8.
49 Mistichelli, *Trattato dell'apoplessia*, pp. 99–100.
50 N.G. Siraisi, *History, Medicine, and the Traditions of Renaissance Learning* (Ann Arbor: University of Michigan, 2007).
51 On eighteenth-century Hippocratism and the polemical use of Hippocrates' authority, see D. Cantor (ed.), *Reinventing Hippocrates* (Aldershot: Ashgate, 2001).
52 G.M. Lancisi, *Dissertatio de nativis, deque adventitiis Romani coeli qualitatibus, cui accedit historia epidemiae rheumaticae, quae per hyemem anni 1709 vagata est* (Rome: Gonzaga, 1711), p. 13.
53 Archivio di Stato di Roma, Università di Roma, b. 58, fasc. 51; C. Meyer, *Nuovi ritrovamenti dati in luce ... per eccitare l'ingegno de' virtuosi* (Rome: Komarek, 1689); F. Bianchini, *Opuscula* (Rome: Barbiellini, 1753), vol. 1, pp. 35–50; P.A. Giulianelli, *Essame delle acque di Civita Vecchia, e di Trevi* (Rome: Monadi, 1701). Lancisi's work was referred to by F. Pinelli, *Lettera de' Bagni di Petriuolo* (Rome: De Rossi, 1716), which was part of a dispute on the use of water, especially of cold water, for the preservation of health and the cure of fevers that raged in Italy in the early 18th century, sparked by the reprint of N. Mainardes, *Del bever in ghiaccio* (Venice: Pittoni, 1689).
54 R. Porter (ed.), *The Medical History of Water and Spas* (London: Wellcome Institute for the History of Medicine, 1990).

55 S. Jarcho, 'The "Epidemia Rheumatica" described by Lancisi (1711)', in C.E. Rosenberg (ed.), *Healing and History. Essays for George Rosen* (New York: Science History, 1979), pp. 51–8.
56 G.M. Lancisi, *Dissertatio historica de bovilla peste* (Rome: Salvioni, 1715), reminiscent of Cardinal G. Gastaldi's famous tract on the 1656 plague, *Tractatus de avertenda et profliganda peste politico-legalis* of 1683; Lancisi, *De noxiis paludum effluviis, eorumque remediis* (Rome: Salvioni, 1717).
57 In his book, Lancisi actually devised a regimen for those who ought to travel through the marshlands; see M. Conforti, S. Marinozzi and V. Gazzaniga, 'Delle arie, acque e luoghi: igiene e sanità pubblica a Roma nell'opera di Giovanni Maria Lancisi', *Roma moderna e contemporanea*, 13:1 (2005), pp. 115–32.
58 Archivio di Stato di Roma, Università di Roma, b. 62.
59 A.A. Rusnock, *Vital Accounts: Quantifying Health and Population in Eighteenth-century England and France* (Cambridge: Cambridge University Press, 2002). See also R. Favier, 'Penser le changement climatique au siècle des Lumières', in D. Lamarre (ed.), *Climat et risques: changements d'approches* (Paris: Tec & doc, 2008), pp. 9–24.
60 Their contributions were later included in the 1716 Geneva edition of T. Sydenham, *Opera medica*, and later editions; see also G. Olagüe de Ros, 'La epidemia europea de gripe de 1708–1709', *Dynamis*, 1:1 (1981), pp. 51–86.
61 C.A. Spinage, *Cattle Plague. A History* (New York: Kluwer, 2003); K. Appuhn, 'Ecologies of beef: eighteenth-century epizootics and the environmental history of Early Modern Europe', *Environmental History*, 15:2 (2010), pp. 268–87.
62 G. Rosen, *From Medical Police to Social Medicine: Essays on the History of Health Care* (New York: Science History, 1974); C. Barthel, *Medizinische Polizey und medizinische Aufklärung: Aspekte des öffentlichen Gesundheitsdiskurses im 18. Jahrhundert* (Frankfurt: Campus, 1989). With reference to England, P.E. Carroll, 'Medical police and the history of public health', *Medical History*, 46:4 (2002), pp. 461–94.
63 B. Ramazzini, *Constitutionum epidemicarum mutinensium annorum quinque* (Padua: Conzatti, 1714), p. 170.
64 I refer to J. Wainewright, *A mechanical account of the non-naturals* (London: R. Smith and J. Wale, 1707). G. Millers, '"Airs, waters and places" in History', *Journal of the History of Medicine*, 17:2 (1962), pp. 129–40. On Cheney's later *Essay of Health and Long life* (1724) and its religious inspiration, see A. Guerrini, 'Newtonianism, medicine and religion', in O.P. Grell and A. Cunnngham (eds), *Religio Medici. Medicine*

and Religion in Seventeenth-Century England (Aldershot: Ashgate, 1996), pp. 293–312.

65 A. Emch-Dériaz, 'The non-naturals made easy', in R. Porter (ed.), *The Popularization of Medicine, 1650–1850* (London: Routledge, 1992), pp. 134–59.

66 Some historians consider interest on weather and climate typical of British medical culture, whereas medical topography mostly flourished on the Continent; see Riley, *The Eighteenth-Century Campaign*, pp. 31–47; I. Golinski, *British Weather and the Climate of Enlightenment* (Chicago: University of Chicago Press, 2007).

IV

Spiritual health and bodily health

7

Sleep-piety and healthy sleep in early modern English households

Sasha Handley

> Despise not the Rules for promoting Health and Temperance, the ways of God and Nature are plain and simple, but mighty in operation and effects, the Body is an Instrument to the Soul, and being out of tune no harmony can be expected in the microcosm.[1]

The merchant, campaigner for vegetarianism and author of popular lifestyle guides Thomas Tryon was convinced that a strict regimen of bodily discipline held the key to the long-term preservation of physical and spiritual health.[2] He shared this conviction with many of his peers even though his own commitment to pursuing an ascetic daily routine was more pronounced than most. Tryon's reformed Protestantism had developed through close contact with Baptists, Quakers and mystics and it went hand in hand with his prophylactic health regimen but he nevertheless recommended it for the perusal of others. His pocket-sized and modestly priced *Wisdom's Dictates: or, Aphorisms and Rules Physical, Moral, and Divine, For Preserving the Health of the Body, and the Peace of the Mind* (1696) was designed for everyday use and its extensive set of practical recommendations for maintaining a healthy body and a healthy household epitomised the kind of practical spirituality that suffused devotional culture in late seventeenth- and early eighteenth-century England. A healthy night's sleep played a central role in Tryon's regimen. Restful sleep offered inimitable refreshment for bodies, minds and souls and it also fitted people to pursue their work, domestic affairs and Christian duties with purpose and vigour. It was revered above all else for its unique capacity to safeguard the vitality and virtue of body and soul. Sound sleep was idealised as a gift of God and Nature but this chapter shows that it was also actively pursued within early modern households on a daily basis.

The hours of sleep offered an unparalleled natural restorative but they also represented an oscillatory and perilous threshold between this world and the next. Faithful Christians who consulted scripture and the Book of Common Prayer on a regular basis were only too aware of the earthly and spiritual dangers that might befall them in the night. Perceived perils ranged from household fires, the assaults of bed bugs and accidental suffocation of babies due to overlaying, to the temptations of diabolical spiritual forces in dreams or premature and unprepared death during sleep. God's careful watchfulness offered a protective shield against all of these dangers, and it was to God that men and women gave thanks when they were delivered from near destruction.[3] Sermons, and a proliferating genre of published guides to holy living offered further incentives to prepare body and soul for sleep's onset and practical guidance on how to do it from the late seventeenth century onwards. This advice cut across formal confessional divisions amongst Protestants who shared a common understanding of the relationship between sleep, death and the Christian resurrection. Evidence from personal testimonies reveals how men, women and children struggled to overcome their daily tribulations and enter the transitional state of sleep with a clean bed and a clean conscience.[4] A sleep regimen that incorporated pious bedtime rituals thus satisfied physical and spiritual purposes. The daily practice of sleep-piety, defined here as any bedside or sleep-related practice motivated in part by Christian belief, was also believed to instil prized habits of temperance and virtue that complemented principles of Christian morality. Thomas Tryon indeed spoke for many when he declared that the moderation of sleep's daily practice was 'the True way, or Royal Road to Peace and Happiness, both in this World and the World to come; for without, no Man can observe the Law of God and Nature'.[5]

This chapter shows how the fusion of preventative healthcare practices and devotional habits fostered a vibrant culture of sleep management in English households between 1650 and 1750. It traces the cultural value of sound sleep and how its pursuit ordered the daily rhythms of household life by examining a selection of diaries and spiritual autobiographies, and their interactions with sermons, popular guides to holy living, household advice books and manuscript recipe books. In so doing it reveals the combined physical and spiritual motivations that framed sleep regimens, which included regular performances of bedtime prayer, the assiduous cleansing and material management of sleeping environments and the fastidious preparation of homemade medicaments to prevent and to treat periods of sleep loss. The preventative healthcare principles of Non-Natural medicine underpinned all of these practices.

The chapter also shows how and why the combined physical and spiritual benefits of sleeping soundly became increasingly pronounced in the years after 1650. Non-Natural healthcare principles and practices were enlivened by the fragmented religious terrain of this period, which intensified household devotional practices. The central dictates of Non-Natural advice were also supported by subtle shifts in physiological understandings of sleeping and waking that emerged after 1660, which emphasised sleep's centrality to the healthy functioning of the brain and nerves and in so doing augmented the value of sound sleep.[6] Physician and Sedleian Professor of Natural Philosophy at Oxford Thomas Willis revealed the origin of the nerves that controlled sleeping and waking in the brain in his influential *Cerebri Anatome* (1664); Scottish physician William Cullen classified sleep and its disorders as neurological conditions in the mid-eighteenth century; whilst Cullen's fellow physician George Cheyne publicised the physical and mental debilities posed by nervous disorders in his bestselling medical regimens *An Essay of Health and Long Life* (1724) and *Essay on Regimen* (1740), which blended Newtonian physiological principles with Non-Natural healthcare advice.[7] These physicians shared the conviction that careful management of sleep routines held the key to physical and mental health, which was echoed in many subsequent guides to health management published in eighteenth-century Britain.[8]

Historians have noted the existence of a pervasive interest in the neurological origins of sleep from the late seventeenth century, yet little attention has been paid to the ways in which Non-Natural advice relating to sleep was able to absorb and adapt to this new emphasis and retain a strong place in a lively mixed economy of homemade and commercialised cultures of healthcare.[9] This chapter thus complements and builds on the foundations of recent work that emphasises the relevance and vitality of Non-Natural healthcare principles to daily life across early modern Europe.[10] The chapter begins by tracing the role of sleep management as an embodied expression of faith before moving on to assess how spiritual motivations shaped the make-up and care of sleeping environments within many homes. The final section analyses the precautions taken by householders to prevent and treat intermittent periods of sleep loss in a sample of fifty English manuscript recipe books that span the years 1650 to 1750.

Seasonable sleep and spirituality

Early modern religious culture motivated pious Christians of many shades to carefully manage their bedtimes, their hours of sleep and the cleanliness and security of their sleeping environments. People invested varying degrees of effort into these habits according to opportunity, personality and individual circumstance, but most understood the implicit connection between well-regulated sleep and a well-cleansed body and soul. The close relationship between healthy sleeping habits and godliness was underlined by Richard Allestree, Church of England clergyman, Regius Professor of Divinity at Oxford and author of the bestselling *The Whole Duty of Man*, first published in 1657. Allestree declared that peaceful sleep was ordained by God 'as a medicine to that weariness, as a repairer of that decay, so that we may be enabled to such labours as the duties of Religion or works of our Calling require of us'.[11] In Christian culture the very need for sleep was closely linked to human frailty. Psalm 121 of the King James Bible affirmed that 'he who keeps Israel will neither slumber nor sleep'. Yet humans, by contrast, required the daily refreshment of sleep to fortify their weak bodies and souls. Sound sleep was understood to be a gift from God, but good Christians were responsible for its temperate practice, which was essential for the daily performance of worldly and spiritual duties. Familiar biblical passages thus cautioned against excessive indulgence in sleep, which was routinely linked to sloth, poverty and spiritual apathy.[12] The bedtime prayers and meditations that preceded sleep in daily life clearly drew on these commonplace understandings of sleep as a fragile, yet necessary process of physical and spiritual nourishment.

Nightly devotions offered Christians the chance to confess their sins and to forge a personal relationship with God as they begged for protection and refreshment. The perceived dangers to be met in this unconscious state of repose ranged widely. Periods of disturbed sleep were frequently interpreted as punishment for daily transgressions, whilst scripture confirmed that sleepers were in danger of succumbing to diabolical temptations, or even death. In the Book of Samuel, Ish-bosheth, King of Israel, was beheaded as he lay asleep in his bed, whilst in the Book of Judges, Sisera, commander of the Canaanite army, met a similar fate when his enemy Jael drove a tent peg through his head as he slept beneath a blanket.[13] The close parallels drawn between sleep and death in scripture found expression in textual, architectural and artistic representations, and in everyday vocabularies and practices surrounding sleep.

Some may not have feared their souls to be in imminent danger of damnation if these schedules of sleep-piety occasionally slipped but they still took care to note down their lapses and make resolutions to reform. Sleeping temperately – at the right times, in the right places, and in an appropriate frame of mind – was moreover intimately linked to the management of health. Richard Allestree affirmed that sound sleep was essential to maintain the faculties of body and mind in good health and thereby procure 'happiness' in his *Art of Contentment* (1675).[14] Temperate sleep was likewise valued as a measure of personal morality that was widely adopted as a means of self-fashioning and as a barometer of other people's characters. Sleeping behaviour was thus readily absorbed within contemporary models of educational development and Christian ethics. Temperate sleeping habits were conceived as a means of avoiding vice and as the eighteenth century wore on they were increasingly esteemed for maintaining the intellectual and nervous faculties in good order, thus rendering good citizens 'brisk and alart at their Learning'.[15] Approaching sleep with the right attitude and with the appropriate material apparatus was thus a critical facet of early modern constructions of piety, virtue and good health.

Sleep-piety has a long history both within and beyond early modern England. Christopher Hill illustrated the special significance of household devotional culture amongst nonconformist Protestants in late sixteenth- and early seventeenth-century England although he drew no connection with their sleeping habits. More recent work by Alec Ryrie and Erin Sullivan has redressed this absence and illustrated the myriad ways in which Protestant religious cultures shaped understandings of sleep and dreams across the British Isles before 1640.[16] Phyllis Mack has elucidated the relationship between ascetic sleep regimens, dreams and eighteenth-century evangelical culture yet much remains to be said about the increased significance of sleep-piety in the years after 1650 and about the specific ways in which these beliefs shaped everyday practices within the home.[17]

The pursuit of practical household piety was a well-established tradition within the culture of godliness that shaped Protestant devotional habits. The value of temperate sleep was nevertheless forcefully evidenced from the late seventeenth century as the household assumed unprecedented significance as the hub of devotional life for a wide cross-section of Protestants. Sleep-piety and other forms of practical piety were characteristic features of the religious culture of English society after 1660. This culture was formally ruptured by the provisions of the 1662 Act of Uniformity, which required conformity to the Church of England and to the 1662 Book of Common Prayer. The Act led to the ejection of more than 2,000 clergymen from the Church of England who refused to conform and who were thereafter labelled as 'nonconformists'. These men were forbidden to hold civil or military office and their public worship was further curtailed by the Conventicle Act of 1664, which forbade unauthorised gatherings of more than five people who did not belong to the same household. The value of household devotions thus grew in direct response to the proscription of public worship for many of these people, especially before the 1689 Act of Toleration allowed limited freedom of worship to some nonconformists if they agreed to swear particular oaths of allegiance. Ejected ministers responded to these developments by publishing practical guides to holy living for their followers. The guides offered spiritual succour and practical advice, and set forms of prayer that could be used within the home on a daily basis; sleep-piety was a central feature within these texts. Fresh impetus for adopting forms of household piety was not just confined to nonconformists, however, and recent work has shown that the boundaries between conformists and nonconformists were highly porous.[18] Sleep-piety was strongly promoted by Church of England ministers who engaged in pastoral reform initiatives, including the publication of guides to holy living, to improve the devotional habits of their parishioners and to cement their loyalty to the Church of England. The guides were intended to enrich Anglican devotional culture by forming a bridge, or a 'fellowship of prayer', between private, family and public forms of worship.[19] Taken together, these shifts positioned the household as the principal site of devotion for a wide variety of Protestants, and indeed for English Catholics for whom public worship remained strictly prohibited.[20] The material enhancement of English homes in these years moreover offered practical support for this development.[21]

Pious prescription and daily practices of sleep were closely related in the homes of committed Anglicans like Yorkshire woman Alice Thornton. Alice learned the virtue of early morning prayers from her parents at an early age and she regularly engaged in bedtime reading and prayer after she married William Thornton on 15 December 1651. Alice described how she took charge of her own, and of her husband's, schedule of sleep-piety; she made her husband read parts of 'some good booke' as he lay in bed until he was overcome with sleep as she constructed a posthumous and pious reputation for him in her autobiography. Alice connected her husband's well-disciplined sleep routine, which allowed him to rise at five or six o'clock each morning, with his spiritual fortitude and thereby underlined the reciprocal relationship that she conceived between a healthy body and a healthy soul.[22] William Coe was a successful farmer from Suffolk, and like Alice Thornton he was firmly committed to his local parish church, serving as churchwarden in West Row in the parish of Mildenhall in 1693. Coe's Anglican faith led to him to become a strong opponent of Quakerism in his local area and it also motivated him to pursue a disciplined and consistent schedule of piety. Coe kept a regular diary from 1 April 1694 and he used it as a physical and spiritual account book to record those intermittent occasions when he had overindulged in worldly business, stayed up late drinking and playing cards in company, or when he and his family members had received particular providences that indicated divine favour on the household. Coe regularly resolved to amend his wayward behaviour and he was particularly concerned about those activities that caused him to omit family prayers or his 'owne private devotions', which he believed were detrimental to his relationship with God. Coe's faith also meant that he held the Lord's Supper in great reverence and he hoped that receiving the sacrament would fortify him to fulfil his 'solemn resolution' to keep regular bedtimes and never to play out of his own home after nine o'clock at night.[23]

The physical and spiritual benefits to be gained from a temperate regimen of sleep were similarly articulated in the diary of village shopkeeper Thomas Turner from East Hoathly in Sussex. Turner was a young married man, a committed Anglican and a parish officer who made thirteen resolutions regarding his daily diet and regimen of sleep after hearing a Sunday morning sermon on 8 February 1756. Turner's first and final resolution illustrated his conviction that his sleeping habits were an integral safeguard of his bodily and spiritual health:

> As I by experience find how much more conducive it is to my health, as well as pleasantness and serenity to my mind, to live in a low, moderate rate of diet, and as I know I shall never be able to comply therewith in so strict a manner as I should choose (by the unstable and over easiness of my temper), I think it therefore [right] (as it's a matter of so great importance to my health etc.) to draw up rules of proper regimen, which I do in manner and form following, and which, at all times when I am in health, I hope I shall always have the strictest regard to follow, as I think they are not inconsistent with either religion or morality: First, it be either in the summer or winter, to rise as early as I possibly can; that is, always to allow myself between 7 and 8 hours' sleep, or full 8, unless prevented on any particular or emergent occasion ... And lastly [13th] always to go to bed at or before ten o'clock when it can be done.

The timing of Turner's promise, immediately following public worship, showed that his faith was a critical motivation for maintaining a disciplined schedule of sleep at home, even if he was unable to maintain it at all times.

Bedtime reading formed an integral part of sleep-piety, being intended to conjure serious thoughts of life after death and thus bridge the gap between the natural and spiritual realms. So it did for tailor's daughter Sarah Hurst from Horsham in West Sussex, who worked alongside her father. Sarah kept a diary of her emotional highs and lows from the age of 22 when she was preoccupied by her romantic entanglements with the sailor Henry Smith. It was in her diary that Sarah tried to calm her passions as sleep approached by using her bedtime reading to reflect 'on the Instability of all earthly things' as she read at night to her mother from Pliny's letters and from William Romaine's sermon *A discourse on the benefit which the Holy Spirit of God is of to man in his journey through life,* first published in 1755. Romaine, a Church of England clergyman, was renowned for his personal piety.

The effects of bedtime reading were just as significant as its content. Bedtime reading, like bedtime prayer, had a discernible soporific effect by procuring a calm state of mind and body that was conducive to restful sleep. Manchester barber and wigmaker Edmund Harrold, borrowed and eagerly devoured Church of England clergyman Richard Sherlock's work on death and future judgment in 1712.[24] Sherlock, like Romaine, was known for his fastidious practical piety, which he recommended to Anglican parishioners through his published works. Edmund kept his diary from 1712, when he was aged 34, until 1715 and he used it to record his daily concerns and failings, and as a spur to improve his piety as a dedicated Anglican. Spiritual reading at bedtime was a method of devotion for Edmund but it also consoled him and composed his passions in preparation for sleep. He noted the special comforting powers of bedtime reading on those occasions when he had quarrelled with his wife. On 4 November 1712 Edmund was ejected from the marital bed on account of his drunkenness; he turned for comfort to the sermons of Church of England clergyman and philosopher John Norris, from which he took 'a great deal of comforts to my soul' before falling asleep on the couch chair for three hours.[25] The inseparability of physical and spiritual health was further underlined on those occasions when sleep would not come. It was to divine forces that Sarah Hurst turned for help when she was unable to sleep due to the tumults of her passions. In her diary she beseeched 'Oh Power Supream how awfull, how wonderfull are all they works, look down with pity on me thy poor weak sinfull infirm creature, & restore me to health.'[26]

Antiquary and topographer Ralph Thoresby was born to moderate nonconformist parents who combined attendance at dissenting meetings with a weekly presence at Anglican services in Leeds. Ralph followed a strict regimen of daily worship in secret, with his family and in public, both before and after he fully conformed to the Church of England in 1697. Sleep-piety formed a critical part of Ralph's daily habits when he was at home and when he was removed from it. Indeed, Ralph's commitment to sleep-piety was no more evident than on his tour of the British Isles where he fought hard to find the time and space to perform his secret devotions whilst sharing a room, and sometimes a bed, with his travel companions. When Ralph was at home he was particularly fond of the practical guides to holy living composed by Presbyterian minister Richard Baxter. Ralph read them in bed when he couldn't sleep and as a preparative to prayer. He also turned on occasion to the work of devotional writer Elizabeth Burnet, wife of the Bishop of Salisbury Gilbert Burnet, after a friend gifted him a copy of Burnet's *Method of Devotion*, first published in 1708 and republished in 1709, 1713 and 1738. Burnet recommended temperate sleeping hours and the daily recital of bedside prayers as a preserver of good health and as an expression of faith.[27] Ralph may well have applied her advice to his daily habits and he seems to have been particularly influenced by Richard Baxter's recommendations for attaining 'seasonable sleep' that featured in his *Christian Directory* of 1673 since he conceived of the careful regulation of his sleeping hours and environments as a central part of his Christian duties.[28] Baxter's advice closely approximated the kind of moderate bed rest advocated in Non-Natural health regimens, which recommended six to eight hours of sleep each night and took careful account of variations in age, constitution and illness.[29] Ralph also carefully transcribed a sermon by dissenting minister Dr Sharp in September 1680, since he wished to recall and avoid the 'too common practice' of men who 'can outstare the sun'.[30] Ralph's efforts to safeguard his time to fulfil his Christian duties led him in November 1680 to place an alarm clock at his bedside so that he could 'arise every morning by five, and first to dedicate the morning (as in duty obliged) to the service of God, by reading and prayer'. Ralph had achieved his ambition by December of that year but he was nonetheless sensible that too little sleep was equally damaging to his attempts at spiritual purification and he allowed himself a later hour of rising when he rested badly.[31] Striking the right balance between piety and good health was thus of paramount importance.

In similar fashion to Ralph Thoresby, the dissenting clergyman Henry Newcome kept a near-daily record of his bedtimes in the single surviving volume of his diary from 1661 to 1663. Newcome was ordained a Presbyterian minister in Sandbach, Cheshire in 1648 before moving to a post in Manchester in 1657. He was, however, ejected from his post after refusing to conform to the Church of England. Henry's commitment to a more thoroughgoing reform of the national church set him at odds with many Church of England clergymen, yet he shared with them an understanding of the importance of sound and well-regulated sleep. He wrote of taking physical and spiritual 'refreshment' from sleep, which he considered a divine mercy and begged that the Lord 'continue ye mercy of health' to himself and his family by safeguarding his rest. By contrast, he lamented those occasions when an 'unquiet night of dreams' meant he was 'not so much refreshed by rest'. By and large, Henry rose before eight o'clock each morning. He was well aware of the physical and spiritual inconvenience of too little sleep and indeed of excessive sleep. When he arose 'by a mistake' at five o'clock one winter's morning he noted that this was 'too soone' and his overtiredness made him cold and careless in his devotions. In the following month, Henry resolved to forego sociable company one Saturday evening and get an early night, observing that 'much better I hope it is for mee'. It is uncertain what he meant by the term 'better', but a later entry in his diary suggests that his concern to fortify his constitution through regular, healthy sleep was inextricably intertwined with the Christian-moral discourse that surrounded seasonable bedtimes. It was in this context that he interpreted 'uncomfortable' or 'indifferent' nights of sleep as a sign of his distance from God, which triggered resolutions to reinvigorate his devotions by keeping better hours. The physical and spiritual dimensions of Henry's sleep were thus inseparable, which was underlined by his feeling 'much out of order' when he had overslept.[32] Henry understood seasonable bedtimes as an act of Christian humility before God and something that he hoped might transform his body and soul into worthy recipients of God's grace. Alice, William, Thomas, Sarah, Edmund, Ralph and Henry each perceived seasonable bedtimes, regular sleeping hours, and the regular practice of bedtime devotions as a means of preserving the health of body and mind that was simultaneously essential for the fulfilment of their spiritual duties. They varied in their commitment and ability to perform these pious duties but they nevertheless strove hard to integrate them within their busy schedules of work and sociability.

Sleeping environments

Sleeping in a hygienic and secure environment was just as important as regular bedtime devotions within prophylactic regimens of sleep-piety. Principles of Non-Natural healthcare played a formative role in shaping the make-up and management of household sleeping environments and they offered a reassuring sense of safety and sensory satisfaction that helped ease minds and bodies into sleep.[33] Most important of all was maintaining the cleanliness of the bedstead, bedding textiles and bedclothes that lay closest to the skin and guarded sleepers during the night. The shifting cultural value of sleep as a safeguard of the brain and nerves sparked unprecedented efforts to optimise its material environments and minimise potential disruption in these years.[34] This development was typified by widespread preferences for bedding textiles that looked and felt healthy. White linen bed sheets that felt cool to the touch and were able to withstand vigorous and regular cleaning were highly prized by householders throughout the eighteenth century despite the growing availability and affordability of cotton bedding textiles.[35]

People carefully managed the materials used in sleeping chambers to minimise the potential dangers that could be met in them particularly since accidental fires were not uncommon due to the reliance on fires and candles for warmth and light at night. Candles were easily knocked over by sleepy hands and deliverance from these near calamities was regularly interpreted in a providential light, which underscores the widespread understanding of sleeping chambers as sanctified spaces that were penetrated by benevolent and harmful spiritual forces at particular times of the day and night.[36]

The methods employed to maintain a healthy sleeping environment varied in degree, kind and cost. Thomas Tryon echoed earlier health regimens by praising the benefits of building homes in appropriate places and locating sleeping chambers in the most apposite and airy parts of the house. English physician Andrew Boorde's health regimen *A Compendyous Regyment, or Dyetary of Helth* (1547) recommended situating houses in pure and fresh air, away from standing water, and with the house oriented in an east–west direction to avoid the south wind that 'doth make euyl vapours'. These measures were all intended to fortify the constitution and thereby lengthen life.[37] At the time that Thomas Tryon wrote, the principal bedsteads in many English households were gradually being relocated, being removed from multifunctional ground-floor parlour chambers and placed above stairs.[38] Considerations of status and household circumstance principally guided this relocation yet the architect Isaac Ware judged that the further away that sleepers lay from cold and damp ground floor chambers, the better for their health.[39] The specific location of the bedstead within the chamber was just as important as the chamber's location in the wider household.

Tryon noted that bedsteads 'for the most part stand in Corners of Chambers', which limited the free circulation of air and exposed the sleeper to disease from the cold and damp walls. He recommended instead that they should be set 'as near as you can in the most Airie Places of your Rooms, exposing them to the Air the most part of the day'.[40] The bed itself should be made of simple straw or chaff with canvas ticks and woollen or flock quilts. These simple and cost-effective materials were preferable to luxurious feather beds because they were easier and cheaper to clean and replace. They had the added benefit of preventing the body from overheating and thereby retained the tension of the nerves and muscles. In so doing, Tryon judged that they offered a 'certain Means and Way … to preserve Health and Strength' that was widely approved by churchmen and medical practitioners alike.[41]

Aside from fires and cold, damp fumes, sleepers were regularly disturbed by the incursions of bed bugs. Medical writers and householders complained constantly about infestations of bed bugs, flies and fleas, especially during the summer months. Diaries and correspondence teem with references to the pains that these creatures caused, particularly in travel narratives, where they were a constant cause of broken sleep and general discomfort.[42] This problem could be traced to the fabric of many houses, whose walls were plastered with a mixture of hogs hair and lime that attracted bugs. Wooden bedsteads also predominated and exacerbated the problem. Bedsteads were the most expensive items of household furniture and often dated back many generations, being routinely gifted between family members as cherished heirlooms or given as practical and symbolic gifts when setting up home. There also existed a vibrant second-hand trade in bedsteads and bedding textiles that extended the lifecycle of these objects still further. Bedsteads represented the symbolic heart of early modern households and indeed of marriage, but their physical make-up also presented health hazards.[43]

Commentaries on the unclean nature of lodgings highlight the ordinary expectations that people had of the standards of cleanliness of sleeping environments. Although the eighteenth century saw the emergence of professionalised extermination services for bugs, household recipe books in both manuscript and print featured a wide range of recipes to rid sleeping chambers of bugs that could be prepared at home.[44] A family 'Booke of divers receipts' that spanned several generations from

1660 to 1750 included a comprehensive set of instructions for washing and cleaning wooden bedsteads with soap, aqua fortis and a homemade paste made of quicksilver, black soap and tobacco dust that was to be left in the holes and joints of the bedstead where bugs were believed to congregate. A second recipe for exterminating bugs was added that was recommended by a local physician who had 'told it to scores of families' who all affirmed its efficacy. The book combined these guidelines with advice on how best to cleanse the bed curtains and valences that encased sleepers in middling- and upper-sort households.[45] Recipe books of this kind were routinely given and bequeathed across generations of families and they provided continuity of care for loved ones that accompanied the giving of treasured bedsteads, sheets and other family bedding textiles. Alice Thornton no doubt wished to preserve the good health of her family for future generations when she bequeathed to her 'dear daughter Comber all my Phisicall books and Recepts, together with my stock of salves and oyntments' in her will dated 1705.[46] Books were updated over time with new recipes drawn from local networks and copied from published advice books and household guides that proliferated in these years. Hannah Glasse's popular *Servants Directory, or Housekeeper's Companion* boasted a long list of subscribers and it included no less than eight separate recipes for keeping sleeping chambers and bedsteads free from flies, fleas and bugs of different kinds: one of the recipes was provided by a 'Lady' who claimed to have 'cleared a Hundred Beds from those troublesome Vermin'.[47] The cleansing process that Glasse described was both time-consuming and messy: in extreme cases the bedchamber had to be completely repainted. The dramatic nature of this recipe nevertheless underlined its importance and the variety of recipes allowed readers to personalise Glasse's advice to suit their particular needs.[48] Vigorous attempts were thus made to predict and to prevent sleep disruptions occasioned by the material composition of sleeping environments, which show the pervasive influence of preventative healthcare culture in shaping household sleeping practices and cleansing routines.

Alongside maintaining the cleanliness of sleeping environments, householders were equally keen to moderate their temperature and to ensure the free circulation of air during the night. This ambition became increasingly prevalent after 1650 as the importance of fresh air, which had long been advocated in Non-Natural health regimens, was augmented by new physiological research into the properties and perils of breathing noxious air. Sleepers were exposed on a nightly basis to the noxious excretions of vegetation and indeed of their own lungs as they breathed in their fetid recycled breath. This perception was confirmed by the mechanical experiments of Dutch botanist and physician Jan Ingen-Housz, published in the *Philosophical Transactions of the Royal Society*, and later by the Yorkshire born physician William Alexander who studied medicine under William Cullen at the University of Edinburgh.[49]

The eighteenth-century medical marketplace was increasingly sensitive to the dangers of bed bugs and noxious air, offering devices and professionalised services to expel them, which complemented the concerted efforts of householders to do the same. A wide variety of preventative measures were available that aimed at keeping the night air pure; they ranged from keeping chamber windows open to the use of specially designed ventilators for those that could afford them.[50] Efforts to secure the free circulation of air during sleep reveal a holistic understanding of healthy sleep that drew on more than one category of Non-Natural healthcare advice. At night householders were advised 'not to have your Window-Curtains drawn, nor your Curtains that are about your Beds; for it hinders the sweet refreshing Influences of the Air'.[51] Lighting fires in sleeping chambers drew similar criticism for it overheated sleeping bodies and exacerbated their sweaty excretions.[52] Household recipes suggest that this kind of advice bore a close relation to daily practice. The recipes arranged by Francis Elcocke, author of a commonplace book featuring household recipes, prized the virtues of sprinkling 'Coleing hearbes' such as lettuce, purslane, willow leaves and water lillies between the bedstead and the walls of the chamber to keep a cool and temperate climate. If a fire had to be lit then sprinkling 'special good rose vinegar' on the green boughs of a chamber fire was believed to temper the hot air and emit 'a cool and fresh sent, all over the chamber'.[53] Householders were keen to ensure the temperate air of their own sleeping chambers but they also made sure that the beds of guests were well aired upon arrival. Routine ventilation of beds and sleeping chambers intensified from the late seventeenth century within the emerging culture of household sociability where it became esteemed as a token of decency, civility and affection between friends as well as a means of securing good health.[54]

Treating sleep loss

If prophylactic cleansing regimes and prayer schedules failed to secure peaceful rest then all was not lost. People possessed many ways of summoning sleep that extended from the recital of special prayers to a change of sleep posture, yet only fleeting glimpses of these habits survive.[55] More visible are the pre-prepared stocks of medicaments to which householders could turn that combined an array of homemade and purchased remedies so as to treat periods of sleep loss. Close analysis of fifty manuscript recipe books that span some or all of the period 1650–1750 show just how important it was to secure healthy sleep. Of the fifty books examined twenty-three feature at least one recipe specifically designed and named to procure sleep; fifteen of the twenty-three contain multiple recipes, with one book including no less than seven. This number is swelled by adding the number of books that include recipes for preparing syrups, distillations or conserves of poppies, violets, roses or water-lillies that were commonly attributed with the power to beckon sleep.[56] An additional seventeen of the remaining twenty-seven books feature at least one recipe for these needs. When these figures are combined, forty of the fifty books examined, or eighty per cent of the total sample, include at least one recipe intended to induce sleep, prevent nightmares or to treat people who walked and talked in their sleep so that they could enjoy a peaceful night's rest. Sleep loss was thus an unsavoury prospect that householders sought to prevent or to cure as quickly as possible.

Historical studies of over 400 English manuscript and printed recipe collections also reveal the near universal interest of early modern people in maintaining physical health as well as outlining the extensive range of cordial waters, balms and plasters that a single household prepared and used.[57] Despite important incursions into household medical practices, little attention has been paid to preventative measures related to specific ailments and disorders.[58] No study has yet quantified or explained the pervasive presence and variety of sleep-inducing medicines that populated recipe collections and cabinets.[59] The recipe books analysed here combined cookery recipes with recipes to prevent or cure common ailments and they reveal how householders anticipated and assiduously prepared for periods of sleep loss by making a wide range of medicaments that could be consumed or applied to different parts of the body.

The vast majority of the sleep recipes examined were expressly designed to treat sleep loss that had no identified cause. A small proportion were nevertheless intended to treat sleep loss that resulted from predictable physical conditions and ailments such as pregnancy, childbirth, gout, melancholy, fevers, burning of the arteries and common colds that impeded respiratory function at night. The recipe books were personalised and flexible to attend to the changing needs of a family over the course of life. The book signed by Elizabeth Jacobs, and expanded by later hands between 1654 and 1685, included four separate recipes to procure sleep, one of which was specifically designed 'To make A man sleepe'. The recipe was further adapted to different age groups with the key ingredient of poppy to be mixed with 'sack', or fortified wine, 'for an old body'; with white wine 'for the middle' body; and with beer 'for younger people'.[60] Express references to differentiating sleep remedies according to complexion are rare within the sample, yet they surely indicate a more pervasive concern with such gradations in daily practice to suit the needs of different constitutions. Indeed, careful regulation of dose was especially apparent in recipes that used powerful ingredients. Recipes based on poppy seeds, poppy syrups or laudanum were administered gradually in small drops and consumed slowly over extended periods of time so that their effects could be closely monitored, and no doubt adjusted to suit different complexions. Elizabeth Jacobs's recipe book advised that the 'halfe a grain' of laudanum in a pill designed to procure sleep should not be exceeded 'without good Advice'. This kind of caution likely combined a concern to conserve costly ingredients with a desire to mitigate the potentially damaging effects of heavy, long-term use of powerful medicaments, which individual hands and medical practitioners like George Hartman routinely warned against.[61] The external application of somniferous concoctions could also mitigate their damaging effects; commonplace recipes for poppy cakes included directions for adapting them for medicinal purposes by steeping the cakes in a soporific liquid and laying them onto the temples to bring on sleep.[62]

A wide range of alternative ingredients routinely featured in sleep recipes, whose effects were more gentle and that were often more affordable. They nevertheless required heavy investment of time and labour to prepare, which could extend over several days. Some ingredients could be gathered in the local countryside, whilst others were recommended for kitchen gardens. They included aniseed, cowslip flowers, gillyflowers, lavender, lettuce, roses, chamomile, lemons, violets, strawberries, burrage roots, cucumbers and rosemary. Some ingredients like sugar and blanched almonds were commonly in use in well-stocked kitchens and there was indeed an important overlap between the general preparation of foodstuffs and recipes for sleep loss.[63] A final set of ingredients that included posset ale, nutmeg, barley water, cinnamon, henbane, dates, mace, fennel roots, melon seeds, hog lice, malmsey, elderflowers, elderberries, eringo roots, grains of musk, vinegar and vine leaves, might be sourced from physical herb sellers at local markets or from grocers and apothecaries.[64] Lettuce, cucumber seeds and poppy water had a well-established tradition of use for procuring sleep in Non-Natural medicine because they worked to cool overheated brains and stomachs and thereby restore humoral balance.[65] Similar properties were associated with eringo roots, or *eringium maratimum*: the preserved roots of sea holly. The roots were commonly used as an aphrodisiac but when preserved and candied their moistening effects were recommended for the elderly.[66] A cool, moist and soporific effect may have been produced by many of the other sleep recipes examined since most of them were made as sweetened liquids to be drunk at bedtime or to be applied to the body.[67] A cooling sensation was similarly sought after in two recipes from the Boyle family recipe book. The application of chamomile water to the feet and legs was recommended at bedtime, whilst a mixture of rose water and bruised aniseeds placed in a string bag was believed to give 'a cold smell and procureth sleep' if it was tied onto the upper lip so that its fumes could infuse through the nose during the night.[68]

Methods of preparing these preventative concoctions were straightforward; the most common stipulated was boiling, usually in a chaffing dish, or in earthen or copper pots and pans that were staple features of early modern kitchens.[69] The cost effectiveness of these preparations was further enhanced by the common practice of making and storing large quantities of prepared recipes for long periods of time. This was particularly useful to treat periods of sleep loss that were intermittent and unpredictable. A number of the sleep recipes were deliberately designed to serve a household's needs for months or even years. Lavender flowers and red roses were noted to keep for many years if boiled as conserves, whilst distillations of violets, if boiled to syrup strength, kept for up to two years. A recipe for 'Conserve of violets the Italian manner' was highly praised for procuring rest and for its longevity. This recipe intermingled with an extensive array of sleep-inducing preparations, which underlined the seamless combination of local medical advice, knowledge gathered by visitors to Europe, or poached from published guides to health that included an eclectic range of prescriptions from far-flung locations.[70] Wherever they originated, the preparation and storage of sleep treatments complemented the long-term preventative culture of healthcare that underpinned the principles of Non-Natural medical advice and that attended the prophylactic culture of sleep preservation in early modern households.

Conclusion

A preventative and holistic approach to sleep's daily practice predominated in early modern English households. This was supported by the increasingly high value placed on the physical and spiritual benefits of healthy sleep. The refreshment and satisfaction that peaceful sleep offered was self-evident from embodied experiences of sleep but it began to be articulated ever-more forcefully in regimens of health, household recipe books, and in the wider marketplace of medical publications and guides to household management. These texts confirmed and indeed augmented the importance of moderate sleeping hours and hygienic sleeping environments by praising the value of temperate sleep for maintaining the vigour of the nerves and intellectual faculties as well as for more general health preservation. This advice was widely heeded within many households and adapted to suit individual circumstances.

One crucial motivation for these practices was the religious culture of the decades after 1660. These years witnessed the intensification of household devotional practices as a direct result of the fragmentation of confessional unity. The household became an increasingly pivotal site of spiritual activity, of which sacralised sleep regimens formed a crucial part. The periodic and non-life-threatening nature of disturbed or broken sleep also meant that the household remained the primary location for sleep management on a day-to-day basis. Recourse to paid medical services for sleeping problems was the last resort and household recipe books suggest that many people prepared carefully for occasional periods of sleep loss by producing a wide variety of distillations, syrups, conserves and other medicaments that provoked sleep and that could be stored for months or even years.[71] The prevailing emphasis of sleep management was thus on preventative measures, but if curative treatments were required, they drew heavily on the healthcare principles of the Non-Naturals.

The extent to which individuals linked their sleeping habits to theologies of salvation and resurrection did of course vary widely. The importance of redeeming time was most visible amongst Puritans and Presbyterians, yet most Christians understood that seasonable bedtimes and healthy sleeping environments offered an important means of making good their relationship with God on a nightly basis: something that was underlined by regular performances of morning and evening prayer. A flourishing genre of spiritual advice books also supported practices of sleep-piety as embodied expressions of faith. The emphasis of Church divines on practical theology, both before and after the Toleration Act of 1689, ensured that the immoral nature of unseasonable sleep was consistently emphasised to lay folk who prioritised temperance and restraint in their sleep regimes to preserve their reputations and to safeguard their physical and spiritual health on a daily basis. The long-term temporal approach of preventative healthcare practices surrounding sleep dovetailed neatly with practices of household piety. Sleepers considered their physical and spiritual health as two sides of the same coin and in so doing they ensured the vitality of Non-Natural healthcare principles within English households into the mid-eighteenth century and indeed beyond.

Notes

1 T. Tryon, *Wisdom's dictates: or, Aphorisms & rules, physical, moral, and divine, for preserving the health of the body, and the peace of the mind* (London: Thomas Salisbury, 1691), p. 3.

2 Thomas Tryon's guides to health management were directed at a wide popular audience and they proved influential in the British Isles in the late seventeenth and eighteenth centuries. They included *Healths grand preservative: or, the women's best doctor* (1682); *A treatise of cleanness in meats and drinks* (1682); *Monthly observations for the preserving of health* (1688); *A pocket-companion; containing things necessary to be known, by all that values their health and happiness* (1693); *A discourse of waters* (1696); *The way to health, long life, and happiness* (1697). See also note 1.

3 Alice Thornton gave thanks to God when her daughter was saved from being overlaid by her nursemaid one night. The maid had fallen asleep with her breast in the child's mouth. A. Thornton, *The Autobiography of Mrs. Alice Thornton of East Newton, Co. York*, ed. C. Jackson (Durham: Andrews and Co. for Surtees Society, 1875), p. 91.

4 For detailed exploration of the relationship between religious beliefs and sleeping habits in late seventeenth-century England see S. Handley, 'From the sacral to the moral: sleeping practices, household worship and confessional cultures in late seventeenth-century England', *Cultural and Social History*, 9:1 (2012), pp. 27–46.

5 Tryon, *Wisdom's Dictates*, p. 87.

6 T. Willis, *Cerebri anatome: cui accessit nervorum description et usus* (London: Ja. Flesher, 1664). On the classification of sleep and sleep disorders as neurological conditions see S. Handley, 'Sleepwalking, subjectivity and the nervous body in eighteenth-century Britain', *Journal for Eighteenth-Century Studies*, 35:3 (2012), pp. 305–23.

7 William Cullen's most influential publication was *First Lines of the Practice of Physic* (Edinburgh: W. Creech, 1777–84).

8 See for example Francis de Valangin's *A Treatise on Diet, or the management of human life; by physicians called the six non-naturals* (London: J. and W. Oliver, 1768), and James Makittrick Adair's *Essays on Fashionable Diseases* (London: T. P. Bateman, 1790).

9 Growing links between sleeping patterns and the anatomy of the brain and nerves in the medical culture of late seventeenth- and eighteenth-century Europe and the British Isles are explored in K.H. Dannenfeldt, 'Sleep: theory and practice in the late Renaissance', *Journal of the History of Medicine and Allied Sciences*, 41:4 (1986), pp. 415–41, and in Handley, 'Sleepwalking, subjectivity and the nervous body'.

10 S. Cavallo and T. Storey, *Healthy Living in Late Renaissance Italy* (Oxford: Oxford University Press, 2013); S. Cavallo, 'Secrets of healthy living: the revival of the preventive paradigm in late Renaissance Italy', in E. Leong and A. Rankin (eds), *Secrets and Knowledge in Medicine and Science, 1500–1800* (Farnham: Ashgate, 2011), pp. 191–212; E. Leong, 'Medical recipe collections in seventeenth-century England: knowledge, gender and text', PhD dissertation, Oxford University, 2005; A. Withey, *Physick and the Family. Health, Medicine and Care in Wales 1600–1750* (Manchester: Manchester University Press, 2011); M. Stolberg, *Experiencing Illness and the Sick Body in Early Modern Europe* (Basingstoke: Palgrave Macmillan, 2011).

11 R. Allestree, *The Whole Duty of Man* (London: Robert Harford, 1680), p. 203.

12 Proverbs 20:13, 'Love not sleep, lest you come to poverty; open your eyes, and you will have plenty of bread'; Proverbs 6:9, 'How long will you lie there, O sluggard? When will you arise from your sleep?' (KJV).
13 2 Samuel 4:5; Judges 4:18–21.
14 R. Allestree, *The art of contentment* (Oxford: The Theatre, 1675), pp. 67–8.
15 T. Tryon, *A new method of educating children* (London: J. Salusbury and J. Harris, 1695), p. B1, 72. J. Locke, *Some thoughts concerning education* (London: Churchill, 1693), pp. 23–4.
16 C. Hill, 'The spiritualization of the household', in C. Hill, *Society and Puritanism in Pre-revolutionary England* (London: Secker & Warburg, 1964), pp. 382–416. A. Ryrie, 'Sleeping, waking and dreaming in Protestant piety', in J. Martin and A. Ryrie (eds), *Private and Domestic Devotion in Early Modern Britain* (Farnham: Ashgate, 2012), pp. 73–92. E. Sullivan, 'The watchful spirit: religious anxieties towards sleep in the notebooks of Nehemiah Wallington (1598–1658)', *Cultural History*, 1:1 (2012), pp. 14–35.
17 P. Mack, *Heart Religion in the British Enlightenment, Gender and Emotion in Early Methodism* (Cambridge: Cambridge University Press, 2008). P. Mack, 'The unbounded self: dreaming and identity in the British Enlightenment', in A.M. Plane and L. Tuttle (eds), *Dreams, Dreamers and Visions. The Early Modern Atlantic World* (Philadelphia: University of Pennsylvania Press, 2013), pp. 207–25.
18 W.M. Jacob, *Lay People and Religion in the Early Eighteenth Century* (Cambridge: Cambridge University Press, 1996), p. 6.
19 *Ibid.*, p. 95.
20 The significance of devotional literature for Catholic communities is examined in J. Bossy, *The English Catholic Community 1570–1850* (London: Darton, Longman & Todd, 1975).
21 T. Hamling, 'Old Robert's girdle: visual and material props for Protestant piety in post-Reformation England', in Martin and Ryrie (eds), *Private and Domestic Devotion*, pp. 135–63. T. Hamling, *Decorating the Godly Household: Religious Art in Post-Reformation Britain* (New Haven and London: Yale University Press, 2010).
22 Thornton, *Autobiography*, p. 190.
23 *Two East Anglian Diaries 1641–1729, Isaac Archer and William Coe*, ed. M. Storey (Woodbridge: Boydell Press, 1994), pp. 217–18.
24 Edmund Harrold likely read one or both of Richard Sherlock's popular texts: *A Practical Discourse concerning Death* (1689) and *A Practical Discourse concerning a Future Judgement* (1689).
25 S. Hurst, *The Diaries of Sarah Hurst 1759–1762, Life and Love in Eighteenth Century Horsham*, ed. S.C. Djabri (Stroud: Amberley, 2009), p. 83. *The Diary of Edmund Harrold, Wigmaker of Manchester 1712–15*, ed. C. Horner (Aldershot: Ashgate, 2008), pp. 10, 22–3, 43–4.

26 Hurst, *Diaries*, pp. 210–11.
27 R. Thoresby, *The diary of Ralph Thoresby, F.R.S. author of The topography of Leeds (1677–1724)*, ed. J. Hunter, 2 vols (London: Henry Colburn and Richard Bentley, 1830), vol. 2, p. 147. E. Burnet, *A Method of Devotion: or Rules for Holy & Devout Living* (London: Joseph Downing, C. Smith, & A. Barker, 1709).
28 Thoresby, *Diary*, vol. 2, pp. 12, 15, 94.
29 R. Baxter, *A Christian Directory* (London: Simmons, 1673), p. 405.
30 Thoresby, *Diary*, vol. 2, p. 58.
31 *Ibid.*, pp. 71–3, 85.
32 *The diary of the Rev. Henry Newcome from September 30, 1661 to September 29, 1663*, ed. T. Heywood (Manchester: Chetham Society, 1849), pp. 7, 10, 25–6, 38, 44, 62, 103.
33 Cross-cultural desires for security during sleep are explored in B. Steger, 'Cultures of sleep', in A. Green and A. Westcombe (eds), *Sleep. Multi-Professional Perspectives* (London, Philadelphia: Jessica Kingsley, 2012), pp. 68–85.
34 For further information see S. Handley, *Sleep in Early Modern England* (New Haven: Yale University Press, 2016).
35 J. Styles, 'What were cottons for in the early Industrial Revolution', in G. Riello and P. Parthasarathi (eds), *The Spinning World. A Global History of Cotton Textiles* (Oxford: Oxford University Press, 2009), pp. 307–26.
36 Thornton, *Autobiography*, pp. 49, 122–3, 134. Newcome, *Diary*, p. 83.
37 A. Boorde, *A compendyous regyment or a dyetary of healthe* (London: Wyllyam Powell, 1547), pp. A3–4. Boorde was also the likely author of the anonymous *Boke for to Lerne a Man to by Wyse in Buyldyng his Howse for the Helth of his Body* (London: Robert Wyer, 1540).
38 On the removal of beds from parlours see L. Weatherill, *Consumer Behaviour & Material Culture in Britain, 1660–1760*, 2nd edn (London: Routledge, 1996), pp. 11–12; F.E. Brown, 'Continuity and change in the urban house: developments in domestic space organisation in seventeenth-century London', *Comparative Studies in Society and History*, 28:3 (1986), pp. 558–90.
39 I. Ware, *A Complete Body of Architecture* (London: T. Osborne and J. Shipton, 1756), pp. 346–7.
40 Tryon, *Treatise on cleanness*, pp. 5, 7.
41 *Ibid.*, pp. 10–11. See also Locke, *Some thoughts*, pp. 23–4 and J. Wesley, *The duty and advantage of early rising* (London: J. Paramore, 1783), pp. 6–7.
42 L.T. Sarasohn, '"That nauseous venomous insect": bedbugs in Early Modern England', *Eighteenth-Century Studies*, 46:4 (2013), pp. 513–30.
43 A. McShane and J. Bailey, 'Making beds, making households: the domestic and emotional landscape of the bed in early modern England'

(pre-publication copy); L. Gowing, '"The Twinkling of a bedstaff": recovering the social life of English beds 1500–1700', *Home Cultures*, 11:3 (2014), pp. 275–304.

44 J. Southall, *A Treatise of Buggs* (London: J. Roberts, 1730).

45 'A booke of divers receipts', MS 1322, Wellcome Trust Library (hereafter WT), *c*.1660–1750, fols 50–1.

46 M. Berg, 'Women's consumption and the industrial classes in eighteenth-century England', *Journal of Social History*, 30:2 (1996), pp. 415–34. Thornton, *Autobiography*, p. 333.

47 H. Glasse, *The Servant's Directory, or House-Keeper's Companion* (London: printed for the author, 1760), pp. 38–42, 427. Comparable advice featured in Glasse's earlier work, *The Art of Cookery, made Plain and Easy* (London: printed for the author, 1747). See also recipe 'Buggs to destroy in a dwelling house', MS 3295, WT, fol. 209.

48 Glasse, *Servant's Directory*, pp. 39–40. The ways in which medical advice was appropriated by individual consumers has been explored in E. Leong and S. Pennell, 'Recipe collections and the currency of medical knowledge in the Early Modern "medical marketplace"', in M.S.R. Jenner and P. Wallis (eds), *Medicine and the Market in England and Its Colonies, c.1450–c.1650* (Basingstoke: Palgrave Macmillan, 2007), pp. 133–52, on pp. 133, 145.

49 W. Alexander, *Plain and easy directions for the use of Harrogate Waters* (Edinburgh: A. Kincaid & W. Creech, 1773), pp. 53–4; Adair, *Essays*, p. 52.

50 In a letter of 1750 to Horace Mann, Horace Walpole described a device with two silver tubes that was kept by the bedside and used to expel polluted air. *Horace Walpole's Correspondence with Sir Horace Mann*, ed. W.S. Lewis, W.H. Smith and G.L. Lam (New Haven: Yale University Press, 1960), vol. 20, p. 203. On the invention and availability of ventilators see S. Hales, *A Description of Ventilators* (London: W. Innys, 1743); *The London Magazine, or, Gentleman's Monthly Intelligencer*, 23 (1754), pp. 126–7.

51 Tryon, *Treatise on cleanness*, p. 7.

52 *Ibid*., p. 10; Newcome, *Diary*, p. 222.

53 'Francis Elcocke, List of diseases arranged astrologically', MS Sloane 2287, British Library, fol. 21. 'Culinary Receipts', MS Sloane MS 703, British Library, fols 8, 99.

54 For more detailed explanation see S. Handley, 'Sociable sleeping in Early Modern England, 1660–1760', *History*, 98:39 (2013), pp. 79–104.

55 For examples of dedicated prayers to be said when waking unexpectedly in the night see R. Warren, *The Daily Self-Examinant* (London: printed for Edmund Parker, 1720), pp. iv, 54–5; anon., *Crumbs of Comfort and Godly Prayers* (London: publisher unknown, 1726), p. 56; Newcome, *Diary*, p. 111.

56 For example recipes for poppy water see MS 1796, WT, *c.*1685–1725, fol. 97; 'A booke of useful receipts for cookery', MS 1325, WT, fol. 183 verso.
57 Leong, 'Medical recipe collections'.
58 An important exception is Stolberg, *Experiencing Illness.*
59 Leong notes the close relationship between Elizabeth Freke's medical recipes and the medicines listed in her inventory of 1711, which suggests an important synergy between these collections and daily practice. Leong, 'Making medicines', pp. 148–9.
60 'Receipt book of Elizabeth Jacobs & others', MS 3009, WT, 1654–85, fol. 96.
61 'Elizabeth Jacobs', MS 3009, fol. 57; Sloane MS 3295, BL, fol. 101, verso; 'Book of Phisick', MS 1320, fol. 109. G. Hartman, *The Family Physitian* (London: Richard Wellington, 1696), pp. 65–6. Hartman's remedies to prevent 'the Watching Evil' cautioned against overuse of these ingredients.
62 'A Booke of Phisick', MS 1320, WT, 1710–25, fol. 107; 'Anne Brumwich, Book of Receits in Medicines', MS 160, WT, *c.*1625–1700, fol. 54.
63 L. Meager, *The English gardner* (London: J. Dawks, for M. Wotton and G. Conyers, 1699), pp. 85–113. A recipe for 'A very good conserve of roses' advised its preparer to gather rose buds seasonally when the buds were 'not blowne out, after the sunne hath drawen up the deawe'. 'Culinary Receipts', Sloane MS 703, fol. 3.
64 Harvey, *Family Physician*, pp. 4–5, 134–5. On the availability of individual ingredients see J. Stobart, *Sugar and Spice: Grocers and Groceries in Provincial England, 1650–1830* (Oxford: Oxford University Press, 2012).
65 'Receipt Book', MS 1796, WT, *c.*1685–1725, fol. 97.
66 N. Culpeper, *The English physitian* (London: Peter Cole, 1652), pp. 48–9.
67 'Collection of Receipts', MS 634, BL, fols 37, 122; Sloane MS 2203, BL, fol. 164.
68 'Boyle family recipe book', MS 1340, WT, *c.*1675–1710, fols 17, 122, 132.
69 'Culinary Receipts', Sloane MS 703, BL, fol. 6 verso; S. Pennell, '"Pots and pans history": the material culture of the kitchen in early modern England', *Journal of Design History*, 11:3 (1998), pp. 201–16.
70 MS 3295, BL, fols 102, 133; BL Sloane MS 703, BL, fol. 4.
71 'Book of Receites', MS 144, WT, *c.*1650–1739; MS 634, BL; 'English Medical Receipt Book', MS 809, BL, *c.*1635, fols 231, 232 verso; MS 809, BL, fol. 192 verso; MS 3295, BL; MS Sloane 2203, BL.

8

English and Italian health advice: Protestant and Catholic bodies

Tessa Storey

One of the most successful and influential vernacular medical works in early modern England was Thomas Elyot's *Castel of Helth*, first published in 1534.[1] Not the first such text to be published in England, it explained the principles underlying the preservation of good health and, most importantly, contained a diet or *regimen* for the daily management of the six Non-Naturals, as well as advice on bloodletting and caring for the sick.[2] Elyot was initially criticised for writing the *Castel of Helth* on the grounds that as a 'knight' he was not qualified to write a work of medicine. He responded, in the preface to the next edition, by acknowledging that although he had not studied at 'Montpellier, Padua or Salerne', he had read Galen, Hippocrates, and the Salernitan *Regimen Sanitatis*, and that he had been tutored by a 'worshipfull phisition' – widely presumed to be Thomas Linacre.[3] Linacre was the foremost English medical humanist and, having studied medicine in Padua, presumably told Elyot of the importance of dietetic tracts in both university curricula and contemporary medical practice in Italy. Indeed, Linacre's first medical translation from Greek to Latin was of Galen's *De Sanitate Tuenda*, in 1517.[4] Thus Elyot's defensive preface was surely articulating his awareness of the unquestioned superiority of an Italian medical education and Italian medical theory, whilst locating his work in the classical medical tradition.[5]

However, despite having its roots in antiquity, the regimen genre was far from static, and it is with Elyot's *Castel of Helth* that the history of Italian and English regimen start to diverge, despite their shared medical genealogies. As Sandra Cavallo and I have shown for Italy, the contents of texts providing preventive health advice responded not only to developments in medical theory, but also to social and cultural change.[6] This essay extends this notion geographically, based on the assumption that anomalies and differences would have arisen between the various 'national' traditions which developed along with the vernacularisation of the genre during the sixteenth and seventeenth centuries. Taking the Italian regimen as a comparison this chapter explores the proposition that the English regimen took on characteristics which were particular to the national and religious context in which it evolved.

This is not entirely new territory. Virginia Smith has shown the ways in which discussions of bodily hygiene were influenced by Protestant rhetoric and brought our attention to the existence of a 'cold' regimen which developed in England in the late seventeenth century.[7] Moreover, Andrew Wear has drawn our attention to the ways in which a range of early modern English texts, including regimen, constructed English national identity through reference to the Hippocratic *Airs, Waters, Places* tradition, thereby embedding the good health and positive national characteristics of the English in their home environment.[8] This chapter will examine, from a comparative perspective, ways in which aspects of three of the Non-Naturals were discussed. This helps us discern the national specificities of the regimen and to consider the extent to which medical ideas about these Non-Naturals were manipulated in order to shape or conform to an English Protestant identity, or an English, as opposed to a Catholic, Mediterranean body. The chapter will consider the 'ideological' framework of the regimen in the two countries; perceptions about the impact of climate and air on the body and of the role played by the pores in maintaining health; advice on eating; and discussions of coitus.

Appealing to the common English reader

As noted in Chapter 1, recently scholars have engaged in lively debate on the likely readership of such vernacular medical texts. Murray Jones for example has suggested that the success of Elyot's *Castel* was largely its appeal as a demonstration of 'judgement and taste'.[9] However, even if the *Castel* did subsequently accrue 'status' appeal, it was certainly intended to be used as a practical guide for healthy living and – following our arguments in Chapter 1 – most likely was also widely employed for this purpose.[10] Elyot's declaration that he intended his book to serve the 'common-weal' was accompanied by formal, stylistic and paratextual choices which represented an attempt to reach out beyond courtly circles, at the very least to members of the professions, the gentry and merchants interested in preserving their health. Moreover the small, slim format (8vo or 4° with under 100 pages) implied a low-cost volume.[11] It was a typical example of the astute publishing practices of Thomas Berthelet, who had strong commercial reasons for making the regimen more widely accessible.[12] The layout was designed to make it easier for a lay readership to navigate the text. The typeface was black-letter, with which the less able readers would have been familiar as it was used in primers, proclamations and public bills.[13] There was an opening index, there were breaks between paragraphs with small headings for new topics and short printed references to the sources being discussed placed in the margins.[14] Moreover much of the more detailed information on complexions and humours in the first part of the text was stripped down to a series of innovative 'tables' or headings, which gave the necessary information at a glance. Interestingly, these paratextual methods were adopted in England several decades earlier than in Italy.

Later authors would employ other strategies in their quest to make regimens more accessible, such as employing a conversational dialogue form. Moreover, in the *Government of Health* by William Bullein, a fervent Protestant physician (1559), the questions posed are in roman type, whilst the actual medical advice is in black-letter print, as if to make it clearer for the user to understand the crucial content.[15]

Similar measures were also adopted in Italy, however, whilst an English peculiarity was the adoption of a Hippocratic approach to maintaining health. Charles Webster has argued that in Puritan England Hippocratic medicine was considered to be purer and to 'possess spiritual and scientific merits' not present in the works of Galen and later Galenic authors.[16] This perhaps explains why rather than adopting the doctrine of the six Non-Naturals, which had only assumed 'canonical status' in Galenic medicine at the end of the middle ages, some vernacular authors in Protestant England drew on Hippocrates' *Epidemics* IV/

VI for an alternative way of organising their regimen.[17] Hippocrates had referred to five (not six) aspects of life 'upon which our health is based': diet, living conditions, exertion, sleep, sexual intercourse and mental activity. As early as about 1547 Christopher Langton, soon to be a qualified physician, wrote a short regimen based on what later were referred to as the 'Hippocratic Five words'. He also cites Hippocrates and never Galen in his advice, despite his ardent embrace of Galenism in the preface.[18] Another regimen to adopt this kind of structure was by Guglielmo Grataroli, an Italian Protestant physician who lived in exile in Basle.[19] First published there in 1555, it was then translated into English in 1573–74 by the scholar Thomas Newton. Grataroli explains that the Hippocratic topics are 'laboure or exercise, meat, drinke, sleep and the arte of carnall copulation'.[20] He does not explain his preference for these five factors, but, given his fervent Protestant convictions, it is possible that he sought to contextualise his advice for the city fathers in Basle in terms of a rejection of the complexities of Galenism (without, however, entirely rejecting Galen's authority), and of a return to a more 'pure' Hippocratic approach for his Protestant readership and, by extension, the Protestant body.[21]

Another possible explanation for Grataroli's choice comes ten years later when a Mancunian physician named Thomas Cogan published his regimen for students. It also took the Hippocratic 'five words' as his source for the structure and these are prominently placed in his title, emphasising the significance of this decision: *Amplified upon five words of Hippocrates, written Epid. 6. labor, cibus, potio, sumnus, venus.*[22] Cogan provides a justification for this with reference to Thomas Elyot, on the grounds of simplicity and the particular needs of his 'common' English readership. On the one hand, he explains, the Hippocratic five words provide a structure simple enough and memorable enough that even the 'dull of understanding' can understand and remember them: 'In my judgement, this aphorism of Hippocrates, which I purpose … to declare, is more evident for the common capacitie of men, and more convenient for the diet of our English nation. For who is so dull of understanding that cannot remember these five words'?[23] He argues that these 'five words' are easier to remember because the order in which they are given is the natural order in which one experiences them. In order to live, one must first labour (i.e. exercise, in medical terms), and that makes one hungry, so, one needs to eat and then drink;

then one feels tired, and so goes to bed to sleep, and there, finally, one indulges in Venus. He also notes that beginning 'the preservation of health with labour' is in some measure part of an 'old English fashion' and ultimately 'more convenient for the diet of our English nation', although the reason for this is not explained. However, he does note that this choice allows for a further simplification of the structure, due to the elimination of separate topics such as 'air' and 'affections of the mind' which are integrated into the discussions of the other topics.

Airs, waters, places and bodies

Analyses of air temperature and air quality had often appeared in the more popular late medieval regimen.[24] However, the translation of the entire Hippocratic corpus, particularly *on Airs, Waters and Places* and *Epidemics*, into Latin in 1525 and Greek in 1526, had a considerable impact on these discussions. Hippocrates had insisted that physicians could not treat their patients successfully without first understanding how their bodies were affected by local winds, local waters and local soils. This advice was taken so seriously by Italian physicians that increasingly it was considered evident that advice on climate could not be meaningfully applied across the entire Italian peninsula. From the mid-1550s, regimens appeared which were tailor-made for the needs of people living in individual cities. Indeed, even within this local context, physicians then analysed the prevailing winds, various water courses and micro-climates of the different districts of the city.[25]

This concern to accurately map bodies onto localities meant that whereas the body discussed in the late medieval and early sixteenth-century regimen had been in a sense a 'universal' body, albeit differentiated by complexion, age and sex, after the mid-sixteenth century Italian regimens increasingly add this new set of distinctions, which corresponded to the geographical and political divisions within Italy. They effectively fragmented the subject into multiple 'local bodies', writing regimens for the people of Venice and the people of Genoa and of Rome.[26] In his advice to the inhabitants of Rome for example, translated from the Latin in 1592, Petronio warned that they were particularly subject to three 'local' ailments. These derived from the variations in climate caused by the seven hills, from the humidity in its air which rose from underground and was brought by south winds, and from local food which absorbed this moisture, negatively affecting everyone's digestion.[27]

By comparison, the impact of the new Hippocratism amongst English physicians was far less dramatic. Air and water are analysed, but discussions do not run into extensive chapters, or independent publications, whilst analyses of different winds and water courses barely feature. Mention is made of problematic marshy areas, but overall, regional and geographical variation is virtually ignored. Instead, the English took a much broader perspective, discussing their climate within a global context, by invoking comparisons not only with places in Europe but also looking much further afield – at Peru, Africa, Asia, the Tropics and North America. One of the concerns here was to establish the English climate as ideal, that is, temperate, in a fiercely nationalistic political climate. It is a theme first established by Elyot, who writes of the 'just temperature' of the realm, and it was subsequently taken up by Bullein in 1559 and later authors.[28]

In keeping with this sense of a singular 'English' climate, there is also the corresponding sense of a single English body. We do not encounter different health advice for Yorkshire men, the men of Devon, Cumberland or Wales – even though they might be mentioned in passing. We find instead the reiteration of phrases like 'English men's natures', or 'the dyet of our English nation' or 'our islanders of Great Britaine'. Indeed, one author feels able to describe English men as a whole as 'comely of body, well coloured in the face … and joyful in their prosperous health'.[29] Moreover, this view that there was just 'one' distinctively English body, adapted to the English climate, was then used to dismiss some of the rules of healthy living which had been elaborated with a Mediterranean body in mind: particularly when these rules conflicted with well-established English customs. Thomas Elyot had set this trend when he wrote, 'And here I wil not recite the sentences of authors which had not experience of English men's natures or of the just temperature of this realme of England.'[30]

Whilst on the one hand English authors were concerned to establish the English climate as being 'temperate', at the same time sixteenth-century regimens accepted without demur that it was a 'cold' climate – where cold was perceived as a positive quality. It was indeed this cold which resulted in the excellent health and particularly positive character attributes of the English, such as vigour, hardiness and bravery, as

Andrew Wear has shown.[31] So, although the dangers of cold and hot air and particularly of sudden temperature changes were recognised by English authors, there is a significant difference in emphasis and the nature of the debate. On balance, as Tobias Venner summarises, it seems to have been agreed that 'for sound bodies' the cold 'is more convenient and agreeable than air that is over hot', since it 'is healthfull, because it impelleth the natural heat into the inner parts, and so causeth a strong digestion'.[32] This long-standing positive characterisation of the cold in English regimens prepared the way for the subsequent development of the so-called 'cold regimen' in England as discussed by Virginia Smith; a regimen based on cool air, cool beds and cool drinks and promoted by Sydenham in the last decades of the seventeenth century.[33] However, it is in sharp contrast to the attitude found amongst Italian authors for whom cold air, especially cold damp air, represented a very serious threat to health throughout the period in question.

One element which seems key to the differences in attitudes towards the climate, lay in the different emphases placed on the functions of the pores in the two countries. In Galenic physiology the pores were considered to play a crucial role in the maintenance of health, as a porous layer of exchange between the body and the outside world. In repeated discussions of them in Italian regimens, physicians were most concerned about their role as a conduit for the expulsion of waste products from the third 'concoction' or digestion, whether in the form of vapour or sweat.[34] There are also consistent, scattered, but less well-explained references to their role as an entry point for air which 'restores' the body and tempers the body heat.[35] An Italian physician for example advises one to stand after sunrise before an open window which faces north or west, and 'having at this time opened all the pores, one will draw into oneself the purest air'.[36] However, there were also dangers associated with both these functions of the pores. Given that they could also *admit* air into the body, corrupted air was likewise believed to penetrate the skin. We find references to this threat in discussions of plague from the late fifteenth to mid-seventeenth century in England and Italy, as readers are advised against vigorous exercise or hot baths at times of plague, both of which opened the pores excessively wide, allowing corrupted air to flow into the body.[37] In English regimens the dangers associated with widened pores gradually become a significant consideration even in general healthy living advice – to the point that in 1650 the physician

Brooke, writing of sweating, warns that 'though it frees the body from internal causes of diseases, yet it *more* disposes it [the body] to receive wrong from external sharpness and penetration of the aire of wind, by opening the spiracles, and so giving admission thereunto' (my italics).[38]

Physicians were also concerned with another of the consequences of pores which are over-widened by heat; mainly the loss of vital spirits which escaped through these open channels. In England over the seventeenth century this notion was increasingly used to account for national differences, explaining the Englishman's 'vigour' and the southerners' lassitude. Francis Bacon for example expressed the belief that people lived longer 'in cold and northern countries' because 'the skinne is more compact and close; And the juices of the body less dissipable.'[39] Indeed, he even discusses numerous ways of closing and filling the pores against the external environment – whether with mastick, myrrh, myrtle, astringent mineral waters or 'filling up the pores, paintings and such like unctous dawbings' using oil and fat; something quite unthinkable in Italian regimens.[40]

By comparison, in Italy the danger of succumbing to illness as a result of the entry of putrid air through the pores was a concept which received far less attention than inhalation through the nose and mouth, particularly amongst the welter of provisions and warnings given in Italian plague tracts. Moreover in general health regimens the overriding concern for Italian physicians was, on the contrary, the need to keep the pores open.[41] One physician notes that the benefits of this evacuation are so great that 'the preservation of health depends largely upon this'.[42] To the Italians any blockage or narrowing of the pores, particularly by cold air which 'constipates the skin', could lead to the dangerous accumulation of wastes within, which would then 'putrify' inside the body 'from which derive infinite numbers of illnesses'.[43] Added to this were the dangers posed by damp air, viewed as 'thick' and heavy, liable to block the pores as it tried to pass through them, as well as filling the head and chest, causing 'obstructions' which lead ultimately to 'catarrhs and coughs'. Coastal areas with their 'fat, dense, hot air' were particularly suspect, as were mists and the damp night air in general.[44]

The particular anxieties which surrounded the quality of the air explain why Italian authors paid such close attention to the nature of local airs and particularly winds. For, although certain light, pure and especially dry winds were greatly approved of for health, and welcomed during the sweltering summer, those which were damp and warm, or very cold, were regarded with great suspicion. This was largely because of their impact on the pores as discussed above, since winds could 'hit' the body's apertures with inescapable vehemence. Italian authors also worried about the impact of cold winds on the brain. This was understood as a 'cold' organ and, as they repeatedly point out, the head being elevated above the rest of the body, 'round and eminent', it was particularly vulnerable to the impact of such winds.[45]

All the elaborate detail on the dangers of cold air and winds which fill the pages of Italian regimen from the 1560s seems to be almost entirely missing from English regimens.[46] Due attention is paid to the dangers of environment, and there is passing mention of the dangers of cold 'blasts', but in some cases the Italian fear of the cold was completely reversed. In 1633 William Vaughan wrote that those living 'with cold northerly Air' as in northern Ireland, or other 'hilly windy, dry places' where sheep are grazed and 'where winds abound', will 'live untill their sonnes waxe weary of them'.[47] James Hart's 1633 discussion also challenges some traditional topoi on the subject, particularly the ancient prejudice against damp sea-winds, citing the health and vitality of Venetians and the appetites of sailors from the north of England to support his argument.[48] And in English regimens there seems to be almost no concern about dangers to the brain from external air, although they seem to have focused instead on the threat from putrid vapours rising from the stomach.

Eating in a cold climate

Contextualising the English body in a 'cold' climate also had important implications for discussions of eating and drinking. One of the key debates on eating within the regimen genre concerned how often one should eat – whether one meal a day was sufficient or two excessive – and whether one should eat more at midday or in the evening. All these questions, however, had to be considered in relation to one's complexion and the other Non-Naturals, particularly sleep and exercise – and the latter was inevitably related to class.

Although Thomas Elyot covers the subtleties of the debate over several pages he then establishes, as his point of reference for 'generall' use, that the healthy average 'English' body can be defined as having a 'hot lusty' complexion, with much choler in the stomach' – a complexion which results from the coldness of the climate.[49] Importantly, as part of patriotic rhetoric, heat carried positive implications, considered as the most prized quality in one's complexion and associated with the male body. This notion was then taken up by successive authors. Thomas Cogan clarified the issue and its implications for the English Diet: 'And doubtless the temperature of this our countrie of England is such that our stomachs for the more part, are hotter, by reason of the coldnesse of the clime, and therefore may digest better and naturally require more meate, and sooner, than other nations who inhabite hotter countryes'.[50]

At the heart of this debate seemed to lie the need to justify the English preference for eating a third meal: breakfast. This was a meal which in late sixteenth-century Italian regimens was not generally medically condoned, although, given the variation in local climates, the region where one lived influenced how often one should eat. There was, however, a broad consensus that, ordinarily speaking, for the non-labouring classes two meals, if moderately sized, were the ideal.[51] However, in his 1551 tract the English physician Wingfield cited Elyot closely, before explaining that 'breakfasts' were 'neessarye in thys Realme', on the grounds that 'perilous syckness' is likely 'if the heate inclosed in the stomacke have not convenient matter to worke on'.[52] And in 1600 William Vaughan noted as standard practice that one should 'eat three meals a day until you come to the age of forty years'.[53] Physician James Hart in 1633 legitimised the consumption of different foods and drinks as well as different eating practices in England on the same grounds.[54] Moreover, Vaughan seems to have used the cold climate to explain why the English (and other northern nationals) should not fast, unlike the Israelites, Spanish and Italians whose stomachs 'thanks to the vehement heat' of the climate were better able to go without food.[55] It is interesting, then, to see how only twenty years after the first publication of Elyot, this understanding of English men's 'cholericke' bodies bred by the distinctive climate, and, implicitly or explicitly distinct from southern bodies, had come to be accepted as the 'standard' healthy English body, and was reiterated over the coming decades. Indeed, as Anita Guerrini has shown, debates around which kind of diet was most appropriate for the English body in the English climate were rekindled at the end of the seventeenth and into the eighteenth centuries.[56]

Moderation and diet

Notions of moderation had formed the cornerstone of all aspects of healthy living advice ever since antiquity and, intersecting with ethical and religious ideals, were seen as particularly relevant to discussions of food and drink.[57] In view of this it is not surprising that in the context of the religious fervour of the sixteenth and seventeenth centuries, and given that gluttony was the first of the seven deadly sins, diatribes against immoderate eating and in favour of self-discipline, sobriety and temperance were common to authors across the religious divide. Yet, from relatively early on English authors focused more on the dangers of gluttony and went to greater lengths to embed correct eating practices firmly in religious rhetoric.

Bullein's 1559 *Government of Health* is an example, opening with a number of verses on the theme of the dangers of Bacchus, feasting, gluttony and unbridled lusts, and in praise of moderation. Moreover the first part of the dialogue starts with a debate on food as the 'foolish' speaker argues that abstinence is an enemy, and the 'wise' speaker counters this view, by explaining the rules of health.[58] Just two decades later Cogan uses eating practices to articulate a clear sense of a post-Reformation identity, as he refers back to the lengthy and overabundant meals of pre-Reformation prelates, taken as a cipher for all that was bad in the Catholic Church. 'In time past, when prelates were as princes, I mean before the suppression of Abbeys, as their fare was great, so they sate a great while at meate.'[59] And the belief that the Reformation had brought about some kind of fundamental change in dietary practices also emerges in the Puritan James Hart's 1633 regimen, when he claimed that the diet prescribed by Hippocrates 'differs greatly from that of our times … especially of this our land', particularly after 'the revolution of so many yeers'.[60] Although he does not elaborate on how that 'revolution' had altered the English diet, we can perhaps assume he was referring to an already familiar trope which constructed the ideal Protestant/Puritan body as being controlled and moderate in its food intake.

A common introductory topos to English discussions of food, which is entirely absent in Italy, is that of the fall of Adam and the link between food, sin and the body. In the introductory matter to *The Englishman's Doctor* (1608), allegedly a translation of the *Regimen Sanitatis Salernitanum*, the reader is reminded that the fall of Adam was occasioned through a fateful act of gluttony: as he walked through the garden of Eden 'He long'd for fruits unlawfull, fell to riots / wasted his god-like bodie by ill dyets.'[61]

The Flemish physician Ghesel who lived in England, and whose *Rule of Health* was translated into English in 1631, reminds the reader that 'Adam, by eating sinning, by sinning transmitting an inordinate appetite to all posterity.' This religious critique is then framed in a medical perspective as he explains how this act made humanity 'prone to surfeit, by surfet to gather noxious and hurtful humours, by these to lay the foundation of innumerable diseases ... and thus to death.'[62] Not dissimilarly, writing at around about the same time, Vaughan's comments on overeating drew on powerful religious imagery: that 'all men which respect their bodies as the temple of the holy ghost labour to keep themselves pure, without repletion or surfet.'[63] In Italy, by comparison, although gluttony was also routinely condemned, the tone is rarely as strident as anything we find in England, with the exception of one extremely moralising mid-seventeenth-century text which devotes nearly fifty pages to the dangers of immoderate eating.[64]

This said, there were two Catholic writers who if anything exceeded this Protestant emphasis on temperance. One was Alvise (also called Luigi) Cornaro, an Italian patrician who wrote four short tracts in Italian on sobriety in 1558, 1561, 1563 and 1565 which were then posthumously printed as a collected edition in 1591.[65] Cornaro was then translated into Latin in 1613 by Leonardo Lessius, a Flemish Jesuit, and printed as an 'appendix' to his own tract on eating, entitled the *Hygiasticon*. Both tracts were then translated into English and published in 1634.[66] This introduces an obvious complexity into a discussion of 'Catholic' and 'Protestant' bodies, particularly as these tracts appear to have had far greater impact on debates about eating in England than in Italy.

The basis of Cornaro's advice is that what gives the body the ability to withstand illness is the management of one's diet. Hence, if one's diet is above all Spartan (and he specifies twelve ounces of food, and fourteen of drink a day), the body can withstand almost any alterations of the humours derived from imbalances produced by 'heat and cold, wearinesse, watching, ill aire, overmuch use of the benefit of marriage'. In other words, the other Non-Naturals are deemed to have 'no great power' over bodies 'kept in good order by a moderate diet'.[67] The complex rules on food types, qualities and combinations which characterised traditional regimen are ignored, and he pointedly denied the late medieval belief that pleasure in eating was an indication that a food was beneficial to the body.[68]

Lessius's text was a more elegant elaboration of Cornaro's thesis which engages more directly with the fact that his advice, at a stroke, dismisses hundreds of years of debate regarding which foods men of differing complexions could and should eat, when, and how much. He criticises those regimen which 'charge men with so many rules' that they 'bring men into a labyrinth of care', indeed, 'perfect slavery' in their attempts to observe them.[69]

We can see how these two tracts – although penned by foreign Catholics – could have had such resounding success in Protestant/Puritan England.[70] Both stressed the virtues of living soberly and in the case of Lessius, which was aimed at men of letters, students at the Jesuit colleges and 'divines', explicitly addressed an increasingly vocal strand of criticism that some men devoted too much time to the care of their bodies, when what really mattered was the care of their souls. They both offered a wider public simple rules which enabled a 'self-help' approach to health suitable even for the 'common man' and offered men the chance to demonstrate self-discipline and temperance in a way which harmonised with Protestant ethics. Moreover, in its relentless focus on the role of the stomach in health Cornaro was possibly echoing and appealing to a kind of simplified 'popular' notion of illness causation, based around the stomach, of a kind described by Stolberg in his analysis of mid-sixteenth-century German lay and medical culture.[71] Both authors also dispensed with the complexities and obfuscations of Galenism, something which may have appealed particularly amongst more zealous religious sects, for whom Galenism was equated with anti-Christianism.[72] Indeed, prior to publication both texts had almost certainly been circulated within the strict religious community of Little Gidding given that it was Nicholas Ferrar, priest and founder of the community, who first translated Lessius into English. Moreover, his close friend George Herbert, the deeply religious poet and priest, was responsible for translating Cornaro for the first edition.[73]

Many references to these two authors in later seventeenth-century England testify to their popularity. In 1650 the physician Humphrey Brooke omits discussing the benefits of temperance since it has been 'so largely and plainly recited' in Lessius and Cornaro, 'both of which are almost at every booksellers to be had in English'.[74] Others refer to them as if their names were a byword for moderation: in 1659, Gayton advises his female patron to 'be your own *Lessius*, be to your self a *Cornara*'.[75] There were also more subtle influences: large chunks of Nicholas Culpeper's popular *Health for the rich and poor by dyet without physick* (1656) are actually passages copied directly from Lessius and slightly reworded, whilst the popular author Thomas Tyron's focus on the stomach and food as the main sources of health or illness accords well with the premises laid down by Cornaro and Lessius.

Yet there was also resistance to the strictness of their proposed diets and their disregard for individual complexions. Venner's 1620s regimen opens a discussion of diet with the topic of 'Whether a precise and exquisite manner of diet be best for the preservation of health?' He answers that those 'wholy addicting themselves to a curious and accurate kinde of diet are more likely to fall ill', and argues, contrary to Cornaro, that food 'taken with delectation is more welcome to the stomach, more firmly detained, and consequently better digested'.[76] Hart's 1633 regimen dismissed Lessian principles, particularly in a colder climate, except for those with very weak stomachs. Brook, pointing to the fundamental Galenic principle that one cannot prescribe the same diet to all bodies, given the differences between individual constitutions, wrote, 'I cannot approve of that *Arithmeticall Proportion* or *Dieta Statica* the allotment of a *certain weight and measure of meat and drink not upon any tearms to be exceeded* ... for how should the same shoo fit every foot.' He concludes they should leave 'the strictness of Lessius and Cornaro to speculative and monastick men'. Maynwaring's regimen dismisses it altogether.[77]

Marisa Milani has traced the success of Cornaro's texts with Anglo-Saxon readers and taken Gerolamo Cardano's praise of him in his 1580 regimen as a sign of his acceptance in Italy. Yet she also describes the debate and criticism with which they met, implying that his fame was partly a result of the polemical discussions sparked by his tracts.[78] If Cornaro was popular amongst the Italian public, this popularity was not echoed in vernacular health advice. All eight of the best-known Italian regimens were published in or after 1565 – after the last of Cornaro's had been printed – yet none of them emulated his approach. Indeed, it is hard to find any references to him or his ideas other than in Paschetti who implicitly dismisses Cornaro when he notes drily how 'difficult, serious and boring it would be' to have to weigh one's food.[79] On the contrary, all engaged in a more or less 'traditional' discussion of the proper place of eating in relation to the other five Non-Naturals with no obvious intrusion of 'new' approaches to eating.[80]

Coitus

Not surprisingly, the topic known as either 'venery' or 'coitus' provides some clear differences in treatment between the two confessional areas. In Galenic physiology semen was regarded as a 'useful' excrement – produced by abundant nutrition and which, like all excrements, had to be voided regularly for the good of one's health. The difficulty with venery was getting the right balance. Whilst retention – as with all excrements – was considered very damaging, it followed that moderate evacuation was associated with a range of benefits, exciting natural heat, lightening the body, mitigating passions, reviving the senses and the spirits and so on.[81] On the other hand, excessive 'use' brought with it an even longer list of dangers. Weakness, dissipation of the spirits, heart attacks, loss of sight, damage to the nerves and kidney stones, to name just a few.[82] Though women were not often mentioned, this was understood to be true for both sexes.[83]

The discussions surrounding how often it should be voided from the body generally came under the rubric of 'evacuations', sometimes that of exercise. Either way, it was rarely granted a separate chapter in Italian regimens and on the whole, Catholic authors tended to downplay discussions of venery, de-emphasising it and medicalising it. Boldo for example in 1575 lists in exhaustive detail the essential rules regarding when one could have coitus, at what time of day, in which season, how long after meals and so on.[84] The most extreme example of this is Traffichetti who, writing at the height of the Counter-Reformation, slips discreetly into the topic after a discussion of bloodletting, then provides an analysis of the physiology, with guidelines for use, 'neutralised' of any immodesty to the maximum. Thus, the particularly 'hot, damp, lively nature, of semen' means that 'it quickly boils and then putrefies, thereby becoming like poison … damaging the vertues and destroying natural heat'.[85] As a result it must be 'expelled, like something toxic and contrary … into the woman's belly'.[86]

Regulating the frequency of coitus was the central issue and there were different ways of presenting the solutions. One was to frame it in terms of avoiding 'artificial' stimuli, such as 'lascivious talk', on the understanding that left to itself 'nature does not often provoke this excrement'.[87] Another tack was to condemn those who allowed their senses to prevail over reason, thereby having coitus when they wanted to, rather than when they should do. This would result in ignoring the crucial rules regarding timing and frequency in relation to meals, bed-times and the climate, all of which acted as a framework within which one could 'expel' these wastes without endangering health or incurring questions of moral laxity.[88]

Presumably Catholic authors were also conscious of the difficulties of the debate given the generally unacknowledged fact that Catholic clerics, being celibate, were supposed also to be continent. Moreover, such men were very likely to be amongst their readers. Authors therefore navigate a subtle course between medical necessity and morality; between the fact that semen was a 'useful' excrement and one which should not be retained, and the dangers of excess. Perhaps for this reason few used discussions of venery as an opportunity to over-moralise the issue.[89] One of the few authors who referred, albeit obliquely, to this matter was Salando, in his short popular-style pamphlet printed in 1609. He avoided all explanations of the health imperatives of coitus, and concluded by commenting that 'a paucity of venereal acts benefits the soul, making man almost divine and benefits the body infinitely, lengthening life and preserving him from illness'.[90]

By contrast, regimens published in English tended to favour a more prominent, 'stand-alone' discussion of coitus, which was perhaps partly a result of the trend for following the Hippocratic structure in which 'Venery' was a category of its own as the last of the Hippocratic 'five words'. This also offered the perfect opportunity for authors to moralise, one which was seized on by most Protestant authors as they sought to downplay, even dismiss, the medical benefits of sex. Ghesel for example condemns those (implicitly, Galenists) who think 'we are about the business of health, when we are about the drudgery of carnall pleasure', and carries dire warnings about the multiple dangers of excess venery.[91] Moreover, after a brief introductory section, he announces that he will omit further discussion of the Non-Naturals in order to give himself more space to discuss 'Venus', which he notes, 'is of all the rest [of the Non-Naturals] the most dangerous'.[92]

Thomas Cogan had also undermined the delicate balance of factors inherent in the Galenic physiological framework by stating that the only area of a daily regimen in which excess would actually damage one's health was venery.[93] Cogan also openly expresses scepticism about the possibility of continence. Having listed the standard advice on the frequency of sexual activity with respect to one's age, he asks whether coitus could in fact be necessary for one's health, given that priests in the past had been forced to remain celibate with no detriment to their health. Moreover, students, despite being of an age when intercourse was considered medically essential, were unable to marry and by implication, were continent, yet also essentially healthy.

In keeping with this shift in emphasis to the morality of coitus, Protestant writers also tended to muster far more exhaustive lists of the many ways in which men should try to avoid the lusts and desires which lead them to any illegitimate expulsion of their seed. Going far beyond the advice on moderate eating and drinking familiar from Italian texts, they recommend a range of coolants, since venery was associated with excessive heat: men could cool their kidneys with ointments and their testicles by sitting on cold marble or by plunging them in cold water. Prayer and mediations on chastity were also highly recommended.[94]

Conclusion

This chapter suggests that despite the many obvious and necessary similarities between English and Italian regimens, we need now to pay far greater attention to the fact that they also differ in many significant ways. Despite their shared genealogy, starting with Thomas Elyot the often reiterated desire to help the 'commonweal' and speak to a Protestant commonwealth is a particularly English/Protestant feature which suggests that the intended readership, even of more serious regimens written by physicians or scholars, as opposed to just popular almanac-style texts, was at least *notionally* broader than that of comparable Italian regimens. The frequent recourse in texts in English to a Hippocratic classification of topics rather than a Galenic one is perhaps the most striking structural and conceptual embodiment of this attempt to present the advice in a new guise, ostensibly distancing it from the complexity of Galenism on the grounds that it was simpler and more suited to a wider readership. Likewise, the popularity of dialogue and question-and-answer formats even in lengthy regimens exemplifies this search for a more comfortable prose style. The trend towards simplification of content is also presumably one of the most significant reasons why Cornaro and Lessius and later Culpeper and Tyron were so popular. However, it must also be acknowledged that claims for a wide intended public were also marketing strategies in both countries. Ideally an analysis of the linguistic strategies used in the regimen in both countries would help ascertain the comparable 'ease' with which these texts could actually be read, whilst only a comparative study of evidence of readership and possession will enable us to offer broader observations on the extent to which the aspirations for a wider readership were matched in practice in both England and Italy.[95]

Over and above questions of readership, we also find that a Protestant/Puritan body was, in subtle but important ways, often constructed in English texts. However, it is interesting that authors engage more with notions of national identities than they do with religious identities, as the English body is constructed in opposition to a southern body, defined largely by the heat of the Mediterranean, particularly in discussions of climate, the air, even the porosity of the skin. Specific references to a distinctively Catholic body were very rare: if they appear it was most likely in relation to food and sex. Yet for all this, the fact that the southern body was also a Catholic one was implicit.[96] By contrast, Italian regimens barely ever define their subject in relation to an external 'other'. The body they discuss is neither Catholic nor Italian, but universal; that is, until the fascination with local differences causes this overarching model to fragment, allowing the appearance of distinctive 'local' bodies.

There is also a huge difference in the extent to which Protestant authors used health advice to moralise: the preserving of health was a 'Christian duty', for author and reader alike.[97] This shaped the actual text, its appearance, and sometimes its structure as well as giving space to authors to frame medical debates on food and sex within discussions of morality rather than merely health. Religion also had a tremendous impact on the 'passions', a Non-Natural which I have chosen not to discuss here, given the vast amount of scholarship on the topic.

Whether we pay specific attention to the minutiae of the advice, such as attitudes towards the cold or the pores, or whether we consider broader trends, such as the differing receptions of Cornaro and Lessius, these differences and discontinuities in the genre are striking. They lead us to the conclusion that rather than assuming that we are dealing with a common European 'body' of knowledge, we now need to pay more attention to the ways in which medical advice can illuminate the different national 'bodies' and the quite specific evolutions of medical ideas which underpinned them.

Notes

1 M. Fissell notes that the text went through at least seventeen editions. See 'Popular medical writing', in J. Raymond (ed.), *The Oxford History of Popular Print Culture*, 9 vols (Oxford: Oxford University Press, 2011), vol. 1, *Cheap Print in Britain and Ireland to 1660*, pp. 418–31.

2 An example of an earlier text is *The Governayle of Helthe* (Caxton, 1490 and 1506).

3 T. Elyot, *The Castel of Helth* (London: T. Berthelet, 1541, first ed. 1534). For a detailed discussion of Elyot's preface see A. Wear, 'The popularisation of medicine in Early Modern England', in R. Porter (ed.), *The Popularisation of Medicine 1650–1850* (London: Routledge, 1992), pp. 17–41, on pp. 20–4.

4 W.D. Sharpe, 'Thomas Linacre 1460–1524: an English physician scholar of the Renaissance', *Bulletin of the History of Medicine*, 34 (1960), pp. 233–56. On his time in Italy, pp. 238–9. On Elyot and Linacre, p. 242. On translations, p. 250. On regimens in Italian universities, see M. Nicoud, *Les régimes de santé au Moyen Âge: naissance et diffusion d'une écriture médicale (XIIIe–XVe siècle)* (Rome: École Françaíse de Rome, 2007), pp. 15–18 and chapter 7.

5 Elyot, *Castel*, preface. On Italian medicine as viewed from England and Linacre's contribution see V. Nutton, 'John Caius and the Linacre tradition', *Medical History*, 23:4 (1979), pp. 373–91, esp. pp. 377–9.

6 See S. Cavallo and T. Storey, *Healthy Living in Late Renaissance Italy* (Oxford: Oxford University Press, 2013), pp. 270–9.

7 V.S. Smith, *Clean. A History of Personal Hygiene and Purity* (Oxford: Oxford University Press, 2007).

8 See in particular A. Wear, 'Place, health and disease: the *Airs, Waters, Places* tradition in Early Modern England and North America', *Journal of Medieval and Early Modern Studies*, 38:3 (2008), pp. 443–65. See also his 'The popularisation'. He discusses other aspects of the English regimens in

'Making sense of health and the environment in Early Modern England', in A. Wear (ed.), *Medicine in Society: Historical Essays* (Cambridge: Cambridge University Press, 1992), pp. 119–47.

9 P. Murray Jones, 'Medical literacies and medical culture in early modern vernacular medicine', in I. Taavitsainen and P. Pahta (eds), *Medical Writing in Early Modern English* (Cambridge: Cambridge University Press, 2011), pp. 30–43, on p. 32.

10 On the use of vernacular regimens see J. Richards, 'Useful books: reading vernacular regimens in sixteenth-century England', *Journal of the History of Ideas*, 73:2 (2012), pp. 247–71.

11 In 'Medical literacies', p. 32, Murray Jones argues that at the cheapest end of the market volumes of prognostications cost about 2d. In 'Mirrors', p. 247, Slack notes that a copy of *The Castel* could be had for 6d in the decades around 1600 whilst other medical textbooks cost from 4 shillings to 48 shillings. From this I suggest that *The Castel* could also have circulated amongst readers at the poorer end of the spectrum.

12 On Berthelet see H.S. Bennett, *English Books and Readers*, 3 vols (Cambridge: Cambridge University Press, 1970), especially vol. 1 (1474–1557), pp. 42–3, 103, 153.

13 This distinction is explained by P.M. Jones. However, although *The Castel* is in this typeface he then assigns it to the category of texts which required the greatest degree of cultural literacy to read it. 'Medical literacies', pp. 32–3.

14 Compare this to the layout of A. Boorde's *Compendyous Regiment* (London: Thomas Colwell, 1542), clearly addressed to those able to build their own house 'or any mansion place': it has no margins, no breaks on the page, few subheadings and barely any use of space to visually articulate the text.

15 W. Bullein's *Government of Health* went through two editions (1559, 1595), as did his *Bulwarke* (1562, 1579). W. Vaughan (1602) and T. Venner (1620) also adopted the dialogue form. For an innovative approach to analysing medical texts for clues to their intended readership, see V. Marttilam, 'New arguments for new audiences: a corpus-based analyses of interpersonal strategies in Early Modern English medical recipes', in Taavitsainen and Pahta (eds), *Medical Writing*, pp. 135–57.

16 On Paracelsus' beliefs and their impact, C. Webster, 'Paracelsus. Medicine as popular Protest', in A. Cunningham and O.P. Grell (eds), *Medicine and the Reformation* (London, New York: Routledge, 1993), pp. 57–77, on p. 86. Also *The Great Instauration: Science, Medicine and Reform 1626–1600* (London: Duckworth, 1975), p. 247.

17 On the evolution of the doctrine of the 'six Non-Natural things' see Luis García-Ballester, 'Galen and Galenism on the origins of the "six Non-Natural things" in Galen', *Galen and Galenism* (Aldershot: Ashgate, 2002), pp. 105–15. On this periodisation Pedro Gil-Sotres, 'The regimens of

health', in M.D. Grmek (ed.), *Western Medical Thought from Antiquity to the Middle Ages* (Cambridge, MA: Harvard University Press, 1998), pp. 291–396, on p. 295.

18 Christopher Langton, *An Introduction into Physycke with an universal dyet* (London: Edwarde Whytchurche, *c.*1547). See http://0-www.oxforddnb.com/view/article/16039 for biographical details.

19 See the entry for Grataroli by A. Pastore in *Dizionario Biografico degli Italiani*, www.treccani.it/enciclopedia/ricerca/grataroli/Dizionario_Biografico/.

20 Both from the author's preface in G. Grataroli, *A Direction for the Health of Magistrates and students* (London: William How, 1574, first pub. Latin 1555).

21 D. Cantor argues that by the seventeenth century Hippocrates had become a symbol of empiricism and practice against Galenism, which stood for rationalism and theory; see *Reinventing Hippocrates* (Aldershot: Ashgate, 2002), p. 6. See also H. Mikkeli, *Hygiene in the Early Modern Medical Tradition* (Helsinki: Finnish Academy of Science and Letters, 1999) on the shift in favour of Hippocrates during the sixteenth century, pp. 26–7, 57.

22 T. Cogan, *The Haven of Health* (London: Thomas Orwin, 1589).

23 *Ibid.*, 'To the Reader'.

24 For example Aldobrandino da Siena, *Le Régime du corps*; Ugo Benzi, *Tractato Utilissimo*; Maino de Maineri, *Opera Utilissima di Arnaldo da Villanova.*

25 See Cavallo and Storey, *Healthy Living*, pp. 79–80.

26 T. Giannotti Rangoni, *Thomaso philologo da Rauenna. Come l'huomo può viuere piu de CXX anni* (Venice: Matheum Paganum a Fide, 1556). A.T. Petronio, *Del viver delli Romani, et di conservare la sanità* (Rome: Domenico Basa, 1592). B. Paschetti, *Del conservar la sanità* (Genoa: Giuseppe Pavoni, 1602). See also the chapter by Maria Conforti in this volume for her discussion of texts relating to the climate of Naples.

27 Petronio, *Del Viver*, pp. 1, 199–270.

28 Elyot, *Castel*, c. 41r. W. Bullein, *A newe boke of phisicke called ye government of health* (London: John Day, 1559), p. 79. Cogan, *Haven*, p. 4. H. Ronsovius, *The English Man's Doctor or The Schoole of Salerne* (London: W. Stansby, 1617), p. 14, and, by implication, E. Maynwaring, *Vita Sana e Longa: The Preservation of Health and Prolongation of Life* (London: J.D., 1669), p. 45.

29 Respectively, Elyot, *Castel*, p. 41; Cogan, *Haven*, p. 4; W. Vaughan's, *Directions for Health, naturall and artificial* (London: Bradock, 1602), p. 63; J. Archer, *Everyman his own Doctor* (London: printed for the author, 1673), pp. 16–17.

30 Elyot, *Castel*, p. 42; Cogan, *Haven*, preface to reader, p. 2; J. Hart, *Klinike or the Diet of the diseased* (London: J. Beale, 1633), p. 25.

31 Wear, 'Place, health and disease', pp. 448–51. This understanding of the impact of cold air is based on a passage from the Hippocratic *Airs, Waters, Places.* See also Frances Gage's chapter in this volume citing Panaroli's reference to this matter (pp. 239–43).
32 T. Venner, *Via Recta ad Vitam Longan Pars Secunda* (London: G.Eld, 1623), pp. 4–5. For other examples see Elyot, *Castel,* p. 40; Cogan, *Haven,* p. 3; Vaughan, *Directions,* pp. 7, 11; T. Moffett, (London: T. Newcombe, 1655), p. 83.
33 For a full account of this shift see Smith, *Clean,* pp. 212–23.
34 On understandings of the role of the pores in this period see M. Te Hennepe, 'Of the fisherman's net and skin pores. Reframing conceptions of the skin in medicine 1572–1714', in M. Horstmanshoff, H. King, and C. Zittel (eds), *Blood, Sweat and Tears: The Changing Concepts of Physiology from Antiquity into Early Modern Europe* (Leiden, Boston: Brill, 2012), pp. 523–48. Also M. Stolberg, 'Sweat. Learned concepts and popular perceptions, 1500–1800', in *ibid.,* pp. 503–22.
35 These are the functions of inhaled air, however it enters the body.
36 'Havendo in quell'hora aperti tutti li meati, tirarà a se l'aere più puro.' Petronio, *Del Viver,* p. 301. Te Hennepe explores this function in the context of Mercuriale's discussion of the skin in *De Morbis Cutaneis* (1572), 'Of the fisherman's net', pp. 526–7.
37 For example the tracts by M. Ficino and G. Daciano, both in *Consiglio di Marsilio Ficino Fiorentino contro la pestilentia. Insime con ... altri Autori* (Florence: I. Giunti, 1576), pp. 8 and 5, respectively.
38 H. Brooke, *Ugieine: Conservatory of Health* (London: R.W., 1650), p. 120.
39 F. Bacon, Viscount St Albans, *History Naturall and Experimentall of Life and Death, or of the Prolongation of Life* (London: Lee and Mosely, 1651), p. 21. Maynwaring also notes that cool air 'keeps the spirits vigorous', whilst the great heat of 'southern climates' causes 'so great a transpiration that exsiccates and ennervates the body', accounting for lethargic temperaments; *Vita Sana,* p. 2.
40 Bacon, *History Naturall,* p. 36 item 8.
41 An exception as regards discussions of breathing putrid air is B. Pietragrassa, *Politica medica per il governo conservativo del corpo humano* (Pavia: Gio Andrea Magri, 1649). He notes it is 'breathed and attracted by the pores' ('respirata e attratta per le cutanee aperture'), p. 454.
42 'Et è così grande il beneficio che ... vien affirmato dipendere in gran parte di qua la conservazione della sanità.' V. Viviani, *Trattato del custodire la sanità* (Venice: Girolamo Piuti, 1626), p. 114.
43 Pietragrassa, *Politica medica,* p. 198.
44 Petronio, *Del Viver,* p. 299.

45 Paschetti, *Del Conservare*, p. 86. For a detailed discussion of all these issues see Cavallo and Storey, *Healthy Living*, pp. 73–5.
46 The most interested author seems to be Venner, *Via Recta*.
47 Vaughan, *Directions*, p. 11.
48 Hart, *Klinike*, p. 18.
49 This emerges from his extended discussion on when to eat; Elyot, *Castel*, pp. 40–1 in the 1541 edition.
50 Cogan, *Haven*, p. 183 and a similar passage on p. 4.
51 See for example B. Boldo, pp. 288–91, and Paschetti, *Del Conservare*, pp. 65, 85.
52 H. Wingfield, A *Compendious or Short Treatise* (London: R. Stoughten, 1551), in chapter 2. See also Elyot, *Castel*, p. 41. As a contrast, in the 1602 regimen by the Italian physician Paschetti, the author points out that the climate in the region around Genoa is so healthy that all who live there only ever need to eat twice a day. *Del Conservare*, p. 65.
53 Vaughan, *Directions*, p. 73.
54 Hart, *Klinike*, p. 37.
55 Vaughan, *Directions*, p. 63. The way it is phrased is, however, ambiguous.
56 A. Guerrini, 'Health, national character and the English diet in 1700', *Studies in History and Philosophy of Biological and Biomedical Sciences*, 43:2 (2012), pp. 349–56, on p. 350.
57 See S. Shapin's extended discussion of this topic in 'How to eat like a gentleman: dietetics and ethics in Early Modern England', in C.E. Rosenberg (ed.), *Right Living: An Anglo-American Tradition of Self-help Medicine and Hygiene* (Baltimore: Johns Hopkins University Press, 2003), pp. 21–58.
58 Bullein, *Government*, pp. 1–2.
59 Coghan, *Haven*, p. 187.
60 Hart, *Klinike*, p. 25.
61 Ronsovius, *The English Man's Doctor*, n.p.
62 John Ghesel, *Rule of Health* (Cambridge: Printers to the Universitie, 1633), p. 2.
63 Vaughan, *Directions*, p. 62.
64 E. Frediano, *Arca novella di sanità* (Lucca: Iacinto Paci, 1656), pp. 89, 92–3, 103–4.
65 L. Cornaro, *Discorsi della vita sobria* (Padua: Miglietti, 1591). On Cornaro see the introductory essay by M. Milani to *Writings on the Sober Life: The Art and Grace of Living Long*, ed. M. Milani, G. Critser and H. Fudemoto (Toronto: University of Toronto Press, 2014), pp. 3–71.
66 L. Cornaro, *A treatise of Temperance and Sobrietie*, published with L. Lessius, *Hygiasticon: or The right course of preserving life and health unto extream old age* (Cambridge: R. Daniel and T. Buck, 1634).

67 Cornaro, *A Treatise*, pp. 10–11.
68 *Ibid.*, p. 8. On pleasure in eating see Nicoud, *Les régimes*, pp. 367–77.
69 Lessius, *Hygiasticon*, pp. 1–2.
70 On their impact see also K. Albala, *Eating Right in the Renaissance* (Berkeley: University of California Press, 2002), pp. 37–41.
71 Michael Stolberg, '"You have not good blood in your body". Oral communication in sixteenth-century physicians' medical practice', *Medical History*, 59:1 (2015), pp. 63–82.
72 See P. Elmer, 'Medicine, religion and the puritan revolution', in R. French and A. Wear (eds), *The Medical Revolution of the Seventeenth Century* (Cambridge: Cambridge University Press, 1989), pp. 10–45, on p. 13.
73 In Italy there were only three more editions in the early seventeenth century. After this it was published as an addendum to the *Regimen Sanitatis*. On this circle and the translation see M. Milani, 'How to attain immortality living one hundred years, or, the fortune of the *Vita Sobria* in the Anglo-Saxon world', in *Writings on the Sober Life*, pp. 183–213, pp. 193–7, and entries on George Herbert and Nicholas Ferrar in the *ODNB*. www.oxforddnb.com.view/article/9356?docPos=1 and www.oxforddnb.com.view/article/13025?docPos=1. Also J.F.M. Carter, *Nicholas Ferrar His household and His Friends* (London and New York: Longman, 1892), pp. 226–9.
74 Brooke, *Ugieine*, p. 12.
75 E. Gayton, *The Art of Longevity or a Diaeteticall Institution* (London: printed for the author, 1659). A physician and religious ascetic, Gayton claimed in the introduction that he could live on even less food than Lessius.
76 Venner, *Via Recta*, pp. 169, 174.
77 Brooke, *Ugieine*, pp. 101–2, italics in the original. The quote also refers to Ars Sanctorii Sanctorii de statica medicina (Venice: Nicolò Polo, 1614) and to Santorio's theories on measuring metabolic processes. Maynwaring, *Vita Sana*, preface and p. 54.
78 On Cornaro's rebuttals of criticism, M. Milani, 'Introduction to Cornaro', in *Writings on the Sober Life*, pp. 14, 15, 17, 19, and 'How to attain immortality', in *ibid.*, pp. 183–213, on pp. 187–9. See also comments in Cavallo and Storey, *Healthy Living*, pp. 16–17.
79 'Difficile, così grave e noiso sarebbe …dovendo da una banda il cibo, dall'altra la bilancia tenere'. Paschetti, *Del Conservare*, p. 88.
80 This contrasts with Albala's view that regimens after the 1570s 'tend' to engage in criticism of traditional food rules. Perhaps this is only true of England or the shift is more deeply embedded in the discussions of individual foods. *Eating Right*, pp. 37–41.
81 C. Durante, *Il tesoro della sanità* (Venice: Andrea Muschio, 1586), p. 43.

82 Paschetti, *Del Conservar*, p. 215.

83 See for example Hart, *Klinike*, p. 328, and R. Fonseca, *Del conservare la sanitá* (Florence: Semartelli, 1603), p. 87.

84 Boldo, *Libro della Natura*, p. 261.

85 'Calda e humida, e spiritosa onde facilmente ne seguita bullitione, e putrefatione di essa la quale quale cosi putrefatta acquista natura di veneno e fa sevissimi accidenti, simili alli accidenti del veneno, che prosternono la vertù, e mortificano il calor.' Traffichetti, *L'arte di conservare la salute tutta intiera* (Pesaro: Girolamo Concordia, 1565), p. 132.

86 *Ibid.*

87 *Ibid.*

88 Paschetti, *Del Conservar*, pp. 214–15. For a discussion of venery in regimens see also Cavallo and Storey, *Healthy Living*, pp. 268–9.

89 The exceptions were L. Lennio (a Flemish Catholic physician and astrologer), *Della complessione del corpo humano* (Venice: Domenico Nicolino, 1564), and *Scuola salernitana del modo di conseruarsi in sanità* (Perugia: Petrucci, 1587), edited and translated by Serafino Razzi, a Catholic friar.

90 'Paucità delle cose veneree prima giova all'anima facendo l'uomo quasi divino, giova anche infinitamente al corpo, prolungando la vita e preservando l'uomo da infermità.' F. Salando, *Trattato sopra la regola del vivere nelle sei cose chiamate da' Medici non naturali* (Verona: Angelo Tamo, 1607), p. 15.

91 Ghesel, *Rule of Health*, p. 4.

92 *Ibid.*, p. 11.

93 Cogan, *Haven*, p. 278.

94 *Ibid.*, pp. 285–6.

95 See for example Martilla's analysis of language use in 'New arguments for new audiences', pp. 135–57.

96 The direct attack on Catholic sexuality in Hart, *Klinike*, is probably unique.

97 P. Slack notes the blurring of boundaries between medical and religious language and concerns in publications in England in general. 'Mirrors of health', p. 255.

V

Spaces, paintings and objects: performing and portraying health

9

Chasing 'good air' and viewing beautiful perspectives: painting and health preservation in seventeenth-century Rome

Frances Gage

For early moderns, good air was synonymous with good health. The iconographer, Vincenzo Cartari, in his *Immagini degli dei degli antichi* (1571), quoted the ancient geographer Pausanias as having remarked that Aesculapius, the god of medicine, was 'nothing other than air, which is purged by the sun in a way that offers health to mortals'.[1] The importance of breathing 'good air' was regularly stressed by early modern physicians; those tending the princess Olimpia Aldobrandini when she found herself in delicate physical and mental health in 1668 urged her to enjoy 'fresh air, "which should be clear, benign, and healthy, and of that kind, as the air of Frascati"'.[2] Early modern physicians and laymen agreed that air quality affected health and that distinct locations might be associated with 'good air' (as at Frascati) or bad, but how men and women went about identifying air as pure and healthy in actual practice and how closely their efforts corresponded to conventional health recommendations is far less clear. An examination of early modern letters and Roman news reports demonstrates that men and women not only performed qualitative judgements about the relative warmth, humidity or purity of the atmosphere itself, but also observed those factors thought to indicate a region's air quality, particularly its topography and agriculture. If these tangible signs of 'good' or 'bad' air, investigated at the outset of this essay, were regularly invoked in the quest for the healthiest air, they nevertheless sometimes proved to be misleading. This underscores the difficulty early moderns encountered first in ascertaining what constituted healthy air, and second the potential health effects of a given environment upon an individual or group. Additional complications could also arise when they sought to identify healthy air by location, as in a city such as Rome. Its varied topography was associated with opposing types of air and their contrary health effects, thus leading to conflictual judgements about Rome's air. Yet residents of Rome developed a distinct medical practice – moving between their different lodgings – in order to secure access to healthy (or at least healthier) air. Although this has been widely acknowledged in the scholarly literature, I will demonstrate that the frequency and pervasiveness of this practice was far greater than has hitherto been recognised. At the same time, the Roman habit of continually relocating to other areas in the city or countryside was evidently still considered inadequate in the quest to ensure constant access to healthy air. Roman physicians therefore recommended, and laymen developed, techniques to mitigate the negative effects of 'bad air' when staying put. Among these was the recommendation which will be examined in the second half of the essay, that material adornment of interior spaces, particularly through pictorial perspectives, might preserve overall health. The positive effect of perspectives on the spirits governing the passions was obtained through the faculties of sight and the imagination, which could produce the passions of delight and cheerfulness fundamental to a healthy body.

Good air or bad air

In 1613, Giovanni Battista Bandi, the nephew of Giulio Mancini, a Sienese physician at Rome's Hospital of Santo Spirito, wrote to his uncle Deifebo after arriving to take up the governorship of Veroli, a town in the Roman *campagna* (countryside). Boasting of the location's natural benefits, Bandi remarked that the land around Veroli was fertile and abundant and that the city was favoured with 'very good air'.[3] Three weeks later, Bandi wrote again, having reached the opposite conclusion:

> [I]n the past I have been oppressed by vapours to the head, most vehement towards the teeth and ears with almost continual sorrow, at the

> present I find myself rather liberated; all [of these symptoms] I attribute to the change of air, which is most cold, most subtle and most inclement, this city being positioned on a hill that is rather rugged [*sgreste*], so that it is most ugly within [town], although the *campagna* shows much that is pleasing, accompanied with the most good size fruit of all kinds.[4]

To describe what now turned out to be the very bad air on this particular hill, Bandi linked it to the poor quality of the soil (which many writers thought was conditioned by air), describing the terrain with the term 'sgreste', or 'agreste', a word suggesting a pungent, acidic flavour and associated with a grape that does not ripen fully. Lending further weight to his description of what caused his recent ills was a worrisome attribute of the town's current climate. At that moment, Veroli's air was *sottillissima,* a characteristic typical of 'good air' and suggesting the pure, light, dry air enjoyed on high ground – the opposite of the heavy, thick, dusty, humid 'bad air' in low-lying places.[5] In this case, however, the elevated position of Veroli and its most subtle air did not ensure its salubriousness. Describing the air as *inclementissima,* Bandi underscored the extreme temperatures Veroli was experiencing, cold air and wind being pressing health concerns among sixteenth- and seventeenth-century medical writers and laymen. Not everyone would attribute health dangers to cold air, however. François-Auguste de Thou, a French diplomat residing on the hilly area around the French church of Santa Trinità dei Monti in Rome, remarked in 1627 on the 'great healthfulness' of the season on account of the 'great cold' and the Tramontana blowing from the north.[6] Hailing from northern Europe, he was undoubtedly more accustomed to cold temperatures than others, but Domenico Panaroli, a physician at the Roman hospital of San Salvatore and later professor of anatomy and botany at the Sapienza, argued in his 1641 treatise *Aërologia* that northern climes, provided they are not excessively cold, are better than southern ones (especially for Romans considering travel), for they make men robust, strong and prolong life.[7] In Bandi's case, however, the dry and extremely cold air of Veroli was unseasonal. Given that it was late April, spring should have arrived with its warming temperatures and humid air, both qualities which the physician Bartolomeo Pietragrassa thought made this season 'healthy and sympathetic to the complexion of living beings'.[8] The air of Veroli was particularly dangerous because it was out of sync with customary spring weather.

Bandi discovered he was unable to substantiate Veroli's reputation for good air, but the inverse problem occurred when the physician Scipione Mercurio was called to a town reputed for its terrible air: Peschiera, near Lake Garda. Notwithstanding the unhealthy locals, who 'are all without colour', and who, during winter, are either languishing or convalescing and in summer are like 'infected dying sheep', Mercurio himself found the region healthy.[9] In his account, he set out for Peschiera ill and immediately regained his strength.[10] Consequently, he purchased an estate 'upon a pleasant, gracious hill top, with optimum air, a most fruitful place, rich in olives, abounding with vines, endowed with the most pleasant fruit, where the air is most pure, and the sky serene'.[11] Significantly, he persuaded his readers of his estate's 'optimum air' by linking it to the abundance of olives and vines.[12] Although Mercurio and Bandi discovered they could not rely on mere regional or local reputation when characterising a location's air quality, both considered it a reasonable supposition that a site would enjoy good air if it were elevated, fertile and produced abundant, sweet or large fruit or was embellished with vines and olives. Indeed, the strong links observed here between air, fertile soil, the abundance of foliage and rich agricultural land finds substantial support among contemporary writers on meteorology. For instance the writer Stefano Breventano from Pavia remarked that air makes 'the cereal [*biade*] and grass grow and directs trees to send forth branches', doing so, in part, through the agency of Favonius, or Zephyr, the West Wind, which Panaroli called 'the father of life', and whose warmth and humidity drapes the earth with 'rather beautiful flowers' (*lascivetti fiori*) and green plants.[13] The association between trees, plants and pure air was long-standing; some early modern writers remarked, for instance, that air quality was improved when the winds blew over trees, while others argued that trees softened or refined the air.[14]

Agriculture was championed in sixteenth- and seventeenth-century treatises for contributing to health and longevity overall, while fruit and flowering trees, vines and olives were celebrated for their salubrious effects upon the air.[15] The political theorist Giovanni Botero would even recommend that the air of the Roman *campagna* could be ameliorated if local forests were cleared and the land turned over to apple orchards (and other fruit trees) and gardens, suggesting that fruit trees and cultivated zones were more beneficial than green trees or wild plants.[16] The physician and professor Vincentius Alsarius Crucius, carrying on an ancient literary tradition, argued that trees (presumably flowering and fruit trees) in gardens purified the air through their aromatic qualities.[17]

Attention to the health benefits of agriculture in this period may have been additionally fostered by a constellation of associated factors which bolstered claims for the utility and pleasure that cultivation afforded landowners, regions and nations. Although Mancini disapproved of noblemen engaging in agriculture for any reason other than pleasure and health, he did not fail to remark on its financial rewards, noting that in Lombardy trees were planted upon the birth of a daughter in anticipation that their sale would provide her dowry when she reached marriageable age.[18] Moreover agriculture was increasingly promoted by writers across the Continent and beyond as a wise investment for men of varied classes. Vincenzo Tanara in his treatise *L'economo del cittadino in villa* (1674) recommended this profession as a desirable alternative for a man who possessed neither the talent nor inclination for the traditional Renaissance paths of arms or letters.[19] Other writers, too, remarked on the fact that it promised virtuous profits acquired through honest labour and without the taint of court or trade. Yet success in planting depended upon a householder's careful consideration of the appropriate site (especially for vines), terrain, elevation, soil quality, climate and winds.[20]

Stay put

Judging whether a location enjoyed good air, either theoretically or empirically, required consideration of numerous contingencies and sometimes gave rise to quite conflicting assertions, particularly at a time when this Non-Natural was receiving increased attention in vernacular health manuals and in practices of health preservation and convalescence.[21] As Panaroli noted, the options for managing the effects of air on the body were far less well known than those regarding other Non-Naturals.[22] One could avoid a particular food or renounce a given habit, but one must necessarily take in air even if finding oneself in an undesirable location.[23] Seventeenth-century documentation bears out Panaroli's claim that managing this Non-Natural posed unusual difficulties, particularly in the Eternal City. There was often significant disagreement concerning air quality among medical practitioners and thus a collective uncertainty about how to regulate health with regard to it.

Judgements that a particular site was healthful were passed upon ever-smaller zones and sites, as though this might yield a modicum of certainty about a mobile, changeable element. Montaigne, in a famous passage in his Roman journal, remarked about the fine distinctions made not only between quarters of the city, but also between apartments: hence the Roman habit of moving among various residences according to the season.[24] And subtle divisions were also drawn between districts in the countryside. Giovanni Battista Agucchi, secretary to Cardinal Pietro Aldobrandini, remarking on the air in the location of the papal family's Villa Belvedere at Frascati, declared that 'only *this spot* remains free of harmful properties and is practically the only refuge … [from] Rome'.[25]

Not only did Bandi attribute his recent ailment, described as 'vapours to the head' to the extreme cold, but also to the 'change of air', another widespread preoccupation of early modern medical writers. Bandi's letter leaves it unclear, however, whether he was attributing his health problems to local climate changes or to his recent move from one town with a distinct climate to another, or perhaps to both circumstances at once. The first of three interrelated issues addressed by writers considering the health effects of local changes in air was the mutation in its quality, depending upon winds, season and the time of day. Indeed, air was 'never immobile' and 'never so firm or so quiet that it is not in some sort of agitation'.[26] That mobility, as Breventano assured his readers, 'renders it helpful and vital to whomever breathes it', but seasonal and climatological alterations might pose benefits or dangers to health.[27] In 1627, for instance, Cesare Perini, another of Giulio Mancini's nephews, cautioned Deifebo against venturing out of his room until 'he felt a more temperate season', at which point he could anticipate recovering from illness.[28] A second consideration was the effects of the interaction between the ambient temperature and the changing temperature of a mobile body. In the same letter, Perini expressed concern that Deifebo found he had to ascend and descend stairs, prompting sudden and marked fluctuations to bodily temperature, particularly when the climate had already contributed to Deifebo's ailments.[29]

The third and final consideration pertained to the effects of encountering a distinct type of air when travelling to a new location (whether a city, region or zone). This concern intersected with the growing attention paid to regional climates following encounters with hitherto unknown regions of the world (spurring attention to questions of human diversity) and as a consequence of the dissemination of Hippocrates' *Airs, Waters and Places*. This text, which set forth a geography of regional climates and the corresponding temperaments of their inhabitants, was to exert a significant impact in the sixteenth and seventeenth centuries, serving as a foundation for writers of health regimens to disseminate medical advice according to classifications by regional or national rather than individual complexions.[30] With respect to air, that of one's native territory was considered the most healthy, even if it could not be classified absolutely as 'good air'. Panaroli cautioned his readers that 'the man who does not leave the climate of his fatherland finds a location rather proportionate to health'.[31] In light of this, the best approach to preserving one's health, he added, is to 'stay put'.[32] At the same time, if one no longer resided in one's birthplace or if one found oneself ill, one was likely to receive advice to avail oneself of a 'change of air', and often an exhortation to return to one's native soil. Cardinal Caetano, for instance, having been named Legate to Bologna, ascertained for himself that the air there was not suitable to his temperament and renounced the post, insisting upon a new one.[33]

Roman air

Panaroli recognised, of course, that many would have to leave their native lands and travel to distant areas with diverse climates from those in which they had been born and raised.[34] This was particularly true among Panaroli's readers, who filled Rome's ecclesiastical ranks or who were their clients, many having migrated to that 'most universal city', and who often travelled elsewhere on official business. Indeed, diaries and general manuals for travellers confer a prominent place to topography and climate; for Giulio Mancini, they are the first aspects of a region a traveller should observe.[35] It is hardly surprising, then, that when his brother Deifebo contemplated relocating to Rome in 1631, his nephew promised that his house, where Deifebo would stay, is 'airy with good air'.[36]

Identifying a site with good air, suitable to animate a body with a specific disposition and environmental conditioning, was no straightforward undertaking, particularly in Rome with its disparate topographies and sites. Early modern perceptions of Rome's air have been largely represented as negative ever since Francesco Cancellieri in his *Lettera ... al Ch. Sig. Dottore Koreff ... sopra il tarantismo, l'aria di Roma e della sua campagna ...* of 1817, the first broad history of Roman air, argued that the perception of the city as having '*aria cattiva*' (bad air) crystallised during the Renaissance with the resumption of *villeggiatura*.[37] It is true that Renaissance Rome had so come to be associated with ruins and decay that Montaigne could remark that it is nothing but the sepulchre of the ancient city.[38] Medical writers such as Panaroli, moreover, considered tombs and grottoes to be sources of rotting matter, while animal waste and vapours were apt to corrupt the air; ruins would have likely elicited similar concern.[39] An analogous idea is expressed by the Netherlandish printmaker Hieronymus Cock, who drew a direct connection between Rome's hot, humid atmosphere and its overgrown ruins.[40] In his *View of the Palatine with the Septizonium* (1551) the sun's rays seemingly produce exhalations of humid vapours that form thick, heavy clouds (Fig. 9.1). These billow towards the ruins, formally echoing at the same time the bushy shrubs and rising ground enveloping the Septizonium, and suggesting that the atmosphere generates the organic growth that overcomes these ancient structures. In this era of major archeological excavations, the exploration of the catacombs and massive building projects transformed regions of the city into dusty construction sites so that the city could not but be perceived as producing foul air.[41]

Nevertheless, if Roman ruins suggested to some a city of 'bad air', they increasingly promised healthful recreation to others. One of Rome's most significant ruins – the Colosseum – became a site of botanical exploration which led to the discovery of hundreds of species of flora. These were compiled by Panaroli in his 1643 treatise *Plantarum amphitheatralium catalogus*, in which he also noted violets and melissa, the very flowers that he had recommended a year earlier in his *Aërologia* for improving the air in 'intimate domestic spaces' by cooling it. Moreover, the numerous medicinal species growing within the monument made it possible, without Panaroli explicitly saying so, to reconceive of the Colosseum as a garden of simples.[42] A visual argument that Rome's ruins could be similarly revitalised was made by Jean Lemaire in his composite and imaginary *vedute* of Roman ruins as sites for the gathering of flowers, as in *View with a Circular Ruined Portico ... with Two Ancients Who Gather Flowers* (Prado, Madrid), or as a setting for a

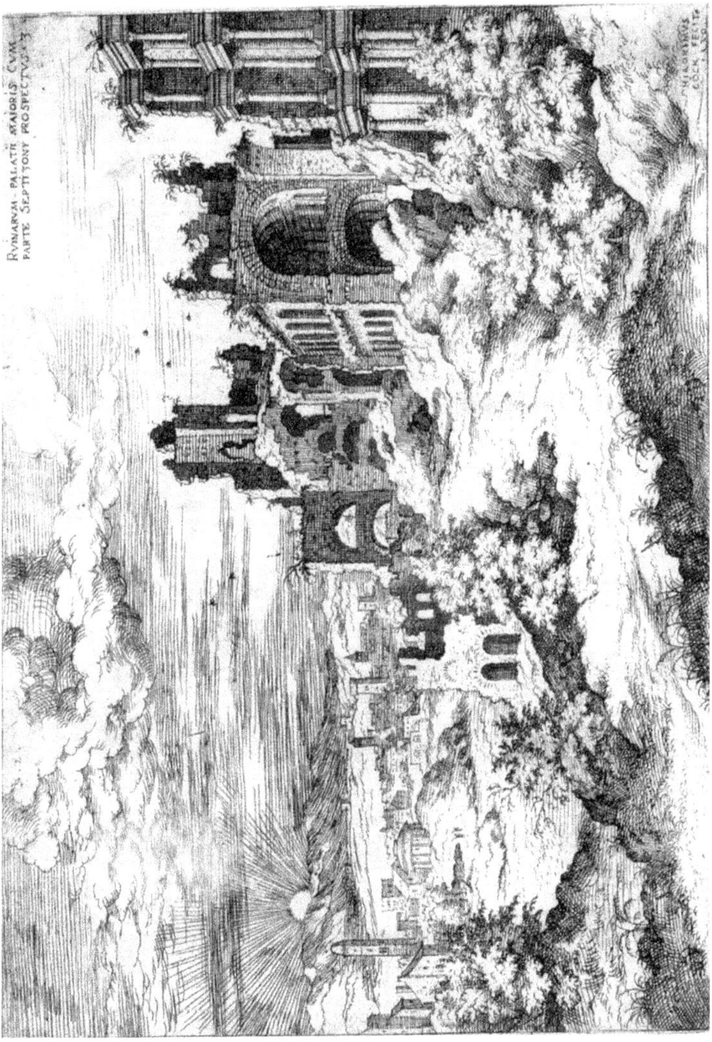

Figure 9.1 Hieronymus Cock, *View of the Palatine with the Septizonium*, 1551

garden, as in *Landscape with a Ruined Edifice in the Wings, a Ruined Theater as a Backdrop with the Story of Vertumnus and Pomona* (National Museum, Stockholm).[43] Here Lemaire challenged conventional images of overgrown ruins (though weeds grow upon the wall at left), transforming these structures into the precinct for a formal garden casually festooned with vines and fruit. Like nature's ever-recurring cycles, these grand ruins suggest renewal rather than decay, the object of human intervention and cultivation, together with the gardens.

Just as Rome's ruins generated conflicting associations, so, too, did its climate, for its drawbacks seemed to constitute its virtues as well.[44] Richard Wrigley demonstrates convincingly in *Roman Fever: Influence, Infection and the Image of Rome, 1700–1870* that in the eighteenth and nineteenth centuries Roman air was an object of conflicting perceptions, both of the dangers it posed to health and its benevolent healing properties.[45] A similar disparity of judgements also characterised the earlier period. The great diversity of topographical features, of its air and winds, which Mancini noted and which the papal physician Alessandro Petroni thought required Romans to regulate their lives more than any other group, could even arguably be regarded as providential.[46] These might attest to Rome's 'universality', with a multitude of climates suitable to a population hailing from sundry parts of Europe. No faithful Catholic could claim that health considerations would deter them from a pilgrimage, when the Eternal City could boast varied climes. Medical writers defended particular quarters of the city, though there was a lively debate concerning many of these sites. Panaroli asserted in his treatise *L'aria celiomontana* (1642) that the healthiness of the air on the Celio was a consequence of the hill's altitude and its gardens, but he was evidently responding to those who disagreed.[47] Even the near consensus among early modern writers that the Quirinal possessed healthy air was disputed; on at least one occasion, a physician to Paul V argued that the air on Monte Cavallo was too cold and it would be better for the Pope to reside at San Pietro, a surprising directive given this site's low-lying ground.[48]

Above and beyond these local debates, there were physicians who defended the overall healthiness of Rome's air, including Marsilio Cagnati, whose treatise *De Romani äeris salubritate* (1599) addressed this matter at length.[49] Montaigne's declaration that 'I found it [the air of Rome] very pleasant and healthy' is well known.[50] Bishop Giovanni Battista Malaspina, when attempting to persuade Deifebo to relocate to

Rome, even audaciously remarked that he regarded as indisputable the view that the air in the Eternal City 'would be rather more beneficial to him' than that in Deifebo's hilltown of Siena.[51] When contemporary medical theory and practice extended to considerations of season, time of day, individual origins and regional or national dispositions, and with cautions such as Tanara's that not 'every type of air is apt to all the complexions', it was especially important for individuals to draw conclusions for themselves on the grounds of apparently empirical evidence as well as to lend an ear to conventional medical advice.[52]

When in Rome, keep moving

The presumed health benefits of both *villeggiatura* (the flight to Rome's suburban hills during hot months) and the transfer of apartments within the city is well known. What has hitherto received inadequate attention is the practice of relocating apartments for reasons other than to mitigate seasonal conditions. Many members of the Roman elite vacated their apartments during illness, either in the hopes of recovery or to receive treatment. Some even relocated to new or borrowed quarters in order to convalesce from the medical treatments themselves. On 5 August 1623, the Roman *Avvisi* reported that Cardinal Gherardi, having just recuperated from a bloodletting in more comfortable rooms (probably his own), had returned to those of the Cardinal Sacrato in the Vatican.[53] Only a few weeks later, the newspapers recounted how the previous week Monsignor Magalotti, having recovered from his indisposition, had been conveyed to Monte Cavallo and assigned rooms formerly belonging to the Cardinal Sacrato, but since Magalotti's condition then worsened he was transported upstairs to an apartment contiguous to the Papal Chapel.[54] The implication was that with this higher elevation, Magalotti could expect to find even purer air (and to have presumably better chances of recovery). Other residents in Rome sought to reside for a time in a particular location because they perceived the air there suitable to their disposition. This occurred in September of 1623, when the *Avvisi* noted that 'the air of Monte Cavallo being appropriate to the Cardinal of Savoy, he has gone to room in the Convent of the Theatine Fathers of San Silvestro for a few days after having been in that of the Novitiate of the Jesuit Fathers'.[55] This may suggest that after an illness passed in the Novitiate, it was particularly important to reinforce his health by spending a few days in a residence where the air was perceived to be ideally suited to his temperament. Individuals therefore moved much more frequently than seasonally, seeking 'good air' of optimal appropriateness to temperament, even for a few days.

Perceptions of the suitability of a type of air to a given individual's temperament often involved no independent analysis of the air itself or even of associated topographical characteristics. Rather, judgements were passed upon the air of a given site if one became sick or experienced recovery there. This seemingly empirical approach even represented a decisive stage in preparations to avail oneself of a particular residence. In 1615,

> Cardinal Zappata, having resolved to rent the palace and garden of Duke Sforza ... at Quattro Fontane, and having wished to try it out, went there last week to live for three or four days, during which period, feeling rather ill, with his nephew, two gentlemen and two staff members, he immediately returned to his regular house in Parione, with the thought to stay there.[56]

(Incidentally, the Sforza palace would later be purchased by the Barberini family, and would be publicised as occupying the healthiest quarter of Rome.[57]) Another example of this trial-and-error approach to identifying air quality occurred when Cardinal Aldobrandini was advised to go reside 'in the palace of Cardinal Farnese, to see if the change of air would liberate him from quartan fever'.[58]

Moving from one zone to another seeking the best air in Rome was a therapeutic method even employed on an institutional level. For patients in the low-lying hospital of Santo Spirito, there are 'certain Coaches and Litters for sick people; wherein they are carryed up and down, in [to] places of more wholsome air of the City; ... that according to the prescript of their Doctors', they may take some freer air', so recorded the translator of *Pietas Romana*, a treatise on Roman charitable institutions written by the Flemish lawyer and writer Theodor Ameyden.[59] These coaches permitted patients with lingering fevers to take the air, to 'exhilarate the spirits and to exhale their disease'.[60] Jaunts from zone to zone seem to have been embedded within Roman medical and cultural practices. After all, pilgrims regularly charted routes to Rome's seven principal churches for the sake of their spiritual health while artists and Grand Tourists wandered the city observing its antiquities and modern glories.[61] But the Roman practice of making frequent moves between their various apartments often ran counter to the advice of medical writers such as Petronio or Mercurio, the latter of whom would even satirise it. 'A hundred times an hour ... the nobles change rooms and beds, which is excessively dangerous, both for the continual agitation of the humors ... which is pernicious during fevers, as for the air taken in when making the passage from one room to the other.'[62] Moving about might be good or bad for one's health, depending upon who one asked, but it certainly demonstrated social privilege.

Painting, *prospettive* and managing bad air

When Cardinal Zappata decided to choose the lesser of two evils, by returning to his excessively hot palace in Parione, he endeavoured to mitigate the situation himself by hanging 'a tent over a courtyard at the level of his rooms and make there a large cannon to throw water onto the tent, which would fall down like rain and rather refresh' the place.[63] Zappata devised an ingenious invention to mitigate dangerous climatological conditions, but the method most often recommended in vernacular medical treatises to minimise the effects of 'bad air' in a chamber was the introduction of specific species of flowers and plants. To so refresh the air, Panaroli recommended cooling flowers such as roses, violets, the species of *semprevivi* as well as lettuce leaves, vines and others, but no yellow flowers, since he considered yellow a hot colour.[64]

Panaroli then established an analogy between the acts of refreshing the air with cooling plants and of recreating the body and soul through delight in colours, images and music; the verb 'rinfrescare' signified not only the act of cooling, but also of taking recreation or restoring oneself generally. Panaroli thereby inferred that the preservation of both body and soul through the manipulation of the perturbations or passions of the soul represented an effective mechanism of resisting the health dangers of 'bad air'.[65] Within the dominant Aristotelian and Galenic medical traditions in which Panaroli and many contemporary physicians were writing, cognition and the emotions were regarded as 'embodied'.[66] The imagination, upon judging an internal image delightful, would have produced the effect of gradually releasing innate heat, the harbinger of life, to the bodily extremities by means of the animal spirits in the brain, which communicated with the body through the nerves.[67] According to Panaroli, this beneficial alteration to the passions could be achieved through the sight of cheerful colours and 'beautiful perspectives' as well as the hearing of harmonies that made one 'forget annoying and grave cares, the mortal enemies of health'.[68] Unusually, however, for medical writers, is Panaroli's apparent promotion of a specific genre of image amongst those arts which he considered to be sources of recreation and preservation. His joint reference to music and 'beautiful *prospettive*' can only denote painted images (not natural ones), given that music and painting were sister arts. Moreover, Mancini, writing in his *Considerazioni sulla pittura* (*c.*1619–after 1624) of the recently developed pictorial genre of *prospettive*, associated it with cheerfulness, the emotion most closely associated with health.[69] Although the greater distribution of spirits throughout the body might moderately warm it even as they stimulated vitality, the cheerful colour of green, presumably prevalent in the pictures Panaroli was recommending, would refresh the body, keeping it cool.

Panaroli's recommendation to view 'beautiful perspectives' compels closer examination of a pictorial genre that has received relatively little scholarly attention. The precise significance of this term *prospettive* is still disputed. It is either interpreted as meaning architectural views, or architectural 'view' paintings (*vedute*) which encompassed landscapes. The historian of topographical painting, Denis Ribouillault, argues that the term *prospettive* refers less to what is painted than to how – either an elevated or bird's-eye viewpoint.[70] But an *Avviso* of 1629 specified that *prospettive* are paintings with colonnades, a remark of some significance, given the importance of pictures of porticoes and *loggie* in the *oeuvre* of Agostino Tassi, one of the painters who was most instrumental in the emergence of this pictorial genre in Rome.[71]

The highly influential *Trattato dell'arte della pittura, scultura et architettura* (1584) by the northern Italian painter and art theorist Giovanni Paolo Lomazzo recommends the placing of *prospettive* on fountains, in gardens and on musical instruments – a text which therefore resonates with Panaroli's suggestions regarding the 'recreative' powers of music. This text gives a strong indication of the kind of images Panaroli may have had in mind and why he introduced them in a medical treatise on regulating the air. Furthermore it is particularly noteworthy that this very chapter by Lomazzo inspired yet another medical writer on air, Bartolomeo Pietragrassa, when he was outlining which wall coverings and decorations would ensure health and good air within delightful urban dwellings.[72] (Like Panaroli, Pietragrassa also recommended the sight of particular colours, which produced warming or cooling effects on the body.[73]) Lomazzo had indicated that 'diverse perspectives' bring objects and spaces 'not [a] little charming beauty'.[74] These paintings specifically 'lengthen porticoes and garden walls, and beyond the columns, in the intervals between them, landscapes that appear to follow nature [are] here coupled' with them.[75] This coupling of architectural elements and landscapes recalls some of the considerations adumbrated by medical writers about how to ensure delightful and salubrious residences by locating them near gardens.[76] They also correspond to several of Tassi's most admired *prospettive*, such as those in the *Sala dei Palafrenieri* in Palazzo Lancellotti (before 1620), where Tassi constructed an illusion that the beholder, with a few short steps, may exit a restricted space and step into a beautiful, tranquil landscape or enjoy a walk along the sea, entering the open air where he will find respiration easier, the air lighter and more pure. The appearance of birds – airy creatures – in the upper register of these porticoes, likewise suggests freely moving air and sweet songs, music being considered an airy medium by the physician and philosopher Marsilio Ficino, whose *De vita libri tres* (1489), a compendium of recommendations to scholars for staying healthy, was tremendously influential in the early modern period. The illusion in Tassi's *Salotto* in Palazzo Odelscalchi is a little different, yet the *oculi* in the vault open up an enclosed space and provide access to fresh, mobile air above. The landscapes in the four lunettes furnish additional suggestions of space and the free passage of air.

Changing skies

Tassi's most famous pupil and one of the most important of European landscape painters, Claude Lorrain, would develop his own style of fully integrating architectural views and landscapes, and distant vistas as in *Pastoral Landscape* (Musée du Grenoble, Grenoble), with its enormous expanse of sky (Plate 1). Claude's skies suggest atmospheric movement and qualitative distinctions in air quality. In the Grenoble painting, the haziness of the mountains and the intensity of the hue of yellow on the horizon give visual expression to a sense of dense, palpable air in the furthest distance. Above the low-lying plain this undistinguished haze begins to form clouds, which suggest lighter air and quicker movement, while the clear and nearly cloudless blue sky, with its suggestion of the lighter, purer, open air of elevated regions, occupies the area above the craggy hill at right. The composition thus suggests that the healthier air is moving towards the foreground (and the beholder) and enveloping the very destination for the eye travelling along the footpath.

Wrigley casts doubt on the degree to which Claude's paintings of the Roman campagna actually resulted from direct observation, but all of the painter's critics have noted his capacity to represent atmospheric conditions with an unparalleled degree of subtlety.[77] According to his fellow painter and biographer Joachim von Sandrart, Claude would lie 'in the fields before the break of day and until night in order to learn to represent very exactly the red morning-sky, sunrise and sunset and the evening hours', times of day in which temperature and humidity are most observable as atmospheric effects change.[78] It can scarcely be accidental that Claude was thought to have observed subtle meteorological changes at a moment and within a geographical location in which similar discernment was considered crucial to the well-being of the class of men constituting Claude's patrons. In fact, according to Sandrart, Claude presented his biographer with a representation of the morning 'in which one can truly recognise how the sun, [is already] risen for some two hours'.[79] The rising sun in *Seaport with the Embarkation of the Queen of Sheba* (National Gallery, London) dispels the dangerous nocturnal clouds, which float away towards the edges of the canvas, opening up the core area to clear skies (Plate 2). Interestingly, morning and evening hours during summer, after nocturnal cold and before and after the day's intense heat, according to both Panaroli and Tanara, are to be preferred for going outdoors in Rome to conduct business or to stroll, though sunrise and sunset may remain dangerous on account of changing climatological conditions.[80]

Claude endows *Seaport* with features denoting 'good air' – tranquil skies and waters, a relative stillness animated by gentle breezes upon which birds take flight, for they, Breventano would remark, soar only in periods of calm, when the air is pure and healthy. Only tranquil seas and the serene earth of the countryside will exhale the pure vapours, producing benevolent winds and air.[81] The gently lapping waves and flowing waters bespeak ventilated air, which does not become stagnant and putrid.[82] Abundant, fertile slopes and plains in Lorrain's *Apollo Guarding the Herds of Admetus* of 1645, attest to the air's wholesomeness (Fig. 9.2). Claude paints elevated viewpoints and open, airy skies

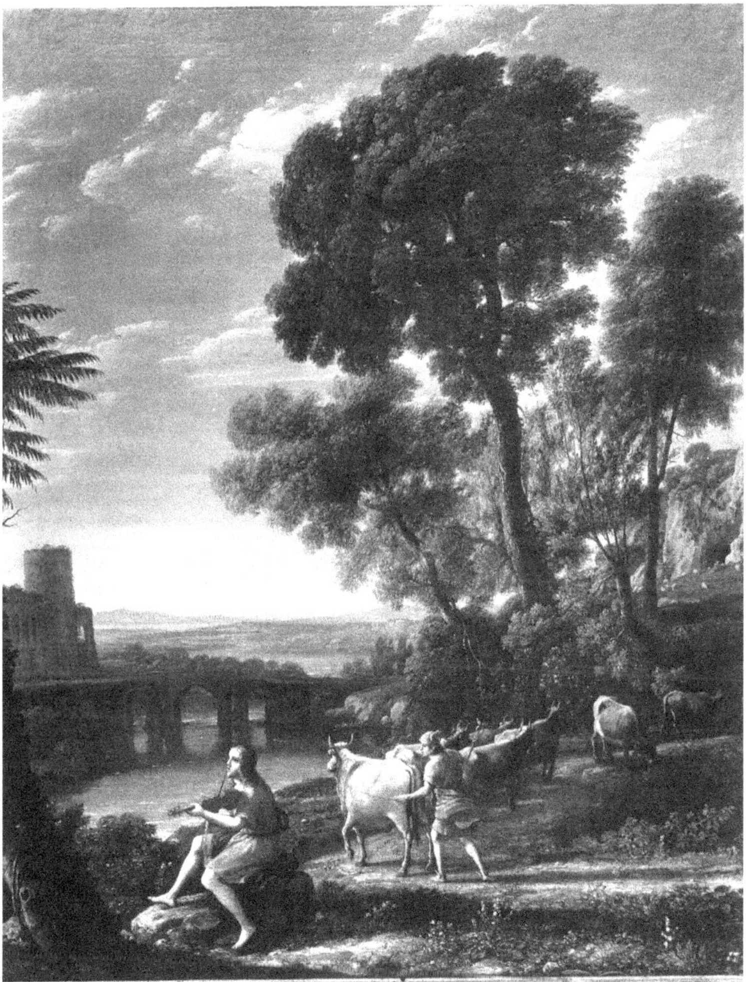

Figure 9.2 Claude Lorrain, *Apollo Guarding the Herds of Admetus*, 1645

and sometimes the destinations of *villeggiatura* such as Castel Gandolfo, Tivoli or the hills of Rome, such as that of Santa Trinità dei Monti, viewed during sunrise.[83] He lends his compositions such as *Landscape with Merchants* of 1629 (National Gallery of Art, Washington, DC) an equilibrium through the conjunction of distant sunshine and foreground areas of shade; warmed by the sun's brilliant illumination, the figures nevertheless occupy cool shady patches (Plate 3). It is as though the perspectival views of the type of open airy spaces associated with 'taking the air', and great distances through which air may travel, being purified and cooled as it does, will give beholders the sensations of breathing more easily, and inhaling wholesome air, and divert their minds from enclosed, dank or stifling rooms. But Claude does not simply present a universal vision of 'good air' as a substitution for what are actual insalubrious sites within the Roman walls or in the Roman *campagna*. Some of the foregrounds of Claude's landscapes picture dusty ports, as in his *View of a Port with the Capitol*, or gypsies, manual labourers (associated with dirt), barren banks or trails devoid of flowers and plants, sites scarcely corresponding to the presumed signs of 'good air' repeated in contemporary medical literature, or sought by laymen (Plate 4). It is as though the beholder's optical movement follows a visually cathartic process of purification in moving out of less wholesome air into that which is freely moving.

It is likely that some of Claude's paintings were appreciated, at least by certain collectors, for their presumed capacity to alter body temperature and respiration. The somatic effects of visual perception via the imagination were explained by the ducal physician Rodrigo Fonseca as a process whereby the immaterial species or images emitted first from an object and transmitted to the eye subsequently enter the internal senses and the imagination retaining some of their natural properties. When beholding an image of fire, a degree of its warmth would thus still be transmitted to the body.[84] Claude's perspectives, avidly collected by the ecclesiastical and diplomatic elite in Rome, the class most engaged in the pursuit of healthy air, were also exported across Europe. It is two of these works sent northward, but sadly lost, that can be likened to *A Seaport* (National Gallery, London) and *View of the Campagna from Tivoli* (Royal Collection, Windsor) that Sandrart cited as exemplifying Claude's atmospheric achievements (Plates 5 and 6). In one, the sun dissipates the mist and dew of sunrise, burning off the nocturnal humidity; in the other, a contrasting piece, he represents a hot and dry summer sun.[85] These prized paintings belonged to the Baron von Mayer in Munich, who reportedly gazed at them in order to divert his mind and alleviate his cares after hours of business. It is tempting to think that von Mayer sought them as a mechanism which would mitigate the effects of the cold, damp German air by igniting his imagination of the dry heat of the Roman sun.

Conclusion

Early modern men and women were preoccupied with securing access to healthy air, going to extraordinary lengths to do so by moving residences, or taking day trips or longer voyages to elevated sites or regions. Claude's paintings, many of which take up themes of travel, present some of the climatological considerations that residents of Rome would have reflected upon when moving between their palaces and apartments, even if only across Rome. That said, Panaroli's advice to view 'beautiful perspectives' certainly underscores the efforts of early moderns to improve air quality when it was believed to be unavailable, and his guidelines may have struck a particular chord amongst those who felt they must stay put, either because of obligations, lack of resources, ill health or simple fear of the 'bad air' abroad. In spite of the fact, however, that conventional attributes of 'good air' – elevated locations, clear, light air and moderate temperatures – were widely repeated in vernacular health manuals, and the abundance or nature of a region's horticulture or agriculture was thought to provide supplementary indications of air quality, men and women often remained uncertain about whether or not air in any given spot might be beneficial to them. This is confirmed by Cardinal Zappata's decision to 'try out' living in a palace before committing to renting it. Here, as well as in the cases of Bandi and Mercurio, early moderns most confidently assessed the relative healthfulness of a city, region, zone or site on the basis of whether or not they fell ill while residing there, even if that experience conflicted with prior expectations or knowledge. Yet the recommendation of physicians to delight the senses and engage in cheerful activities strongly argues that early moderns remained convinced that the pleasure of the senses was a productive compliment to the regulation of other Non-Naturals.[86]

Notes

1 V. Cartari, *Immagini degli dei degli antichi* (1647), p. 45, as quoted in S. Russell, 'Girolamo Mercuriale's *De arte gymnastica* and Papal Health at the Villa Pamphilj, Rome', in Alessandro Arcangeli and Vivian Nutton (eds), *Girolamo Mercuriale: medicina e cultura nell'Europa del Cinquecento* (Florence: Olschki, 2008), pp. 182–3.

2 M. Beneš, 'In sickness and in health: uses of the villa garden by a princess in Baroque Rome, Olimpia Aldobrandini (1623–82)' (1994), unpublished essay. I wish to thank Mirka Beneš for generously sharing her paper and permitting me to cite it here.

3 Giovanni Battista Bandi to Deifebo Mancini, Veroli, 22 March 1613, Archivio della Società di Esecutori di Pie Disposizioni (hereafter ASEPD), CXIX 169, fol. 9r, 'Veroli città in ca[m]pagnia ... di buoniss[im]a aria, abbonda[n]te'.

4 Giovanni Battista Bandi to Deifebo Mancini, Veroli, 16 April 1613, ASEPD, CXIX 169, fol. 11, 'Per il passato sono stato oppresso da co[n]descenzo di testa vehementiss[im]o alli denti et orecchi con dolore quasi continuo, al presente me ne trovo assai sgravato, il tutto attribuisco alla mutatione dell'aria, frigis[sim]a sottiliss[im]a et inc[lemen]tiss[im]a p[er] esser q[uest]a città posta in un colle assai a'[sgreste], onde brutiss[issim]a dentro, se bene alla campagnia mostra molta amenità, acco[m]pagnata co[n] buoniss[im]a grassezza di tutti i frutti.'

5 For air see S. Cavallo and T. Storey, *Healthy Living in Late Renaissance Italy* (Oxford: Oxford University Press, 2013), p. 109.

6 François Auguste de Thou to Paul Dupuy, 9 February 1627, BNF, Coll. Dupuy, fol. 28. '[L]a saison y fair beaucoup, qui est fort froid [et] par consequens fort saine, car quand la Tramontane souffle, il se voir ~~fort~~ peu de gens malades'.

7 D. Panaroli, *Aërologia, cioè discorso dell'aria*. Trattato Vtile per la Sanità (Rome: D. Marciani, 1642), pp. 66, 77.

8 B. Pietragrassa, *Politica medica per il governo conservativo del corpo humano* (Pavia: Gio Andrea Magri, 1649), p. 284: 'l'humido nella Primavera dominante è molto aereo, e perciò salubre, e simpatico con le complessioni de viventi'.

9 S. Mercurio, *De gli errori popolari d'Italia* (Verona: Francesco Rossi, 1645), p. 444: 'li habitatori tutti senza colore ... con il volto giallo, con gl'occhi languidi ... la state poi a guisa di pecore infette morendo'.

10 *Ibid.*

11 *Ibid.*: 'in un colle Ameno, gratioso, d'ottimo aere; luogo fruttifero, ricco d'olivi, abondante di viti preciosissime, dottato di frutti soavissimi; dove l'aere è purissimo, il Cielo serenissimo'.

12 *Ibid.*

13 S. Breventano, *Trattato degli elementi raccolto da varii autori* (Pavia: Girolamo Bartoli, 1571), p. 9: 'ne c'è cosa, che più faccia crescere le biade e l'herbe, ne che indrizzi li alberi, e gli distenda in rami, che l'Aere'. For the West wind, see Panaroli, *Aërologia*, p. 37.
14 For winds and trees, see Cavallo and Storey, *Healthy Living*, p. 72. For the softening effects of trees on the air, see F. Gage, 'Exercise for mind and body: Giulio Mancini, collecting and the beholding of landscape painting in the seventeenth century', *Renaissance Quarterly*, 61:4 (2008), p. 1184.
15 M. Ambrosoli, *The Wild and the Sown: Botany and Agriculture in Western Europe: 1350–1850* (Cambridge: Cambridge University Press, 1997), pp. 232–6.
16 G. Botero, *Discorso intorno lo stato della chiesa* (Venice: Giorgio Varisco, 1605), pp. 114r–v, 116r–v.
17 S. Barker, 'Art in a time of danger: Urban VIII's Rome and the plague of 1629–1634', PhD diss., Columbia University, 2002, p. 181. For trees in Italian gardens, see David R. Coffin, *Gardens and Gardening in Papal Rome* (Princeton: Princeton University Press, 1991), p. 198.
18 Mancini, 'Alcune considerazioni dell'honore', BAV, Barb. Lat. 4314, fol. 84v, concerning trees planted for dowries, and fol. 86v for agriculture practised for pleasure and health.
19 V. Tanara, *L'economia del cittadino in villa* (Venice: Steffano Curti, 1674, first. ed. 1600), p. 77.
20 *Ibid.*, p. 83.
21 Cavallo and Storey, *Healthy Living*, p. 70.
22 Panaroli, *Aërologia*, pp. 73–4.
23 *Ibid.*, p. 73.
24 Cavallo and Storey, *Healthy Living*, p. 84.
25 Tracy Ehrlich, *Landscape and Identity in Early Modern Rome: Villa Culture at Frascati in the Borghese Era* (Cambridge: Cambridge University Press, 2002), p. 83.
26 S. Breventano, *Trattato del'origine delli venti* (Venice: Gioan Francesco Camotio, 1571), p. 3r: 'l'aère non è mai tanto fermo, e queto [*sic*] che non sia in qualche agitatione ... giammai immobile'.
27 *Ibid.*, fol. 5r: 'ma con la continova agitatione lo rendessero e giovevole e vitale à chiunque respire'.
28 Cesare Perini to Deifebo Mancini, 20 March 1627, ASEPD, CXIX, 170, fol. 830r–v, 'VS se abbi cura co[n] no[n] uscir della camera fin tanto che no[n] sente stagion temparata'.
29 *Ibid.*, fol. 830r.
30 S. Cavallo, 'Changing ideas of complexion in the Italian health-advice literature of the long sixteenth century' (2014), unpublished paper. I wish to

thank Sandra Cavallo for sharing her paper and permitting me to cite it here; also Cavallo and Storey, *Healthy Living*, pp. 73–4.

31 Panaroli, *Aërologia*, p. 70, 'non uscendo dal Clima patrio l'huomo si ritrova loco assai proportionate per la sanità'.

32 *Ibid.*, p. 71, 'la migliore è starsene'.

33 *Avvisi*, Rome, 10 May 1623, Biblioteca Apostolica Vaticana, Urb. Lat. 1093, fol. 361r, 'Et il s[igno]r Card[ina]l Caetano non Confacendo alla sua Complessione l'aria di Bologna hà renunciato quella legatione Con voce che si debba fare nuova provis[ion]e.'

34 Panaroli, *Aërologia*, p. 71.

35 Giulio Mancini, 'Modo e regola di far viaggio', BAV, Barb. Lat. 4315, fol. 291r.

36 Cesare Perini to Deifebo Mancini, Rome, 19 April 1631, ASEPD, CXIX 170, fol. 123r, 'casa ariosa di buon aria'.

37 F. Cancellieri, *Lettera ... al Ch. Sig. Dottore Koreff ... sopra il tarantismo, l'aria di Roma e della sua campagna, ed i palazzi ponteficj entro, e fuori di Roma* (Rome: Francesco Bourlié, 1817), p. 38.

38 M. de Montaigne, *Montaigne's Travel Journal*, ed. Donald M. Frame (San Francisco, CA: North Point Press, 1983), p. 79.

39 Panaroli, *Aërologia*, p. 75.

40 R. Zorach, *The Virtual Tourist in Renaissance Rome: Printing and Collecting the 'Speculum Romanae magnificentiae'* (Chicago: University of Chicago Press, 2008), p. 71.

41 D.M. Habel, *'When All of Rome was Under Construction': The Building Process in Baroque Rome* (University Park: Penn State Press, 2013), p. 141.

42 D. Panaroli, *Plantarum amphitheatralium catalogus*, in *Polycarpoponia seu variorum fructes labores* (Rome: J.B. Roblettus, 1647), pp. 356–66. See also, G. Caneva et al., 'Analysis of the Colosseum's floristic changes during the last four centuries', *Plant Biosystems*, 136 (2002), p. 299. See also n. 64, this chapter.

43 M. Fagiolo dell'Arco, *Jean Lemaire pittore 'antiquario'* (Rome: Ugo Bozzi, 1996), pp. 164–5, cat. nos 11–12; p. 218, cat. no. 56.

44 Giulio Mancini, ASEPD, CXIX, 179, untitled, unpaginated manuscript, 'Citta d'Aria ineguale per la gran diversita de i siti et de i Venti'. Also, A. Petronio, *Del viver delli romani, et di conservare la sanità* (Rome: Domenico Basa, 1592), p. 1, 'per la disuguaglianza del sito'. See also p. 6 for a similar declaration.

45 R. Wrigley, *Roman Fever: Influence, Infection and the Image of Rome, 1700–1870* (New Haven: Yale University Press, 2014), pp. 61–80. Wrigley's primary interest in the later period encourages him to lend greater weight to the arguments that it is a city of *mal'aria*, even when treating the earlier.

46 For Mancini on the diversity of sites in Rome, see G. Mancini, ASEPD, CXIX 179, untitled, unpaginated manuscript, 'Citta d'Aria ineguale per la gran diversita de i siti et de i Venti'. For Petroni's opinion, see Petronio, *Del viver*, p. 1.
47 D. Panaroli, *L'Aria Celimontana* (Rome: D. Marciani, 1642), pp. 13–14. Panaroli acknowledges disagreement about the salubriousness of the site (11–12).
48 J.A.F. Orbaan, *Documenti sul Barocco in Roma* (Rome: Sede della Società alla Biblioteca Vallicelliana, 1920), p. 269.
49 For Cagnati, see N. Siraisi, *History, Medicine and the Traditions of Renaissance Learning* (Ann Arbor, MI: University of Michigan Press, 2007), pp. 180–1. See also Orbaan, *Documenti*, p. 478, n. 20.
50 Montaigne, *Montaigne's Travel Journal*, p. 96.
51 Giovanni Battista Malaspina to Deifebo Mancini, Rome, 4 February 1627, ASEPD, CXIX 170, fol. 262r.
52 Tanara, *L'Economia del cittadino*, p. 11: 'ne' ogni aria è atta à tutte le complessioni'.
53 Avvisi, Rome, 5 August 1623, Biblioteca Apostolica Vaticana (hereafter BAV), Urb. Lat. 1093, fol. 590r.
54 Avvisi, Rome, 30 August 1623, BAV, Urb. Lat. 1093, fol. 658r: 'Mons[ignor] Magalotti ... sendo migliorato nella sua Indisposit[ion]e si fece condurre la sett[iman]a pass[a]ta al Palazzo Pontificio di Monte Cavallo, dove gli fù [f. 659r] assegnate le stanze, che vi haveva il Card[ina]le Sacrato, mà per essere poi peggiorato è stato trasportato di sopra nell'Apartam[en]to contiguo alla Cappella pontificia.'
55 Avvisi, 27 September 1623, BAV, Urb. Lat. 1093, fol. 744r: 'Al Card[ina]l di Savoia confacendo molto l'aria di Monte Cavallo è andato à stantiare nel Convento de Padri Teatini di San Silvestro per alcuni pochi giorni dopò essere stato in quello del Novitiato de Padri Giesuiti.'
56 Orbaan, *Documenti*, p. 234, 1615 luglio 22: 'Il cardinale Zappata haveva risoluto di pigliare in affitto il palazzo et giardino del duca Sforza, posto in strada Pia alle Quattro Fontane, et havendolo voluto provare vi andò la settimana passata ad habitare per tre o quatro giorni, nel qual tempo sendosi alquanto amalato con il nipote, doi gentilhuomini et doi staffieri, subito se n'è ritornato alla sua solita casa in Parione con pensiero di fermarvisi et perché li caldi sono eccessivi ha fatta tirare una tenda sopra un cortile, che ha al pari delle stanze et fattovi congegnare canone grande che getta acqua sopra essa tenda, la quale poi cala a basso in forma di pioggia et rinfresca assai.'
57 H. Tetius, *Aedes Barberinae ad Quirinalium descriptae*, ed. L. Faedo and T. Frangenberg (Pisa: Scuola Normale, 2005), p. 181.

58 *Avvisi*, Rome, 2 December 1623, BAV, Urb. Lat 1093, fol. 888r–v: 'Et il Card[ina]l Aldob[i]no per conseglio de Medici hà risoluto d'andar' ad habitare nel Palazzo del Card[ina]l farnese per vedere se con la mutatione dell' aria potesse liberarsi dalla febre quartana.'
59 [D. Ameyden and R.H. Thomas Carre], *Pietas Romana et Parisiensis or a faithful relation of the several sorts of charitable and pious works eminent in the cities of Rome and Paris* (Oxford: publisher unknown, 1687), p. 8.
60 *Ibid.*
61 R. Wrigley, 'Infectious enthusiasms: influence, contagion and the experience of Rome', in C. Chard and H. Langdaon (eds), *Transports: Travel, Pleasure, and Imaginative Geography, 1600–1830* (New Haven: Yale University Press, 1996), pp. 75–116, on 81–2.
62 Mercurio, *De gli errori popolari*, p. 220, 'I Nobili … mutano cento volte l'hora, e letto, e stanze, il che è sopra modo nocivo; così per la continua agitatione dei humori, che si fà nel moversi spesso, il che nelle febri, e pernitioso, come per l'aere, che si prende nel far passaggio dall'una, all'altra stanza.'
63 Orbaan, *Documenti*, p. 234, 1615 luglio 22. See note 53 above.
64 Panaroli, *Aërologia*, p. 87. For the purifying effects of various plants, herbs and flowers, see Cavallo and Storey, *Healthy Living*, pp. 101–3.
65 Panaroli, *Aërologia*, pp. 87–8.
66 E. Carrera, 'Anger and the mind–body connection in medieval and Early Modern medicine', in Elena Carrera (ed.), *Emotions and Health, 1200–1700* (Leiden: Brill, 2013), pp. 95–146, on p. 115.
67 Cavallo and Storey, *Healthy Living*, p. 93; 199–206; see Carrera, 'Anger and the mind–body connection', pp. 109, 118–19.
68 Panaroli, *Aërologia*, p. 88: 'fanno obliare le cure noiose, e gravi, nemici mortali della sanità'.
69 Gage, 'Exercise for mind and body', p. 1188.
70 D. Ribouillault, *Rome et ses jardins: paysage et pouvoir au XVIe siècle* (Lassay-les-Châteaux: CTHS and Institute National d'Histoire de l'Art, 2013), p. 29.
71 Avvisi, Rome, 25 April 1629, BAV, Urb. Lat. 1099. For Tassi's perspectives, see P. Cavazzini (ed.), *Agostino Tassi (1578–1644): Un paesaggista tra immaginario e realtà* (Rome: Iride per Terzo Millenio, 2008), pp. 24–59.
72 Pietragrassa, *Political medica*, p. 411. Though unacknowledged.
73 Cavallo and Storey, *Healthy Living*, p. 93.
74 G.P. Lomazzo, *Scritti sulle Arte*, ed. Roberto Ciardi, 2 vols (Florence: Centro Di, 1975), vol. 2, p. 301, 'posson accommodarvisi con non minor vaghezza … prospettive diverse'.
75 *Ibid.* 'prospettive diverse, le quali facciano allungare i portici e le pareti del giardino, et oltre alle colonne, ne gli intervalli, paesi cosí accompagnati che

paiano seguire il naturale, fingendovi alcune istorie delle dette, che convengano a tali luochi'.

76 Gage, 'Exercise for mind and body', pp. 1185–6, and Cavallo and Storey, *Healthy Living*, p. 174.

77 Wrigley, *Roman Fever*, pp. 110–12.

78 J. v. Sandrart, *Der Teutschen Academie zweyter Theil*, as translated in M. Röthlisberger, *Claude Lorrain: The Paintings*, 2 vols (New Haven: Yale University Press, 1961), vol. 1, pp. 47–8.

79 *Ibid.*, p. 49.

80 Panaroli, *L'aria celimontana*, p. 15; Tanara, *L'economia del cittadino*, p. 12. Mancini, however, in an undated and unpaginated manuscript, cautions against dawn and dusk, ASEPD, CXIX 179: 'i Crespuescoli et in particular q[u]elli del Inverno sieno molto fastidosi et co[n]trarii alla Testa'.

81 Breventano, *Trattato degli elementi*, p. 9.

82 K. Rinne, 'Urban ablutions: cleansing Counter-Reformation Rome', in Mark Bradley and Kenneth Stow (eds), *Rome, Pollution and Propriety: Dirt, Disease and Hygiene in the Eternal City from Antiquity to Modernity* (Cambridge: Cambridge University Press, 2012), pp. 182–201, p. 193.

83 Sandrart, *Teutsche Academie*, pp. 47–8.

84 R. Fonseca, *Del conservare la sanità* (Florence: Semartelli, 1603), p. 112.

85 Sandrart, *Teutsche Academie*, pp. 47–8: 'a reddish morning-piece, where the dew at sunrise is visibly dissolved … in another piece, [one sees] the evening hour before the setting of the sun, which is shown descending in reddish tints over the mountains, so that the red, hot, suffocating atmosphere and the warmth occurring on hot summer days are seen on the mountains, trees, and valleys quite astonishingly and naturally'. The phrase 'hitzige rohte Trückene am Himmel', which Röthlisberger translates as 'the red, hot, suffocating atmosphere', might be read instead as 'the red, hot, dry atmosphere', if one translates 'Trückene' as deriving from *trocken* instead of *drücken* 'to press, push'. I wish to thank Eva Struhal for this suggestion.

86 I wish to thank Professor Vittorio Carnesecchi, Rector of the *Società per Esecutori di Pie Disposizioni* and Doctor Maria Laura Pogni, the Society's director, for permission to consult and publish portions of the Mancini correspondence. I also wish to thank Mirka Beneš, Sandra Cavallo, Patrizia Cavazzini, Tracy Ehrlich, Tessa Storey and Eva Struhal for suggestions on this research and Douglas Basford for reading and commenting on the manuscript.

10

Hot-drinking practices in the late Renaissance Italian household: a case study around an enigmatic pouring vessel

Marta Ajmar

This chapter addresses the relationship and the potential disjuncture between texts, images and objects in the exploration of preventive health practices in the late Renaissance Italian household, focusing on an atypical vessel for the table to open wider questions about the material culture of hot drinking. As Sandra Cavallo and Tessa Storey have clearly articulated in their recent study, a complex set of practices emerging from a medical belief system built around the Non-Naturals accompanied the daily attempts to maintain the physical and mental well-being of the household.[1] At the core of this prophylactic culture sits the genre of regimens, a corpus of treatises, often written in the vernacular by medical authors and available in cheap formats, that from the first half of the sixteenth century contributed to disseminate old and new thinking around health or *sanità* and the prevention of disease, engaging with the ways in which the six Non-Naturals ought to be managed to ensure well-being. These writings offered increasingly detailed advice on these matters and progressively engaged with the employment of material culture in the everyday performance of healthy living. As the genre developed, domestic objects moved gradually towards the forefront of the authors' concerns and texts became more and more specific about issues such as the material, form, colour and design of the artefacts called to participate in the culture of well-being, describing their material properties and defining their purpose with ever-greater accuracy.

Why objects matter

This backdrop is useful for determining whether we need to look at the objects involved in the everyday management of health and why. Why is it important to mobilise the actual objects in the discussion of preventive practices? After all verbal descriptions and sometimes illustrations of artefacts accompany the regimens' guidelines in many cases and feature in the plethora of other literary and archival written sources that might help support this kind of enquiry – from household management and domestic architecture treatises to inventories, wills, account books and private correspondence, to mention just a few. Moreover, how should we approach those objects that are not explicitly included within the written record, but that might nevertheless have been powerful players in the formulation and performance of preventive practices, raising the possibility of a distinctive agency of artefacts in the making of health-related cultures?

Regimens assign an important role to a wide range of objects linked to the maintenance of health, from bedding to heating appliances, from hygiene equipment to clothing.[2] The connection between healthy living advice and material culture is so strong that it is legitimate to think that in some social contexts preventive considerations of some kind might have inhabited nearly every aspect of domestic life. Are there different degrees of 'healthiness' that can be attributed to household material culture? And how can we disentangle the multiple, interwoven meanings embedded within objects and separate out the preventative concerns under discussion from the aesthetic and social values that have been conventionally associated with most domestic material culture? Another problematic area is related to the unpredictable survival patterns of objects. Visual and textual sources may refer to specific objects involved in healthy living that might never have been made or that have not left a record in our collections because they have failed to comply with the various criteria that at any given time have guided the selection and preservation of objects. Conversely, objects that might have been implicated in these practices, but that are not explicitly discussed by the texts, are often difficult to identify for what they might have been and were meant to do.

What are therefore the benefits of an object-based approach to the Renaissance culture of healthy living?[3] In this chapter it will be suggested that artefacts can offer insights into areas of historical enquiry that written sources alone cannot penetrate. At a basic level, material culture can help provide evidence of advice *having been implemented* and therefore of *actual* practice, thus allowing us to move from pure prescription to the realm of historical tangibility, and in the process illuminating aspects of cultural interpretation, use and social dissemination. We should not, however, limit the role of artefacts to that of passive historical executors: objects can be *active* agents in history.[4] Objects can *affect* cultural change, can pre-empt or go beyond the written source and can give material form to ideas and values which are not, not yet or cannot be expressed in writing. Through their material agency artefacts can play a key role in the *production and reproduction* of culture in unique ways, supporting tradition and innovation. Lastly, objects are *embodied*. Their embodiedness aligns them with people, while distancing them from words: like human beings, they exist in space and time and are affected by both, they do not possess the gift of ubiquity, they age and can perish.[5] Of central significance are also their materiality and design, affecting all aspects of our understanding, perception and use: what something is made of and what it looks like are crucial elements in the interface between people and things, physically and culturally. In addition, their being embodied brings about a sensorial relationship with the people who make and use them, involving sight, hearing, touch, taste and smell. It is the job of the historian to attempt to work out the implications of these material and physical interactions (themselves always historically located) in the construction of the wider historical context.

The approach presented in this essay builds on a rich and long-established historiography on material culture.[6] Voices coming from perspectives as diverse as social anthropology, the history of technology and literary studies have highlighted the significance of the material, physical and sensorial properties of things, moving on from the limitations of 'contextual' methods for the understanding of objects, which tend to reduce artefacts to 'meanings' and social relations.[7] Thanks to the 'material turn', in recent decades a renewed attention to the role of objects in interpersonal relationships, and to our own relationship to artefacts, has emerged within the humanities and the social sciences. Literary theorists have emphasised the human ability of forming and transforming themselves through inanimate objects.[8] Objects are increasingly presented as central to 'emotional, sensual, representational and communicative expression' and as an irreplaceable source, key to providing insights into the lives of those with little access to words.[9] Historians have been especially vocal in arguing for the need to inscribe material culture within their own scholarly endeavours, not as mere 'illustration' but as 'exploration' of 'practice, ideology or emotion'.[10] Meanwhile anthropologists have provided some of the most effective interpretive tools for affirming the significance of objects, with the concept of 'agency' – whereby 'things' can be understood as agents of cultural, political or social change – shaping the debate in significant ways. Agency has shifted the emphasis from a dominant understanding of objects as nothing more than a manifestation or representation of intentional human production and meaningful human use, to one in which, in the processes of use and consumption, humans give agency to existing things, attributing autonomous power to them. Thus things can be seen as able to 'act' upon social situations and objects might be interpreted not merely as 'the product of history but also active agents in history'.[11] For others, this notion of agency, whereby an inanimate object is attributed animate properties is precisely what prevents objects from participating in life. What is proposed instead is the idea that we should see all *objects* ('dead') as *things* ('alive'), not because of being endowed with specific 'living' powers, but by virtue of being part of the constant flow of processes and materials that constitute life, and as such always engaged in dynamic becoming rather than static being.[12]

This reaching out towards material culture from a number of different disciplinary perspectives brings into even sharper focus the often-remarked-upon difficulty inherent in 'reading objects'. As landscape historian John Dixon Hunt has famously put it, while in language the different components of a metaphor 'subtly yet crucially modify each other', artefacts cannot easily substitute or adequately represent the contexts within which they operated: 'teapots as objects stay irredeemably teapotish'.[13] Archaeologists, however, have offered illuminating articulations of the ability of objects to work as metaphors, thus reinforcing the notion that they are able to participate in a register of communication as rich as that of language, though possibly more complex.[14] Other scholars too have seen the poetic opening inherent in objects' complex and often enigmatic ontology. As W. David Kingery puts it,

> No one denies the importance of things, but learning from them requires rather more attention than reading texts. The grammar of things is related to, but more complex and difficult to decipher than, the grammar of words. Artifacts are tools as well as signals, signs and symbols. Their use and functions are multiple and intertwined. Much of their meaning is subliminal and unconscious. Some authors have talked about reading objects as texts, but objects must also be read as myths and as poetry.[15]

Beyond the 'teapotishness' of a 'proto-teapot'

This essay will explore and question the 'teapotishness' of what might be named, inaccurately but evocatively, a Renaissance 'proto-teapot'. It will do so by not only exploiting the richly referential, vocally allusive properties of the object under scrutiny, but also by bringing to the table an understanding of artefacts that aims to replace a *reading* with a multisensory *experiencing* of them. By removing objects from a passive, disembodied apprehension based on 'being read', and from a reductive idea that their interpretation can follow a predetermined 'grammar', and instead restoring the physicality, performativity and *aliveness* embedded in their design and materiality, this essay aims to contribute to a growing literature that foregrounds objects as potent, dynamic, transformative cultural agents and sees them as active, alive things.[16]

To illustrate this approach the essay will focus on an enigmatic sixteenth-century earthenware pouring vessel for the table and propose that this object might have been involved in hot-drinking rituals. Supported by a number of contemporary texts discussing and presenting visually a wide range of utensils – some new, some well established, some a revival of ancient classical designs – which can rarely be identified with surviving objects, hot drinking provides an illuminating context for assessing the complex relationship between text, image and object. This object will be inscribed within a hypothetical framework centred around hot drinking and explored in relation to its performative properties, as an artefact that would have come to life – materially, decoratively and operationally – when filled with liquid and mobilised within the rituals involved in drinking at the table. In that performative context the artefact is transformed from inactive receptacle into dynamic tool – whether as table fountain, drinking boat or proto-teapot – and powered by the drink within it and its sensorial appeal: visual, haptic, olfactory and aural. By superimposing an operative lens onto what is now a static museum object removed from practice I am hoping to restore meaningfulness to its materiality and design.

Describing an unidentified object 'thickly'

Labelled variously by museum catalogues as 'sauceboat', 'table fountain' or 'pouring vessel for tisanes', this artefact now held in the Milan Musei Civici is a rare survivor (Plate 7).[17] Only one other is known to have survived.[18] Though through stylistic comparison it has been established that it is very likely that this vessel was made in the last quarter of the sixteenth century in the central Italian pottery centre of Castelli (Abruzzo), renowned for the production of tin-glazed earthenware, this type of container does not appear to have contemporary documented ceramic precedents. Thus in our attempt to understand this object we must rely largely on direct observation, on what can be drawn from the artefact itself and from broader comparisons with other vessels displaying some affinities with it. This approach will move beyond a mostly factual, 'thin' description and engage instead in a richer, 'thick' cultural historical analysis.[19] We will attempt not only to look closely at this enigmatic object and aim at identifying the 'synchronic' elements that recur in artefacts of the same era that might share significant features of design, but also to provide explanations for those stylistic features and material properties.[20]

As we focus on its design and structure it becomes evident that the vessel is made up of two superimposed compartments, thus suggesting that it was intended to showcase liquid *in motion*, through a journey that would start at the top, followed by a cascading movement and ending with the flowing out of the drink. The chamber above is endowed with three narrow nozzles (Plate 9), thus probably designed for filtering the liquid, while the wider, lower compartment would allow the liquid to be further filtered and poured out, as with an ewer (Plate 10). The smaller, upper part (Plate 11) with its brickwork decoration and straw-shaped spouts, is evocative of street fountains and creates a high–low drinking hierarchy (Plate 12). Its lower container, with its embossed decoration and shell-like spouts, is reminiscent of contemporary earthenware sauce-boats, traditionally employed at the table for serving sauces and other liquids, which in turn often allude to the ornamental motifs of contemporary metalwork vessels and borrow the natural shapes of creatures connected with water, such as seashells (Fig. 10.1). Thus, when it comes to design, this object hybridises different, earlier forms. Together, these elements produce an incongruous, but animated, dynamic ensemble, morphing together the boat with the fountain.

Vessel as boat

Let us first explore the vessel as boat. It might be suggested that the nearest reference to its design comes from the late medieval metalwork

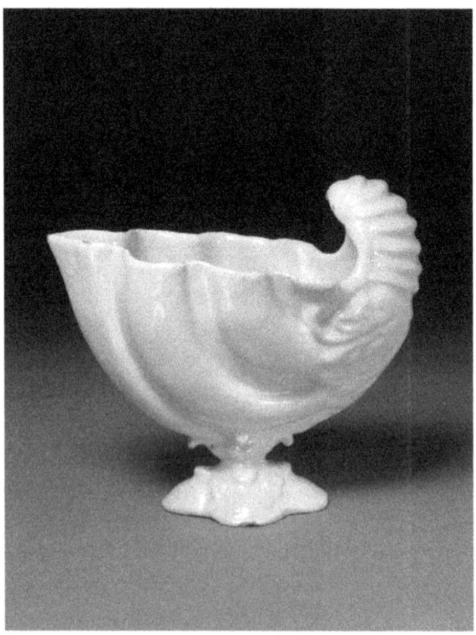

Figure 10.1 Sauceboat, tin-glazed earthenware, possibly made in Faenza (Italy), 1560–80

genre of the *nef*, known in Italian as *navicella* – 'little ship', or *barca* – 'boat'. Nefs were ostentatious table sculptures in the form of ships or boats available from goldsmiths as highly customised or as off-the-peg items, often combining precious materials such as silver and mother-of-pearl (Plate 8). Designed to occupy a position of prestige on the table and signify status, they also fulfilled a practical role either as saltcellars or as containers of individual tableware items, such as napkins, cutlery and trenchers. For one example, the inventory of Charles V of France (1380) describes a lidded 'navette' (little nef) made of gold, which contained his spoon, knife, fork and a 'cup of essay', a vessel used for ceremonial wine tasting at the beginning of the meal.[21] Designs for nefs circulated as drawings from the fifteenth century onwards and soon took printed form, thus providing the potential to travel more widely and inspire imitations across media. Many of these designs, which often also took an *all'antica* idiom with respect to the themes depicted, simultaneously connected the Renaissance nef with its classical precedent, the lamp in the form of a ship, as testified by sixteenth-century bronze examples which made overt reference to Roman prototypes (Fig. 10.2).[22]

By the second half of the sixteenth century objects that resemble nefs appeared in the workshops of potters, as shown in the inventorial record of the highly productive business of Virgiliotto Calamelli in Faenza (1556), where a reference can be found to a tin-glazed and painted *barca da bere* or 'drinking-boat'.[23] This mention marks not only an important 'trans-material' shift in the makeup of the 'barca' – from metalwork to earthenware – but also in its destination, as it is now described as an object involved no longer in the storage of tableware but in *drinking* practices. No surviving object from the large production attributed to the Calamelli workshop fits this description, however, thus leaving us to speculate as to what such 'barca da bere' would have looked like. The ship-inspired shape of the vessel might have brought about allusions to cargos containing spices and other exotic substances and in this way influenced and reflected the kinds of drinks that this object might have contained, for example spiced or scented water-based concoctions, as I will discuss below.

Vessel as fountain

The three-dimensional representation of a fountain that makes up the upper part of this object is also worth focusing on, as this element might

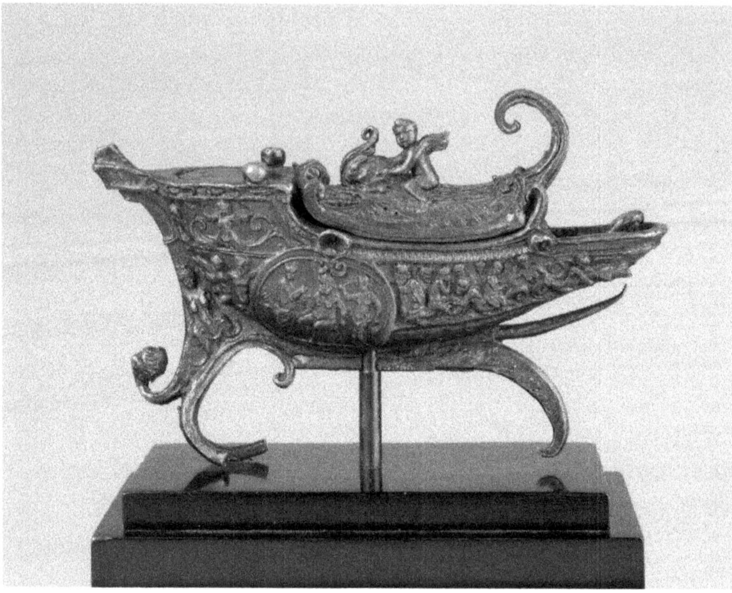

Figure 10.2 Andrea Riccio, 'Cadogan Lamp', bronze, Padua (Italy), 1507–10

provide synecdochally a reference to its possible identity as a table fountain. This interpretation would be supported by another entry in the inventory of Virgiliotto Calamelli's workshop, where a *fontana da bere* or 'drinking fountain' is listed.[24] Going under the modern term of 'table fountains', these playful devices became popular items at banquets and other upper-class dining events from the second half of the fifteenth century. They could take on a variety of forms and material embodiments, ranging from metal to tin-glazed earthenware (Fig. 10.3). Table fountains maximised the visual, and sometimes also aural and olfactory, potential of the journey of the liquid, which might be engaged in performative actions such as activating wheels or ringing bells and eventually come out in the form of a scented drink such as rosewater.[25] Complex table fountains in the shape of a ship populated by a rich series of characters, with the top portion working as a lid and the bottom as a container and able to hold considerable quantities of liquid, have survived, as with an early sixteenth-century German silver and silver-gilt example.[26] These spectacular metal vessels could also take

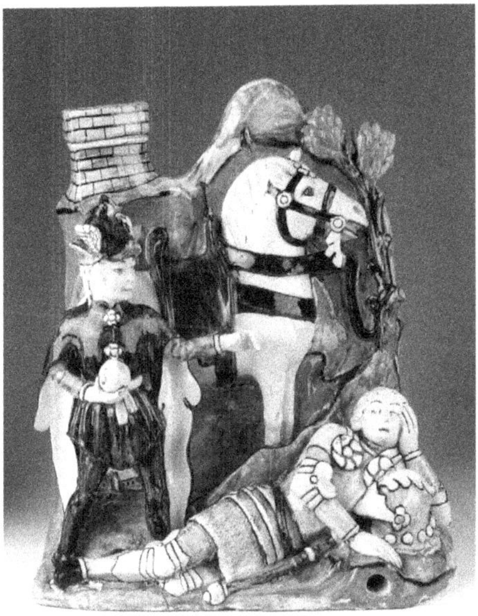

Figure 10.3 Table Fountain, *Mercury and Paris*, tin-glazed earthenware, possibly made in Faenza (Italy), 1500–10

the form of a ship morphing into a carriage mutating into a spouted ewer, as testified by a seventeenth-century example by Esaias zur Linde now at the V&A.[27]

Earthenware table fountains emerged in the sixteenth century, materialising in a wide range of different designs: they often included complex mythological scenes populated by figurines involved in the fountain's wondrous hydraulics, as in the case of the liquid exuding from the mouth or penis of one or more characters. Thus, in common with table fountains, this object would have had the performative quality of the liquid flowing visibly from level to level, and the conspicuous design. Within this interpretive framework it is possible that it might have originally sat within a basin designed to capture the liquid spilling out of the lower spout. Unlike some table fountains referring explicitly through their iconography to the pouring out of wine, as in the case of groups including Bacchus (Fig. 10.4), in this instance the lack of any

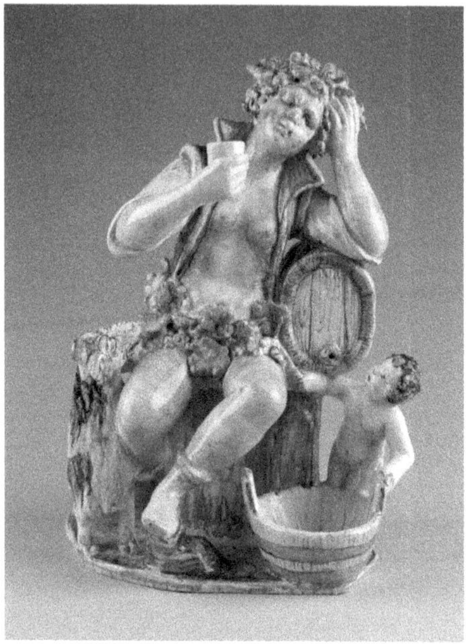

Figure 10.4 Fontana Workshop, table fountain, *Drunken Bacchus*, tin-glazed earthenware, Urbino (Italy), 1560–75

visual reference to the inebriating drink suggests that this might have been an object destined to the pouring out of a non-alcoholic drink, perhaps a water-based concoction, an 'artificial water' where herbs, flowers or spices might have been added, as will be explored below.

What singles out this object, however, making it possibly also differ in purpose and function from conventional table fountains, is the presence of what might be interpreted as a filtering system, as the double layer of triple narrow nozzles would have acted, to some extent, as a strainer. This feature is highly distinctive, and embodies the key difference between our object and its closest parallel, another contemporary boat-shaped earthenware vessel also attributed to Castelli. The latter carries striking affinities with ours in the overall design, constituted of two levels and of a pouring system in two stages. However, in this other example the boat is represented with greater naturalism, as the upper and lower deck and the poop and prow of the ship are clearly outlined and the balustrade marks out the boundaries of the vessel. Moreover, in this object the lower spout does not morph into a filter, but maintains a wide opening, thus ruling out a straining effect. The inscription 'CUSTODI, REGE ET GUBERNA' ('Protect, Rule and Govern') – a quote taken from the Catholic prayer *Angele Dei* – runs across the lower spout, just above an unidentified coat of arms, suggesting perhaps a ritualised use, reinforced by the presence of two angel figurines on both sides of the vessel. The two angels can also be found on the object under examination, pointing perhaps to these vessels' participation to devotional practices during the meals.

As we shift into exploring how this object was used, its materiality becomes worthy of attention, as tin-glazed earthenware or maiolica stands out from the early sixteenth century onwards for its growing popularity as the material of choice for dining.[28] By virtue of their relatively low cost and visual appeal, maiolica services increasingly replaced metalwork, even in the houses of the upper classes, as the preferred form of tableware. Allowing for a considerable variety of different forms and shapes to populate the different courses of the meal, maiolica sets also met contemporary hygienic requirements and responded to the concern, supported by regimens, to employ materials that would be clean and odourless and that would not affect the taste of the foods and liquids contained within them. These might include glass, maiolica and tinned metal, as Vincenzo Tanara reminds us in his treatise on country living (*L'economia del cittadino in villa*, 1644), where he emphasises the need to use these materials for vessels used for storing and serving liquids, while also ensuring that they are absolutely clean, to prevent water from absorbing bad smells.[29]

In order to tease out the function and purpose of this vessel, it is worth taking a closer look at its decoration. Far from offering an arbitrary, purposeless visual repertory, the ornamental vocabulary embracing the vessel might be seen to be in line with the pervasive Renaissance notion of *decorum*, whereby every aspect of design, including the decorative surface, might be seen to be 'fit for purpose', thus providing some clues as to how it was meant to be used. In this case, the vessel's iconography is constructed around the principle of animation, whereby all the spouts, both at the upper and lower level, feature dragonheads (Plate 9), while in the lower part the dragonhead takes up the entire design and is enhanced by a series of blazing flames, creating a radiating crown of fire around the spout. This active, vigorous motif carrying widely understood mythological connotations also evokes the elemental encounter of water and fire, something to which I will return below. Thus the overt structural and visual idiom of this object – particularly the filtering system provided at both levels and the dragonhead theme – suggests that we might be dealing with an object involved in the production of *heated* drinks, something that would connect it with the contemporary concerns about the role played by hot drinking in the promotion of good health.

The late sixteenth century saw the emergence of a lively debate on drinking within the context of healthy living. Traditionally conspicuous sections of regimens had articulated ideas around drinking, but from the 1580s onwards a flurry of specialist new texts emerged, devoted exclusively to hot and cold drinking. Cold drinking – involving the use of snow or saltpetre to cool the drink – had been seen as beneficial since antiquity and continued to grow in popularity during the early modern period.[30] Hot drinking was more controversial and attracted extensive new discussion by both supporters and detractors. Hot drinking is embraced as a healthy practice in the first treatise dedicated entirely to it – Antonio Persio's *Del bever caldo costumato da gli antichi Romani,* published in Venice in 1593. Persio was a priest and pupil of the natural philosopher Bernardino Telesio. His tract might be seen as the most vocal effort to revive hot drinking, which is presented as a social practice enjoyed widely within ancient Greco-Roman culture. Persio extols the health benefits ('più utile') and the better taste ('più gustevole') that result from hot drinking – by which he generally means drinking water heated on the fire and added to one's wine – and supports this contention through a sustained use of classical Greek and Latin sources describing this practice.[31] He refers to the seasonal habit of drinking very hot water enjoyed by the ancient Greeks in winter and spring and associates hot drinking with the elites and their pleasurable lifestyle, while cold drinking is seen as pertaining to the populace. Drunk pure or mixed with wine, hot water is described by Persio as a the drink customarily served in convivial contexts (*convivia*) in ancient times and even associated with a purpose-designed glass, the *calix,* whose etymology he (erroneously) associates with the Latin for hot 'calidum'. Persio supports hot drinking not only on the basis of its classical ancestry, but also by virtue of its popularity in his day among other cultures, such as the Chinese and Japanese. The health benefits associated with hot drinking are countless, according to Persio: it helps re-establish one's natural heat, enlivens the natural spirits, aids digestion, cleanses stomach and intestines, placates thirst and has 'a hundred other effects'. In addition, the quality of what one drinks is seen to improve as a result of the heating process, with the water being 'perfected', becoming better, purer and sweeter.[32]

Persio's enthusiastic support for hot drinking would have sounded novel in the late sixteenth century, as until then the only drinks that would have been customarily boiled and consumed hot would have been medicinal concoctions. Because of being generally inscribed in healing practices, until then the utensils employed in the heating and serving of hot drinks would have perhaps not required the trappings associated with sociable drinking. Because of this gap it is not surprising to find that Persio backs up his campaign in favour of hot drinking by describing and illustrating some of the equipment that should accompany the production of hot drinks and their consumption at the table. He collectively terms these devices *dragoni* or dragons because of the hot steam and liquid that they are designed to pour out, in a way that animates the vessels and endows them with mythological connotations. Persio discusses at some length three 'vasi da scaldar l'acqua' or vessels for heating water: a snaky vase or *dragone*, distinctive for its zigzagging shape, which would have been placed inside a source of heat, with the piping hot liquid coming out of the mouth at the lower end (Fig. 10.5); a *miliario* or *vaso da fuoco* ('fire vase'), which might be seen as a precursor to the modern kettle (Fig. 10.6);[33] and a *caraffa* or jug with a long neck, a simple device that Persio claims as his own invention and that involves placing small elongated vessels with a rounded bottom filled with water inside a cauldron of boiling water and having them brought to the table whenever there was a need for adding hot water to one's wine (Fig. 10.7). All three types of device described by Persio are not part of the ordinary domestic heating or drinking kit, but would have involved the making of purpose-made vessels of different designs and technological complexity. The *miliario* is the most elaborate of all three and involved a significant level of experimental technology, alluded to by the word 'experientia' inscribed at the bottom of the illustration. The vessel is a reconstruction of an invention discussed in the *Pneumatica*,

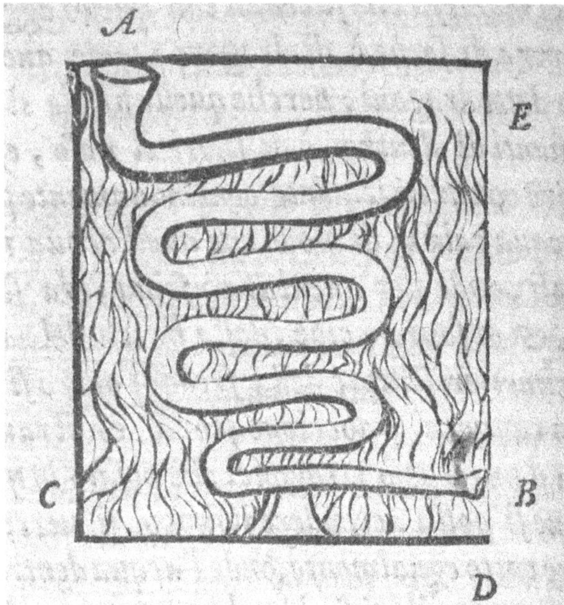

Figure 10.5 *Dragone,* in Antonio Persio, *Del bever caldo costumato da gli antichi Romani,* Venice, 1593

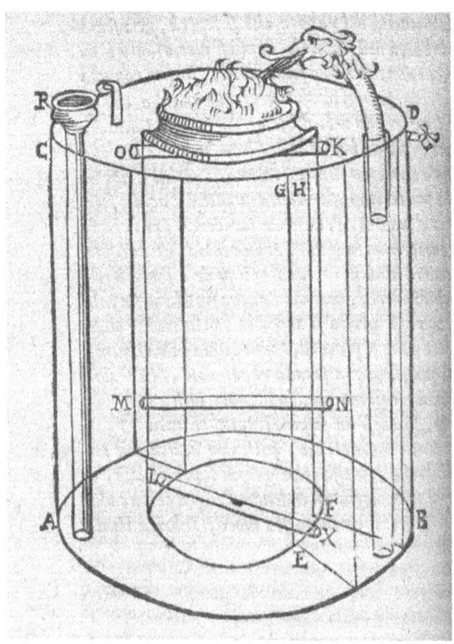

Figure 10.6 *Miliario,* in Antonio Persio, *Del bever caldo costumato da gli antichi Romani,* Venice, 1593

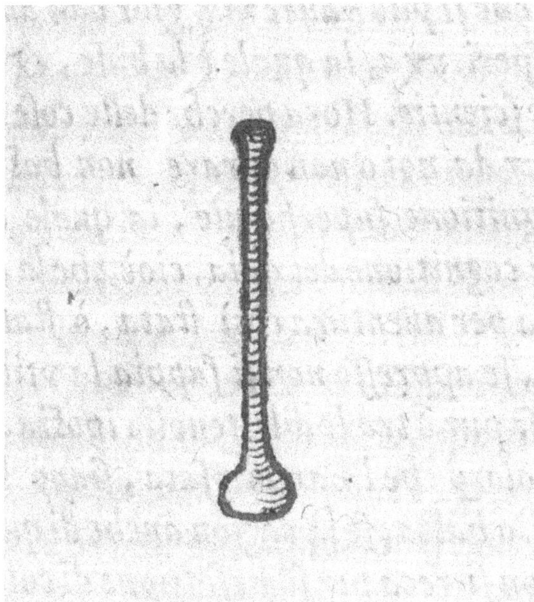

Figure 10.7 *Caraffa*, in Antonio Persio, *Del bever caldo costumato da gli antichi Romani*, Venice 1593

a treatise by the ancient author Hero of Alexandria discussing systems using the energy stored in compressed air to do work and generate movement, most likely known to Persio via the sixteenth-century adaptation by Giovan Battista Aleotti (Fig. 10.8).[34] It is important to point out the convergence that we see here of medical and technological knowledge through the borrowing across these disciplines and the attempted reconstruction of this ancient machine. The complexity of this pneumatic device, built on the principle of the vacuum, made Persio admit that it would have not been a viable solution for everyday water heating. While Persio mentions how he and his humanist friend Ercole Bottrigari – an expert in mathematics and music – had a model made of Hero's *miliario* and a brass prototype commissioned from a master craftsman from Bologna, we have no evidence that this machine was ever made.[35] Although this text is very compelling in his vigorous

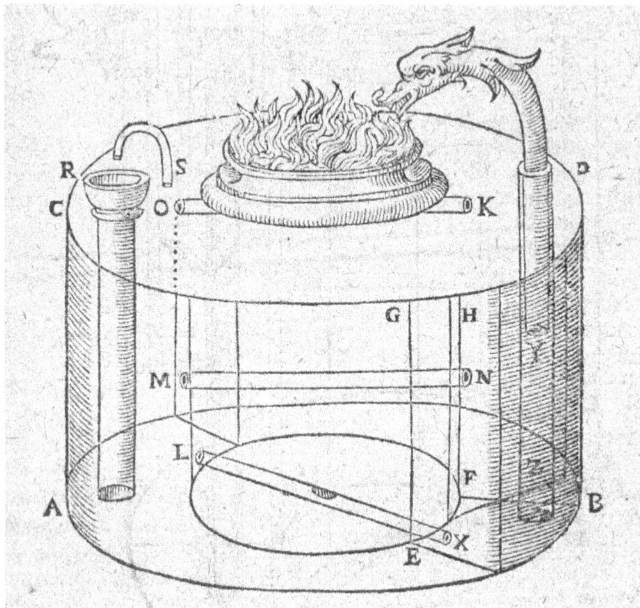

Figure 10.8 *Miliario*, in Giovan Battista Aleotti, *Gli artifitiosi et curiosi moti spiritali di Herrone*, Ferrara (Italy), 1589

promotion of the *miliario* and of other hot-drinking equipment, we are not able to support his campaign with any material survival, thus opening the possibility of a hiatus between the literary debate and technological reality.

Although Persio engages only with the heating of water that one should add to one's wine to obtain a hot drink, he also pays tribute to the Japanese custom of drinking hot tea. He refers to the Jesuit Giovanni Pietro Maffei's description of tea drinking in China in the sixth book of the *Historie delle Indie Orientali* and recalls his encounter with a Japanese delegation to Pope Gregory XIII who used to drink hot tea (*Chia*) during their meals.[36] In a later regimen – *Del conservare la sanita et del vivere de' Genovesi* (1602) – the doctor Bartolomeo Paschetti remarks how in China and Japan it is customary 'to drink a liquor called

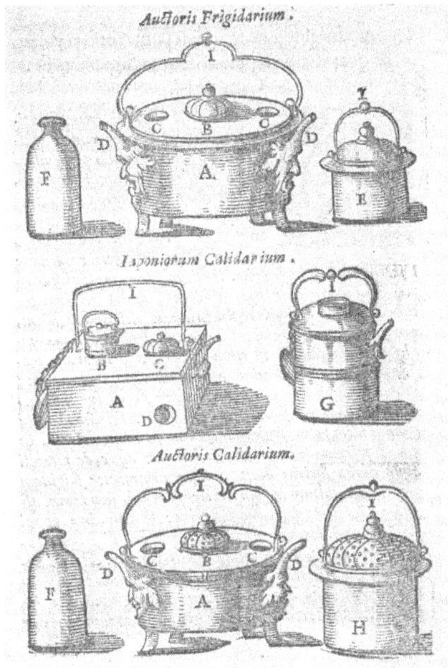

Figure 10.9 *Frigidarium* and *Calidarium*, in Franciscus Scacchus, *De salubri potu dissertatio*, Rome, 1622

Chia which is extracted from a very beneficial herb', as a way to support the drinking of hot herbal drinks and to promote their health benefits.[37] One of the earliest illustrations of tea-making equipment is found in Francesco Scacchi's *De salubri potu dissertatio* of 1622, a text in which the debate around hot-drinking equipment takes a further turn (Fig. 10.9). Scacchi celebrates both cold and hot drinking and includes a lengthy description and detailed woodcut illustrations for a cooling vessel or *frigidarium* and for two different types of hot-drinking equipment or *calidarium*. The first *calidarium* is allegedly inspired by Japanese sources and designed to brew tea and keep it warm, something that Scacchi had seen in operation in Rome in 1615 when Pope Paul V received a Japanese embassy, and also in the household of Cardinal Borghese.[38] The other one is 'invented' by the author and designed not

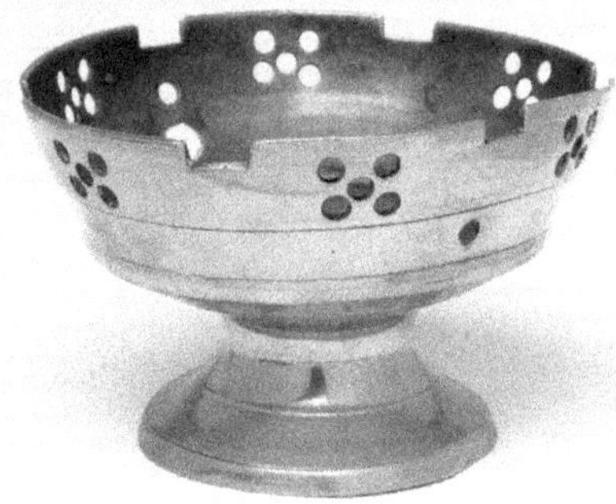

Figure 10.10 Brazier or table heater, brass, Flanders (Belgium), *c.*1550

for tea making, but to heat wine at the table. While this visual evidence is very compelling, these kinds of vessels, to my knowledge, have not left any record within collections. Here we have another detailed textual source, but no corresponding material survival.

When we return to our vessel (Plate 7), it is tempting to associate it with the other hot-drinking devices discussed. Although this object did not contain within itself a heating system, we cannot rule out that it might have been placed on a table heater (Fig. 10.10). In terms of the kind of hot drink that might have been poured out of it, we are also left to speculate. If we associate this vessel with the drinking of wine diluted with hot water, it is possible that this object was used for pouring out *vino mirrato,* a drink of classical descent made up of heated wine mixed with spices, such as myrrh, where the filtering process would have helped to strain the spices. Persio describes conducting an experiment with hot 'vin mirrato' and involving the Bolognese natural philosopher Ulisse Aldrovandi as a consultant in the process of selecting the best myrrh.[39]

Another possible way to identify this artefact is as a container of herbal drinks, a pouring vessel for tisanes, a new type of specialised object, to my knowledge unrecorded by contemporary written sources, allowing herbal drinks to be poured *at the table*. While the term 'tisana' or 'ptissana' is used in the sixteenth century exclusively to refer to a barley-based medicinal concoction and does not seem to have the wide semantic field we associate with it today, regimens offer what might seem like an interesting lead with regard to hot herbal drinks.[40] Paschetti, Petronio and Tanara prescribe 'acque cotte o medicinali', 'boiled and medicinal waters', also known as 'acque artificiose' ('artificial waters'), for the cold months obtained by slowly boiling and brewing hot water with a number of different ingredients.[41] Tanara mentions water infused with honey ('acqua melata'), liquorice, cicory, cinnamon, anise, coriander and 'strawberry water'.[42] The term 'odorata' or scented is often used in association with these waters, thus also alluding to their olfactory qualities.[43] It would have been customary to drink medicinal decoctions hot, and thus it is possible that all these 'heated waters' were consumed hot too. As for the equipment used, Tanara refers to 'glass or tin-glazed earthenware jugs or tin ewers' to make these drinks ('boccali di vetro o vitriato o stagnate').[44] However, according to these writings, the 'filtering' process or 'passatura' of these drinks with a metal sieve or a linen cloth would seem to have happened not on the table, as the vessel under study implied in its design, but in the kitchen.[45]

These suggestions correspond with the written and visual prescriptions provided in an influential cookery book, Bartolomeo Scappi's *Opera*, first published in 1570. In Scappi's treatise the *acque cotte* are heated slowly within large vases kept by the fire, and filtered in the kitchen on a contraption that makes use of a cloth sieve.[46] Thus while discussing the preparation of these tisanes, neither regimens nor cookery books mention vessels specifically designed for preparing or serving these drinks, but simply refer to the standard kitchen equipment, such as pots, jugs and sieves, in which these concoctions would have been made.

The overall design of this vessel, however, seems to conspire against the hypothesis that we are looking at an early European pot for brewing 'acque artificiose' or tisanes, a 'proto-teapot'. These vessels were well established in various parts of Asia, including the Middle East, since at least the early Middle Ages.[47] Their design involving a globular body, a long slim neck and a handle in the upper part – very close to that of an orthodox, 'modern' teapot, except for the absence of a lid, had entered Europe through various routes. By the fifteenth century this shape can be found in various European pouring vessels, including lavers, such as the Flemish examples made of brass, which survive in various collections, and which sometimes featured a dragon's head as the tip of the spout.[48] Given the popularity of this form, it might seem unlikely that such an economical and functional design would have been replaced by the cumbersome and impractical shape of our vessel. On the other hand, this more open vessel would have carried aural performative qualities unavailable in the more practical 'teapot' design and would have aided the cooling of the liquid, while also permeating the air with the pleasant scent of the drink, thus allowing us to associate it more closely to the genre of the table fountain.

While its internal filtering system and its visual allusion to fire and steam through the dragon motif point in the direction of hot drinking, suggesting something definitive about its function is not possible at present. Ultimately, therefore, its relationship with the written debate on hot drinking remains problematic and unresolved. However, although we cannot come to any firm conclusion about the original intended purpose of this vessel, what seems unquestionable is the ingenuity of its complex structure, able to channel the movement of the liquid across different levels, and in the process to highlight the physical and sensorial qualities of the drink, its colour, smell and sound, thus 'bringing it to life'.[49] By bringing the pouring of drinks out of the kitchen and onto the table, this performative object would have certainly emphasised drinking as a social ritual and allowed for any health-related value associated with the drink to be shared. Thus it could be seen as an object not just *responding* in an innovative way to the contemporary debate about drinking, but possibly also *actively shaping* the way in which drinks would have been prepared, served, consumed and ultimately perceived.

This chapter has examined what we might gain from using an object-driven approach in the process of exploring early modern healthy living practices concerned with hot drinking. By foregrounding the materiality, design and decoration of the artefact under scrutiny and locating it within the contemporary medical and technological debate around hot drinking, I hope to have shed some light on its possible purposes, uses and meanings. While the object's identification remains to some extent open, I have shown how, through close object analysis, we are able to locate it within a wider family of table vessels displaying overt performative properties, raising the profile and visibility of drinks on the table and bringing them in close proximity to diners. In addition, by looking closely at a vessel that is not represented in the contemporary written or visual record, but whose tangibility, liveliness and embodiedness are impossible to disregard, we acknowledge the unique contribution of material culture to the expansion and refinement of the questions and answers powering historical enquiry.

Conclusion

In conclusion, this chapter has raised a number of questions concerning the possibilities and challenges involved in the methodologies we employ as historians in the construction and interpretation of the dialogue between written, visual and material sources. Through the focus on an enigmatic, unresolved object, which might be connected to new healthy living practices, it has called for the need to grant objects complex interpretive possibilities. As we continue in the laudable effort of inscribing material culture within the wider narratives informed by early modern healthy living, we must remember that our engagement with objects, rather than offering unambiguous evidence, demands the same inquisitive and critical approaches that we routinely apply to written and visual documentation.

Notes

1 S. Cavallo and T. Storey, *Healthy Living in Late Renaissance Italy* (Oxford: Oxford University Press, 2013).
2 *Ibid.*
3 For an extensive introduction to and bibliography on object-based approaches see K. Harvey (ed.), *History and Material Culture. A Student's Guide to Approaching Alternative Sources* (London and New York: Routledge, 2009).
4 L. Auslander, 'Beyond words', *American Historical Review,* 110:4 (2005), pp. 1015–45, on p. 1017.

5 *Ibid.*, p. 1017.
6 J. Prown, 'Mind in matter: an introduction to material culture theory and method', *Winterthur Portfolio*, 17:1 (1982), pp. 1–19; S. Lubar and D. Kingery (eds), *History from Things: Essays on Material Culture* (Washington, London: Smithsonian Institution Press, 1993); M. Dietler and I. Herbich, 'Habitus, techniques, style: an integrated approach to the social understanding of material culture and boundaries', in M.T. Stark (ed.), *The Archaeology of Social Boundaries* (Washington, London: Smithsonian Institution Press, 1998), pp. 232–63; C. Knappett, *Thinking through Material Culture: An Interdisciplinary Perspective* (Philadelphia: University of Pennsylvania Press, 2005); C. Tilley, 'Ethnography and material culture', in P. Atkinson et al. (eds), *Handbook of Ethnography* (London: Sage, 2001), pp. 258–72; D. Miller, *Material Cultures: Why Some Things Matter* (London: UCL Press, 1997); P. Verbeek and P. Kockelkoren, 'The things that matter', *Design Issues*, 14:3 (1998), pp. 28–42; J.J. Gibson, 'The theory of affordances', in R. Shaw and J. Brausford (eds), *Perceiving, Acting and Knowing: Toward an Ecological Psychology* (New York: John Wiley & Sons, 1977), pp. 127–43; P. Verbeek, *What Things Do: Philosophical Reflections on Technology, Agency, and Design* (Philadelphia: Pennsylvania State University Press, 2005); B. Latour, 'Where are the missing masses? A sociology of a few mundane artefacts', in W.E. Bijker and J. Law (eds), *Shaping Technology / Building Society: Studies in Sociotechnical Change* (Boston: MIT Press, 1992), pp. 225–58.
7 B. Latour, 'The Berlin key or how to do words with things', in P.M. Graves Brown (ed.), *Matter, Materiality and Modern Culture* (London, New York: Routledge, 2000), pp. 10–21; Auslander, 'Beyond words'; B. Brown, 'Thing theory', *Critical Inquiry*, 28:1 (2001), pp. 1–22; B. Brown, *A Sense of Things: The Object Matter of American Literature* (Chicago: University of Chicago Press, 2003).
8 *Ibid.*; Brown, 'Thing theory'.
9 Auslander, 'Beyond words', p. 1017.
10 S. Pennell, 'Mundane materiality, or, should small things still be forgotten? Material culture, micro-histories and the problem of scale', in Harvey (ed.), *History and Material Culture*, pp. 173–91.
11 Auslander, 'Beyond words', p. 1017. For the concept of agency see also A. Gell, *Art and Agency. An Anthropological Theory* (Oxford: Oxford University Press, 1998).
12 T. Ingold, *The Perception of the Environment: Essays in Livelihood, Dwelling and Skill* (London, New York: Routledge, 2000); 'Bringing things to life: creative entanglements in a world of materials', NCRM Working Paper #15 (Realities / Morgan Centre, University of Manchester, July 2010).

13 J. Dixon Hunt, 'The sign of the object', in Lubar and Kingery (eds), *History from Things*, pp. 293–8.
14 C. Tilley, *Metaphor and Material Culture* (Oxford: Blackwell, 1999), p. 6.
15 W. D. Kingery (ed.), *Learning from Things: Method and Theory of Material Culture Studies* (Washington, London: Smithsonian Institution Press, 1996), p. 1.
16 Auslander, 'Beyond words'; T.V. Peterson, 'Introduction: cultural and historical interpretation through nontextual material', *Historical Reflections*, 23:3 (1997), pp. 259–67; T. Fisher, 'What we touch touches us: material affects and affordances', *Design Issues*, 20:4 (2004), pp. 20–31.
17 C. Fiocco and G. Gherardi, *Museo d'Arti Applicate. Le ceramiche*, vol.1, *Musei e Gallerie di Milano* (Milan: Electa, 2000), pp. 386–7. Fiocco and Gherardi call it 'versatoio per tisane'.
18 V. de Pompeis, *La Maiolica Italiana di Stile Compendiario* (Milan: Allemandi, 2010), n. 17.
19 C. Geertz, 'Thick description: toward an interpretative theory of culture', in *The Interpretation of Cultures* (New York: Basic Books, 1973).
20 Prown, 'Mind in matter'.
21 J.A. Levenson (ed.), *Circa 1492: Art in the Age of Exploration*, Washington, DC, National Gallery of Art, 1991 (New Haven and London: Yale University Press, 1991), p. 137.
22 See the entry for Andrea Riccio's so-called Cadogan bronze lamp; Museum no.137-1865 in the Victoria and Albert Museum's *Search the Collections* online catalogue.
23 C. Grigioni, 'Documenti: Serie Faentina. I Calamelli maiolicari di Faenza', *Faenza*, 4–5:22 (1934), pp. 143–53, on p. 148.
24 *Ibid.*, p. 146.
25 M. Belozerskaya, *Luxury Arts of the Renaissance* (Los Angeles: Getty, 2005), pp. 73–5, 230. See also the video of the animated table fountain now at the Cleveland Museum of Art: YouTube video, 'Animated representation of a Medieval table fountain', Getty Museum (www.youtube.com/watch?v=jxAUCdoUTmY, accessed on 16 October 2015).
26 Levenson (ed.), *Circa 1492*, p. 137; Belozerskaya, *Luxury Arts of the Renaissance*, pp. 73–5.
27 Museum no. M.425-1956 in the Victoria and Albert Museum's *Search the Collections* online catalogue.
28 R. Goldthwaite, 'The economic and social world of Italian Renaissance maiolica', *Renaissance Quarterly*, 42:1 (1989), pp. 1–31; M.J. Brody, '"Terra d'Urbino tutta dipinta a paesi con l'armi de' Salviati": The "Paesi" service in the 1583 inventory of Jacopo di Alamanno Salviati (1537–1586)', *Faenza*, 4–6 (2000), pp. 30–46.

29 V. Tanara, *L' Economia del cittadino in villa* (Venice: Bertani, 1661), p. 17: 's'averta in fine, che qual si voglia vaso, che debba servire per fare acque, sia di vetro, o vitriato, o stagnate; in oltre sia polito, e netto, e libero da ogni cosa, che possa porgere mal'odore, perchè l'acqua è facilissima da pigiare ogni tristo odore, si come il fumo.'

30 Cavallo and Storey, *Healthy Living*, ch.7, pp. 209–39.

31 A. Persio, *Del bever caldo costumato dagli antichi Romani* (Venice: Gió Battista Ciotto, 1593), p. 1r: 'ber caldo, cioè l'usar bevanda riscaldata al fuoco, sia più utile e più gustevole del ber freddo'.

32 *Ibid.*, pp. 6r–7v, 8r–11v, 24v, 52r–57v, 53r, 52r–57v.

33 Cavallo and Storey, *Healthy Living*, pp. 233–4 and fig. 7.7

34 G.B. Aleotti, *Gli artifitiosi e curiosi moti spiritali di Herrone* (Ferrara: Vittorio Baldini, 1589).

35 Persio, *Del bever caldo*, pp. 40r and 40v.

36 *Ibid.*, p. 24v.

37 B. Paschetti, *Del conservare la sanitá* (Genoa: Giuseppe Pavoni, 1602), p. 292: 'e se il bever caldo fosse tanto dannoso, e tanto utile il bever freddo, non morirebbono infinite persone in quelle parti da noi tanto remote della China, e del Giapone ove si beve caldo? In molti altri luoghi, e regioni caldissime, dove non si beve in neve, come particolarmente in Siviglia citta principale della Spagna, e patria del Monardes fautore di cosi fatta opinion, il quale scrive, che dal principio di primavera fino alla fine dell'autunno v'ha grandissimo caldo, e sonovi acque quasi bollenti.'

38 F. Scacchi, *De salubri potu dissertatio* (Rome: Alessandro Zanetto, 1622), p. 91.

39 Persio, *Del bever caldo*, p. 21v.

40 For an extensive discussion of this barley-based *ptissana* see Alessandro Peccana, *De' Commentarii della scandella* (Verona: Angelo Tamo, 1622).

41 Paschetti, *Del conservare*, p. 315, 'acque medicinali', made with fennel or anise; A. Petronio, *Del viver delli Romani* (Rome: Domenico Bassa, 1592), p. 46, 'Acque medicinali'; Tanara, *L' Economia del cittadino*, p. 15, 'acque artificiose'.

42 *Ibid.*, p. 15.

43 *Ibid.*, pp. 15–17.

44 *Ibid.*, p. 17.

45 *Ibid.*, pp. 15–16: 'passatura' si fa sempre con 'stamigno' o 'panno di lino'.

46 B. Scappi, *Opera* (Venice: Alessandro Vecchi, 1605); see the caption to the illustration at p. 122: 'bollire piano piano'.

47 See catalogue of the exhibition *Byzantine Palaces in Istanbul* (Istanbul: Istanbul Archaeological Museums, 2010) for examples in the Istanbul Archaeological Museums.

48 See the Victoria and Albert Museum's *Search the Collections* online catalogue, no. M.2669-1931 for a Flemish brass laver with two dragons spouts and no. 411M-1880 for a brass laver made in Northern Europe but inscribed in Arabic, suggesting that it would have been used in Syria. The online catalogue contains other similar examples.
49 Ingold, 'Bringing things to life'.

Bibliography

Primary sources

A., B., *The Sick-Mans Rare Jewel* (London: T.R., 1674).

Adair, J.M., *Essay on Fashionable Diseases* (London: Rateman, 1790).

Aleotti, G.B., *Gli artifitiosi e curiosi moti spiritali di Herrone* (Ferrara: Vittorio Baldini, 1589).

Alexander, W., *Plain and easy directions for the use of Harrogate Waters* (Edinburgh: A. Kincaid & W. Creech, 1773).

Allestree, R., *The art of contentment* (Oxford: The Theatre, 1675).

Allestree, R., *The Whole Duty of Man* (London: Robert Harford, 1680).

Alsario della Croce, V., *Vesuvius ardens siue Exercitatio medico-physica ad rigopyreton* (Rome: Guilelmi Facciotti, 1632).

[Ameyden, D., and T. Carre], *Pietas Romana et Parisiensis or a faithful relation of the several sorts of charitable and pious works eminent in the cities of Rome and Paris* (Oxford, publisher unknown, 1687).

Anon., *The Aphorismes of Hippocrates* (London: Humphrey Moseley, 1655).

Anon., *Crumbs of Comfort and Godly Prayers* (London: publisher unknown 1726).

Archer, I., *Two East Anglian Diaries 1641–1729*, ed. M.J. Storey, Suffolk Record Society, vol. 36 (Woodbridge, 1994).

Archer, J., *Everyman his own Doctor* (London: printed for the author, 1673).

Auda, D., *Breue compendio di marauigliosi secreti rationali ... Con vn trattato ... per conseruarsi in sanità* (Rome: de' Lazari, 1652).

B., T., *The bloudy mother, or, The most inhumane murthers, committed by Jane Hattersley vpon diuers infants* (London: John Busbie, 1610).
Bacon, F., Viscount St. Albans, *History Naturall and Experimentall of Life and Death, or of the Prolongation of Life* (London: Lee and Mosely, 1651).
Baglivi, G., *Opere complete medico-pratiche ed anatomiche* (Florence: Coen, 1842).
Banister, J., *A Needefull, New, and Necessarie Treatise of Chyrurgerie* (London: Thomas Marshe, 1575).
Barret, R., *A Companion for Midwives, child-bearing women, and nurses* (London: Tho. Ax., 1699).
Barrington Family Letters, 1628–1632, ed. A. Searle (London: Royal Historical Society, 1983).
Barrough, P. *The Methode of Phisicke* (London: Thomas Vautroullier, 1583, first publ. 1508).
Basse, W., E. Philips and E. Pond, *A Helpe to discourse: or, More merriment mixt with serious matters* (London: Nicholas Vavasour, 1635).
Baxter, R., *A Christian Directory* (London: Simmons, 1673).
Benzi, U., *Tractato utilissimo circa lo regimento et conservatione de la sanitade* (Milan: Petromartire, 1508).
Bernabei, A., *Dissertazione delle morti improvvise nella quale si ragiona delle perucche e degli acidi* (Rome: Gonzaga, 1708).
Bernier, F., *Abregé de la Philosophie de Gassendi* (Lyon: Anisson, Posuel et Rigaud, 1684).
Bianchini, F., *Opuscula* (Rome: Barbiellini, 1753).
Biggs, N., *Mataeotechnia Medicinae Praxeos, The Vanity of the Craft of Physick* (London: Edward Blackmore, 1651).
Blankaart, S., *A Physical Dictionary* (London: J.D., 1684).
Blount, T., *Glossographia, or, a Dictionary* (London: Thomas Newcomb, 1656).
Boldo, B., *Libro della natura et virtú delle cose* (Venice: Domenico & Gio.Battista Guerra fratelli, 1575).
[Boorde, A.], *The boke for to Lerne a man to be wyse in buyldyng of his howse for the helth of body & to holde quyetnes for the helth of his soule, and body* (London: Robert Wyer, 1540).
Boorde, A., *A Compendyous Regiment* (London: Thomas Colwell, 1542 and Wyllyam Powell, 1547).
Borelli, G.A., *Delle cagioni delle febbri maligne della Sicilia negli anni 1647 e 1648* (Cosenza: Rosso, 1649).
Borelli, G.A., *Historia et meteorologia incendii Aetnaei anni 1699* (Regio Iulio: Ferri, 1670).
Botero, G., *Discorso intorno lo stato della chiesa* (Venice: Giorgio Varisco, 1605).
Braccini, G.C., *Dell'Incendio Fattosi nel Vesuvio a 16. di Dicembre M.DC.XXXI. E delle sue Cause, ed Effetti* (Naples: Secondino Roncagliolo, 1632).

Breventano, S., *Trattato degli elementi raccolto da varii autori* (Pavia: Girolamo Bartoli, 1571).
Breventano, S., *Trattato del'origine delli venti* (Venice: Gioan Francesco Camotio, 1571).
Brooke, S., *Ugieine: or Conservatory of Health* (London: R.W., 1650).
Bruele, G., *Praxis Medicinae, or, the Physicians Practice* (London: John Norton, 1632).
Bruno, M., *Discorsi ... sopra gli errori fatti dall'eccell.te M. Bartolomeo Trafichetti da Bertinoro. Nell'arte sua di conseruar la sanità tutt'intiera* (Venice: Andrea Arrivabene, 1569).
Bryant, A. (ed.), *Postman's Horn: An Anthology of the Letters of Latter Seventeenth Century England* (New York: Privately printed, 1946).
Bullein, W., *A newe boke of phisicke called ye government of health* (London: John Day, 1559).
[Bullein, W.], *Bulleins bulwarke of defence: againste all sicknes, sornes and woundes, that dooe daily assaulte mankind* (London: John Kyngston, 1562).
Burnet, E., *A Method of Devotion: or Rules for Holy & Devout Living* (London: Joseph Downing, C. Smith, & A. Barker, 1709).
Buxton, J., *John Buxton, Norfolk Gentleman and Architect: Letters to his Son, 1719–1729*, ed. A. Mackley, Norfolk Record Society, vol. 69 (Norwich, 2005).
Cancellieri, F., *Lettera ... al Ch. Sig. Dottore Koreff ... sopra il tarantismo, l'aria di Roma e della sua campagna, ed i palazzi pontefìcj entro, e fuori di Roma* (Rome: Francesco Bourlié, 1817).
Capaccio, G.C., *La Vera Antichita di Pozzuolo, Descritta ... A modo d'Itinerario* (Naples: Gio. Giacomo Carlino e Costantino Vitale, 1607).
Castelli, P., *Incendio del Monte Vesuvio* (Rome: Giacomo Mascardi, 1632).
Catalogus librorum quos Exx Italia selegit Robertus Martine Bibliopola Londinensis (London: A. Matthews, 1633).
Ciccolini, B., *L'oro della sanità ritrovato nel clima romano* (Rome: Vannacci, 1697).
Cirillo, N., *Consulti medici* (Venice: F. Pitteri, 1741; first ed. 1738).
Clegg, J., *The Diary of James Clegg of Chapel-en-Frith 1708–1755*, ed. Vanessa S. Doe, 5 vols, Derbyshire Record Society (Matlock, 1978).
Cock, T., *Kitchin-physick: or, Advice for the Poor* (London: J.B., 1676).
Coeffeteau, N., *A Table of Humane Passions* (London: Nicholas Okes, 1621).
Cogan, T., *The Haven of Health* (London: Thomas Orwin, 1589 and Anne Griffin, 1636; first publ. 1588).
Col nome de Dio. Il segreto de segreti (Venice: Zuan Tacuino da Trino, 1538).
Colmenero, A., *Della cioccolata discorso* (Rome: RCA, 1667).
Consiglio di Marsilio Ficino Fiorentino contro la pestilentia. Insieme con ... altri Autori (Florence: I. Giunti, 1576).

Cornaro, L., *A treatise of Temperance and Sobrietie*, published with Lessius, *Hygiasticon*.

Cornaro, L., *Discorsi della vita sobria* (Padua: Miglietti, 1591).

Cowper, M., *Diary of Mary, Countess Cowper*, ed. John Murray (London, Privately printed, 1864).

Cullen, W., *First Lines of the Practice of Physic* (Edinburgh: W. Creech, 1777–84).

Culpeper, N., *Semeiotica Uranica: or, An Astrological Judgement of Diseases* (London: Nathaniel Brookes, 1651).

Culpeper, N., *Health for the Rich and poor by Dyet without physic* (London: Peter Cole, 1656).

Culpeper, N., *Culpeper's Directory for Midwives: or, A guide for women* (London: Peter Cole, 1662).

D'Ewes, S., *The Autobiography and Correspondence of Sir Simonds D'Ewes: During the Reign of James I and Charles I*, ed. J.O. Halliwell-Phillipps (London: R. Bentley, 1845).

Da Sylva, M., *Romanorum lachrymae subitaneis mortibus effusae exsiccantur* (Rome: Herculis, 1706).

[Davenport, G.], *The Letters of George Davenport 1651–1677*, ed. Brenda M. Pask, Surtees Society, vol. 215 (Woodbridge, 2011).

De La Framboisière, N.A., *The art of physick made plain & easie* (London: Newman, 1684).

[De Maineri, M.], *Opera utilissima di Arnaldo da Villanova di conservare la sanità* (Venice: Tramezzino, 1549).

De Mediolano, J., *Regimen Sanitatis Salerni: or, the Schoole of Salernes Regiment of Health* (London: B. Alsop, 1650; first transl. from Latin 1541).

De Montaigne, M., *Montaigne's Travel Journal*, ed. Donald M. Frame (San Francisco, CA: North Point Press, 1983).

De Valangin, F., *A Treatise on Diet, or the management of human life; by physicians called the six non-naturals* (London: J. and W. Oliver, 1768).

Debus, A.G., *Chemistry and Medical Debate: van Helmont to Boerhaave* (Canton, MA: Science History, 2001).

Di Capua, L., *Lezioni intorno alla natura delle mofete* (Naples: per Salvatore Castaldo, 1683).

Di Galeno. Delli mezzi, che si possono tenere per conseruarci la sanità (Venice: Tramezzino, 1549).

Dichiaratione delle virtù della bevanda del caffé (Rome: Bernabò, 1683).

Dionis, P., *Dissertation sur la mort subite et sur la catalepsie* (Paris: d'Houry, 1710).

Donato, M.P., 'La peste dopo la peste. Economia di un discorso romano (1656–1720)', *Roma moderna e contemporanea*, 14:1 (2006), pp. 159–74.

Donato, M.P., *Sudden Death. Medicine and Religion in Eighteenth-Century Rome* (Farnham: Ashgate, 2014).

Donne, J., *Devotions upon Emergent Occasions and Severall Steps in my Sicknes* (London: A.M, 1624).
Durante, C., *Il tesoro della sanità* (Venice: Andrea Muschio, 1586 and Padova: Cezza, 1659).
Durante, C., *Herbario nuovo … hora in questa novissima impressione vi si è posto in fine l'herbe thè, caffè … e cioccolata* (Venice: Hertz, 1684).
Elyot, T., *The Castel of Helth* (London, T. Berthelet, 1541 and Company of Stationers, 1610 as The Castel of Health, first ed. 1534).
Eustachio, G.N., *Opusculum de aere, Situque Beneventanae civitatis* (Naples: Io. Baptistae Subtilis apud Scipionem Boninum, 1608).
Evangelista, A., *Lettera informativa intorno alle cause delle morti improvise* (Rome: Stamperia Camerale, 1706).
Evelyn, J., *Diary*, ed. W. Bray, 2 vols (New York, London: Dunne, 1901).
Evelyn, J., *Fumifugium* (1661) (Exeter: The Rota at the University of Exeter, 1976).
Fanshawe, A., *Memoirs of Lady Fanshawe*, ed. Richard Fanshawe (London: Henry Colburn, 1829).
Ficino, M., *De le tre vite, cioè, a qual guisa si possono le persone letterate mantenere in sanità* (Venice: Tramezzino, 1548).
Fitzwilliam, W., *The Correspondence of Lord Fitzwilliam of Milton and Francis Guybon, His Steward 1697–1709*, ed. D.R. Hainsworth and Cherry Walker, Northampton Record Society, vol. 36 (1990).
[Fleming, S.H.], *The Flemings in Oxford*, ed. J.R. Magrath, Oxford Historical Society, vol. 44 (Oxford, 1904).
Fonseca, R., *Del conservare la sanitá* (Florence: Semartelli, 1603).
Frediano, E., *Arca novella di sanità* (Lucca: Iacinto Paci, 1656).
Freke, E., *The Remembrances of Elizabeth Freke*, ed. R. Anselment, Camden Fifth Series, vol. 18 (Cambridge: Cambridge University Press, 2001).
Fulwood, W., *The Enimie of Idlenesse Teaching the Maner and Stile how to Endite, Compose and Write all sorts of Epistles and Letters* (London: H. Bynneman, 1568).
Furchheim, F., *Bibliografia del Vesuvio: Compilata e Corredata di Note Critiche Estratte dai più Autorevoli Scrittori Vesuviani* (Naples: F. Furchheim di Emilio Prass, 1897).
Gagliardi, D., *Consigli preservativi e curativi in tempo di contagio* (Rome: S. Michele, 1720).
Galeano, G., *Del conseruar la sanitá libri sei di Galeno* (Palermo: Nicoló Bua, 1650).
Galeano, G., *Il caffé con piú diligenza esaminato in ordine al conservamento della salute de corpi humani* (Palermo: D. D'Anselmo, 1674).
Galens Art of Physic (London: Peter Cole, 1652).

Gatta, G., *Di una gravissima peste Che nella Passata Primavera & Estate dell'anno 1656 depopulò la Città di Napoli, suoi Borghi, e Casali, e molte altre Città, e Terre del suo Regno* (Naples: Luc'Antonio di Fusco, 1659).
Gayton, E., *The Art of longevity or a Diaeteticall Institution* (London: printed for the author, 1659).
Georio, F.A., *Flores medicinae theoricae ac fructus medicinae practicae necessarii ad diu vitam prolungandam* (Rome: S. Michaelis ad Ripam, 1726).
Gerard, J., *The herbal or generall historie of plantes* (London: Adam Islip Joice Norton and Richard Whitaker, 1633).
Ghesel, J., *Rule of Health* (Cambridge: Printers to the Universitie, 1633).
Giulianelli, P.A., *Essame delle acque di Civita Vecchia, e di Trevi* (Rome: Monadi, 1701).
Glasse, H., *The Art of Cookery, made Plain and Easy* (London: printed for the author, 1747).
Glasse, H., *The Servant's Directory, or House-Keeper's Companion* (London: printed for the author, 1760).
Glisson, F., G. Bate and A. Regemorter, *A Treatise of the Rickets* (London: Peter Cole, 1651).
Grassi, P., *Mortis repentinae examen ... cum brevi methodo praesagendi et praecavendi* (Modena: apud I. Cassianum, 1612).
Grataroli, G., *A Direction for the Health of Magistrates and students* (London, William How, 1574, first publ. Latin 1555).
Gropretio, R., *Un breue et notabile trattato del reggimento della Sanità*, annexed to D.Romoli, La singolare dottrina (Venice: Tramezzino, 1560).
Guillemeau, J., *Child-birth or, The happy deliuerie of women* (London: A. Hatfield, 1612).
Hales, S., *A Description of Ventilators* (London: W. Innys, 1743).
Harley, B., *Letters of The Lady Brilliana Harley*, ed. Thomas Taylor Lewis, Camden Society (London, 1853).
Harris, J., *The Divine Physician* (London: H.B., 1676).
Hart, J., *Klinike or the Diet of the diseased* (London: J. Beale, 1633).
Hartman, G., *The Family Physitian* (London: Richard Wellington, 1696).
[Hatton, C.], *Correspondence of the Family of Hatton being Chiefly Addressed to Christopher, First Viscount Hatton, 1601–1704*, ed. E.M. Thompson, Camden Society, vols 22–3 (London, 1878).
Heraclitus Christianus, or the Man of Sorrow (London: A.M., 1677).
Hervey, J., *Letter-Books of John Hervey, First Earl of Bristol, vol. 1, 1651–1715* (Wells: Ernest Jackson, 1894).
Hoby, J., *Diary of Lady Margaret Hoby 1599–1605*, ed. D.M. Meads (London: Routledge, 1930).

Hoffmann, F., *Dissertationes physico-medicae curiosae selectiores, ad sanitatem tuendam* (Leyden: Haak, 1708).
Horace Walpole's Correspondence with Sir Horace Mann, ed. W.S. Lewis, W.H. Smith and G.L. Lam (New Haven: Yale University Press, 1960).
Hurst, S., *The Diaries of Sarah Hurst 1759–1762, Life and Love in Eighteenth Century Horsham*, ed. S.C. Djabri (Stroud: Amberley, 2009).
Imperato, F., *Dell'historia naturale* (Naples: Costantino Vitale, 1599).
Jasolino, G., *De Rimedi Naturali che sono nell'Isola di Pithecusa, hoggi detta Ischia* (Naples: Gioseppe Cacchij, 1558).
Jeake, S., *An Astrological Diary of the Seventeenth Century: Samuel Jeake of Rye*, ed. M. Hunter (Oxford: Clarendon, 1988).
Johnstonus, J., *The Idea of Practical Physick* (London: Peter Cole, 1657).
Jones, J., *The Arte and Science of Preserving Bodie and Soule in Healthe* (London: Henrie Bynneman, 1579).
Josselin, R., *The Diary of Ralph Josselin 1616–1683*, ed. A. Macfarlane (Oxford: Oxford University Press, 1991).
Kettlewell, J., *Death Made Comfortable* (London: R. Kettlewell, 1695).
Lancisi, G.M., *De subitaneis mortibus libri duo* (Rome: Buagni, 1707).
Lancisi, G.M., *Dissertatio de nativis, deque adventitiis Romani coeli qualitatibus, cui accedit historia epidemiae rheumaticae, quae per hyemem anni 1709 vagata est* (Rome: apud Gonzagam, 1711).
Lancisi, G.M., *Dissertatio historica de bovilla peste* (Rome: Salvioni, 1715).
Lancisi, G.M., *De noxiis paludum effluviis, eorumque remediis* (Rome: Salvioni, 1717).
Langton, C., *An Introduction into Physycke with an universal dyet* (London: Edwarde Whytchurche, c.1547).
Lémery, L., *Trattato degl'alimenti, e della maniera di conseruarsi lungamente in sanitá; ... secondo i principij chimici, e mecchanici* (Venice: Albrizi, 1704).
Lemnius, L., *The Secret Miracles of Nature* (London: Jo. Streater, 1658).
Lennio, L., *Della complessione del corpo humano* (Venice: Domenico Nicolino, 1564).
Lessius, L., *Hygiasticon: or The right course of preserving life and health unto extream old age* (Cambridge: R. Daniel and T. Buck, 1634).
Lievsay, J.L., *The Englishman's Italian books 1550–1700* (Philadelphia: University of Pennsylvania Press, 1969).
Lister, J., *The Autobiography of Joseph Lister of Bradford, 1627–1709*, ed. Thomas Wright (Bradford: J.R. Smith, 1842).
Locke, J., *Some Thoughts Concerning Education* (London: Churchill, 1693).
Lomazzo, G.P., *Scritti sulle arte*, ed. Roberto Ciardi, 2 vols (Florence: Centro Di, 1975).
Lombardelli, O., *Il giovane studente* (Venice: Francesco Uscio, 1594).

Macollo, J., *XCIX Canons, or Rules Learnedly Describing an Excellent Method for Practitioners in Physic* (London: J. Grismond, 1659).
Macrini, G., *De Vesuvio* (Naples: Hieronymi Fasuli, 1693).
[Magri, D.], *Virtù del Kafe bevanda introdotta nuovaente nell'Italia con alcune osservazioni per conservar la sanità nella vecchiaia* (Rome: Hercoli, 1671).
Mainardes, N., *Del bever in ghiaccio* (Venice: Pittoni, 1689).
Majoli, S., *Dies caniculares, Hoc est, Colloquia physica noua & admiranda* (Mainz: Ioannis Theobaldi Schonnvetteri, 1615, first ed. 1608).
Manfredi, P., *Instruzzione medica ... con la quale s'insinua il modo di osservare il precetto quaresimale, anche da chi patisce qualche indispositione* (Rome: Camera Apostolica, 1703).
Mariani, A., *De peste anni MDCXXX Bononiae. Cuius generis fuit, & an ab aere* (Bologna: Clementis Ferronij, 1631).
Marinello, G., *Le Medicine partenenti alle infermitá delle donne* (Venice: G. Bonadio, 1563).
Martindale, A., *The Life of Adam Martindale*, ed. Richard Parkinson, Chetham Society, vol. 4 (Manchester, 1845).
Mauriceau, F., *The accomplish't Midwife* (London: John Darby, 1673).
Mauriceau, F., *The Diseases of Women with Child* (London: Andrew Bell, 1710).
Maynwaring, E., *Vita Sana e Longa, The Preservation of Health and Prolongation of Life* (London: J.D., 1669).
Meager, L., *The English gardner* (London: J. Dawks, for M. Wotton and G. Conyers, 1699).
Meduna, B., *Lo scolare* (Venice: Pietro Fachinetti, 1588).
Mercurio, S., *La commare o Raccoglitrice* (Milan: G.B. Bidelli, 1618, first. ed. 1595).
Mercurio, S., *De gli Errori Popolari d'Italia* (Venice: G.B.Ciotti 1603).
Meyer, C., *Nuovi ritrovamenti dati in luce ... per eccitare l'ingegno de' virtuosi* (Rome: Komarek, 1689).
Mistichelli, D., *Trattato dell'apoplessia* (Rome: de Rossi, 1709).
Moffett, T., *Health's Improvement* (London: T. Newcombe, 1655).
Mosca, G., *Dell'aria e de' morbi dall'aria dipendenti* (Naples: Alessio Pellecchia, 1746).
Mulcaster, R., *Positions wherin those primitive circumstances be examined which are necessarie for the training up of children, either for skill in their booke or health in their bodie* (London: Thomas Vautrollier, 1581).
Mulsow, M., *Frühneuzeitliche Selbsterhaltung. Telesio und die Naturphilosophie der Renaissance* (Tübingen: Niemayer, 1998).
[Nairone, F.], *Discorso della salutifera beuanda cahue, ò vero Café* (Rome: Hercoli, 1671).

[Newcome, H.], *The diary of Rev. Henry Newcome from September 30, 1661 to September 29, 1663*, ed. T. Heywood (Manchester: Chetham Society, 1849).
North, R., *Notes of Me: The Autobiography of Roger North*, ed. P. Millard (Toronto: University of Toronto Press, 2000).
Orbaan, J.A.F., *Documenti sul Barocco in Roma* (Rome: Sede della Società alla Biblioteca Vallicelliana, 1920).
Panaroli, D., *Aërologia, cioè discorso dell'aria.* Trattato Vtile per la Sanità (Rome: D. Marciani, 1642).
Panaroli, D., *L'aria Celimontana* (Rome: D. Marciani, 1642).
Panaroli, D., Plantarum amphitheatralium catalogus, in *Polycarpoponia seu variorum fructes labores* (Rome: J.B. Roblettus, 1647).
Paragallo, G., *Istoria Naturale del Monte Vesuvio* (Naples: G. Raillard, 1705).
Paré, A., *The Workes of that Famous Chirurgion Ambrose Parey* (London: T. Cotes, 1634).
Paschetti, B., *Del conservar la sanità* (Genoa: Giuseppe Pavoni, 1602).
Passeri, D., *Riflessi consultivi sopra alle cure preservative da farsi in quest'anno 1703 da chi desidera conservare la sanità* (Orvieto: Tosini, 1703).
Passeri, D., *Aeris salubris specimen* (Todi: apud Pascutium & Sambuchium, 1715).
Peccana, A., *De' Commentarii della scandella* (Verona: Angelo Tamo, 1622).
Pechey, J., *A general treatise of the diseases of infants and children* (London: R. Wellington, 1697).
Pechey, J., *A Plain Introduction to the Art of Physic* (London: Henry Bonwick, 1697).
Pellegrino, C., *Apparato alle Antichità di Capua o vero Discorsi della Campania Felice* (Naples: Francesco Savio, 1651).
Persio, A., *Del bever caldo costumato dagli antichi Romani* (Venice: Gió Battista Ciotto, 1593).
Petronio, A.T., *Del viver delli Romani, et di conservare la sanità* (Rome: Domenico Basa, 1592).
Pictorius, B., *Dialogi ... del modo del conseruare la sanitá* (Venice: Bottega d'Erasmo di Vincenzo Valgrisi, 1550).
Pietragrassa, B., *Politica medica per il governo conservativo del corpo humano* (Pavia: Gio. Andrea Magri, 1649).
Pinelli, F., *Lettera de' Bagni di Petriuolo* (Rome: De Rossi, 1716).
Pisanelli, B., *Trattato della natura de' cibi* (Bergamo: Comino Ventura & C., 1587).
Platter, F., *Platerus Golden Practice of Physick* (London: Peter Cole, 1664).
[Plutarch], *The Governaunce of Good Helth by the moste excellent phylosopher Plutarche* (London: R. Wyer, 1549(?) and 1555).
Porrata Spinola, G.F., *Discorso sopra l'origine de' Fuochi gettati dal Monte Vesevo, ceneri piovute, et altri successi, e Pronostico d'effetti maggiori* (Lecce: Pietro Micheli Borgognone, 1632).

Porzio, S., *De conflagratione Agri Puteolani* (Florence: Torrentinus, 1551; first ed. 1538).
Quiñones, J., *El Monte Vesuvio a ora la Montaña de Soma* (Madrid: Por Juan Gonçalez, 1632).
Ramazzini, B., *De principum valetudine tuenda* (Padua: Conzatti, 1710).
Ramazzini, B., *Annotationes in librum Ludovici Cornelii de vitae sobriae* (Patavii: Conzatti, 1714).
Ramazzini, B., *Constitutionum epidemicarum mutinensium annorum quinque* (Padua: Conzatti, 1714).
Rangoni Giannotti, T., *Iulio III Sanctissimo Thomae Philologi De vita hominis ultra CXX annos protrahenda* (Venice: Comin da Trino, 1550).
[Rangoni Giannotti, T.], *Thomaso philologo da Rauenna. Come l'huomo può viuere piu de CXX anni* (Venice: Matheum Paganum a Fide, 1556).
Rangoni Giannotti, T., *De vita principis et Venetorum commoda semper consilium* (Venice: printer unknown, 1558).
Raynalde, T., *The byrth of mankynde, otherwyse named the womans booke* (London: Tho. Ray, 1545).
Rogers, T., *Practical Discourses on Sickness & Recovery* (London: Thomas Parkhurst, 1691).
Ronsovius, H., *The English Man's Doctor or The Schoole of Salerne* (London: W. Stansby, 1617).
Rosaccio, G., *Avvertimenti a tutti quelli che desiderano regolatamente vivere* (Florence: G. Caneo, 1594).
S., J., *Paidon Nosemata. Or, Childrens Diseases* (London: W.G., 1664).
Salando, F., *Trattato sopra la regola del vivere nelle sei cose chiamate da' Medici non naturali* (Verona: Angelo Tamo, 1607).
[Santorio, S.], *Ars Sanctorii Sanctorii de statica medicina* (Venice: Nicolò Polo, 1614).
[Santorio, S.], *De medicina statica libri octo Accedunt Georgii Baglivi* (Romae: haered. L'Hulliè, 1704).
Savonarola, M., *Libreto ... de tutte le cose che se manzano ... e de sei cose non natural* (Venice: Simone de Luere 1508).
[Savonarola, M.], *Il trattato ginecologico-pediatrico in volgare: ad mulieres ferrarienses de regimine pregnantium et noviter natorum usque ad septennium*, ed. L. Belloni (Milan: Industrie Grafiche Italiane Stucchi, 1952).
Scacchi, B., *De salubri potu dissertatio* (Rome: Alessandro Zanetto, 1622).
Scappi, B., *Opera* (Venice: Alessandro Vecchi, 1605).
Scuola salernitana del modo di conseruarsi in sanità (Perugia: Petrucci, 1587).
Sears, J., and F.R. Johnson (eds), *The Library of John Lord Lumley. The Catalogue of 1609* (London: The Trustees of the British Museum, 1956).
Sennert, D., *Practical Physick the Fourth Book* (London: Peter Cole, 1664).

Serao, F., *Istoria dell'Incendio del Vesuvio Accaduto nel Mese di Maggio dell'Anno 1737* (Naples: Novello de' Bonis, 1788).
Sharp, J., *The Midwives book, or, The whole art of midwifery discovered* (London: Simon Miller, 1671).
Southall, J., *A Treatise of Buggs* (London: J. Roberts, 1730).
Spon, I., *Observations on Fevers and Febriguges* (London: Mark Pardoe, 1682).
Svegliarino alli signori veneziani per poter con sicurezza viver di continuo in sanità sino agli anni cento e dieci (Venice: Pittoni, L., 1691).
T., A., *A Rich Store-House or Treasury for the Diseased* (London: Thomas Purfoot, 1596).
Tanara, V., *L'economia del cittadino in villa* (Venice: Bertani 1661 and Steffano Curti, 1674, first. ed. 1600).
Tartaglini, L., *Opera nuoua nella quale se contiene la natura dil sonno cioé come lhuomo debbe dormire per mantenersi sano* (Venice: Tartaglini, 1551).
Telesio, B., *De his, quae in Aere fiunt; & de Terrae motibus, liber unicus* (Naples: Ios. Cacchium, 1570).
Tetius, H., *Aedes Barberinae ad Quirinalium descriptae*, ed. L. Faedo and T. Frangenberg (Pisa: Scuola Normale, 2005).
The Compleat Midwifes Practice (London: Nathaniel Brooke, 1656).
The Diary of Edmund Harrold, Wigmaker of Manchester 1712–15, ed. C. Horner (Aldershot: Ashgate, 2008).
The secrete of secretes of Arystotle … with rules of helthe for body and soule (London: R. Copland, 1528).
Thoresby, R., *The diary of Ralph Thoresby, F.R.S. author of The topography of Leeds (1677–1724)*, ed. J. Hunter, 2 vols (London: Henry Colburn and Richard Bentley, 1830).
Thornton, A., *The Autobiography of Mrs. Alice Thornton of East Newton, Co. York*, ed. C. Jackson (Durham: Andrews for Surtees Society, 1875).
Tozzi, L., *In librum artis medicinalis Galeni paraphrastikē anakephalaiōsis. … Huic adjectum est practicum opusculum de recto usu sex rerum nonnaturalium* (Naples: Porpora, 1710).
Traffichetti, B., *L'arte di conservare la salute tutta intiera* (Pesaro: Girolamo Concordia, 1565).
Traffichetti, B., *Idea dell'arte di conseruare la sanità … et hora per il medesmo diffesa dalle false oppositioni di M. Matteo Bruni* (Venice: Bindoni & fratelli, 1572).
Tryon, T., *A Treatise of Cleanness in Meats and Drinks* (London: Printed for the Author, 1682).
Tryon, T., *A Way to Health, Long Life and Happiness* (London: Andrew Sowle, 1683).

Tryon, T., *Monthly Observations for the preserving of Health* (London: Andrew Sowle, 1688).
Tryon, T., *Wisdom's dictates, or, Aphorisms & rules, physical, moral, and divine, for preserving the health of the body, and the peace of the mind* (London: Thomas Salisbury, 1691).
Tryon, T., *A new method of educating children* (London: J. Salusbury and J. Harris, 1695).
Two East Anglian Diaries 1641–1729, Isaac Archer and William Coe, ed. M. Storey (Woodbridge: Boydell Press, 1994).
Twyne, T., *The Schoolmaster, or Teacher of Table Phylosophie* (London: Richard Johnes, 1583, first publ. 1576).
Valesio, F., *Diario romano*, ed. G. Scano (Milan: Longanesi, 1977).
Van Diemerbroeck, Y., *The Anatomy of Human Bodies* (London: W. Whitwood, 1694).
Vaughan, W., *Directions for Health, naturall and artificial* (London: Bradock, 1602).
Venner, T., *Via Recta ad Vitam Longan Pars Secunda* (London: G.Eld, 1623).
Viviani, V., *Trattato del Custodire la Sanità* (Venice: Girolamo Piuti, 1626).
Wainewright, J., *A mechanical account of the non-naturals* (London: R. Smith and J. Wale, 1707).
Walwyn, W., *Physick for Families* (London: J. Winter, 1669).
Ware, I., *A Complete Body of Architecture* (London: Osborne and J. Shipton, 1756).
Warren, R., *The Daily Self-Examinant* (London: printed for Edmund Parker, 1720).
Watkins, R., *Newes from the Dead. Or A True and Exact Narration of the miraculous deliverance of Anne Greene* (Oxford: Leonard Lichfield, 1651).
Wesley, J., *The duty and advantage of early rising* (London: J. Paramore, 1783).
Willis, T., *Cerebri anatome: cui accessit nervorum description et usus* (London: Ja. Flesher, 1664).
Wingfield, H., *A Compendious or Short Treatise* (London: R. Stoughten, 1551).
Wright, T., *The Passions of the Minde* (London: Miles Flesher, 1630; first publ. 1601).
Zupi, G.B., *Continuazione de' successi Del prossimo Incendio del Vesuvio con gli effetti della cenere, e pietre da quelli vomitate* (Naples: Gio:Francesco Paci, 1661).

Secondary sources

Ago, R., 'Ecclesiastical careers and the destiny of cadets', *Continuity and Change*, 7:3 (1992), pp. 271–82.

Ago, R., 'Giochi di squadra: uomini e donne nelle famiglie nobili del XVII secolo', in M.A. Visceglia (ed.), *Signori, Patrizi, Cavalieri in Italia Centro-Meridionale nell'Età Moderna* (Rome: Laterza, 1992), pp. 256–64.

Albala, K., *Eating Right in the Renaissance* (Berkeley: University of California Press, 2002).

Albala, K., 'Food for healing: convalescent cookery in the Early Modern era', *Studies in History and Philosophy of Science Part C: Studies in History and Philosophy of Biological and Biomedical Sciences*, 43:2 (2012), pp. 323–8.

Ambrosoli, M., *The Wild and the Sown: Botany and Agriculture in Western Europe: 1350–1850* (Cambridge: Cambridge University Press, 1997).

Anselment, R., 'Mary Rich, Countess of Warwick, and the gift of tears', *The Seventeenth Century*, 22:1 (2007), pp. 336–57.

Appuhn, K., 'Ecologies of beef: eighteenth-century epizootics and the environmental history of Early Modern Europe', *Environmental History*, 15:2 (2010), pp. 268–87.

Arbor, A., *Herbals. Their Origin and Evolution. A Chapter in the History of Botany 1470–1670* (Cambridge: Cambridge University Press, 1986).

Arcangeli, A., *Recreation in the Renaissance: Attitudes toward Leisure and Pastimes in European Culture, c. 1425–1675* (Basingstoke: Palgrave, 2003).

Arcangeli, A., 'Del moto e della quiete. Esercizio e igiene nella prima età moderna', *Medicina e Storia*, 8:1 (2004), pp. 35–55.

Aspin, R., 'Illustrations from the Wellcome Library: who was Elizabeth Okeover?', *Medical History*, 44 (2003), pp. 531–40.

Auslander, L., 'Beyond words', *American Historical Review*, 110:4 (2005), pp. 1015–45.

Barker, S., 'Art in a time of danger: Urban VIII's Rome and the plague of 1629–1634' (PhD thesis, Columbia University, 2002).

Barthel, C., *Medizinische Polizey und Medizinische Aufklärung: Aspekte des Öffentlichen Gesundheitsdiskurses im 18. Jahrhundert* (Frankfurt: Campus, 1989).

Bell, R., *How to Do It: Guides to Good Living for Renaissance Italians* (Chicago: Chicago University Press, 1999).

Belozerskaya, M., *Luxury Arts of the Renaissance* (Los Angeles: Getty, 2005).

Bennett, H.S., *English Books and Readers*, 3 vols (Cambridge: Cambridge University Press, 1970).

Berg, M., 'Women's consumption and the industrial classes in eighteenth-century England', *Journal of Social History*, 30:2 (1996), pp. 415–34.

Bergdolt, K., *Wellbeing: A Cultural History of Healthy Living* (Cambridge: Polity Press, 2008).

Bertoloni Meli, D. (ed.), *Marcello Malpighi. Anatomist and Physician* (Firenze: Olschki, 1997).

Bonfield, C.A., 'The Regimen Sanitatis and its dissemination in England c. 1348–1550' (PhD thesis, University of East Anglia, 2006).
Bono, J.J., *Word of God and the Languages of Man: Interpreting Nature in Early Modern Science and Medicine* (Wisconsin: University of Wisconsin Press, 1995).
Borello, B., *Trame Sovrapposte: La Socialità Aristocratica e le Reti di Relazioni Femminili a Roma (XVII–XVIII secolo)* (Naples: Edizioni Scientifiche Italiane, 2003).
Borello, B., 'I segni del corpo: fratelli, sorelle e somiglianze nelle famiglie italiane (XVII–XVIII secolo)', *Quaderni storici*, 145:1 (2014), pp. 9–40.
Bossy, J., *The English Catholic Community 1570–1850* (London: Darton, Longman & Todd, 1975).
Botelho, L., 'Old age and menopause in rural women of early modern Suffolk', in L.A. Botelho and P. Thane (eds), *Women and Ageing in British Society since 1500* (London: Routledge, 2001), pp. 43–65.
Botonaki, E., 'Dissecting bodies and selves in the Early Modern period', in Z. Detsi-Diamanti, K. Kitsi-Mitaka and E. Yiannopoulou (eds), *Flesh Made Text Made Flesh: Cultural and Theoretical Returns to the Body* (New York: Peter Lang, 2007), pp. 75–86.
Bound Alberti, F., 'Introduction: emotion theory and medical history', in *Medicine, Emotion and Disease, 1700–1950* (Basingstoke: Palgrave Macmillan, 2003), pp. xiii–xxviii.
Brayman Hackel, H., *Reading Material in Early Modern England: Print, Gender and Literacy* (Cambridge: Cambridge University Press, 2005).
Brody, M.J., '"Terra d'Urbino tutta dipinta a paesi con l'armi de' Salviati": The "Paesi" service in the 1583 inventory of Jacopo di Alamanno Salviati (1537–1586)', *Faenza*, 4–6 (2000), pp. 30–46.
Brown, B., 'Thing theory', *Critical Inquiry*, 28:1 (2001), pp. 1–22.
Brown, B., *A Sense of Things: The Object Matter of American Literature* (Chicago: University of Chicago Press, 2003).
Brown, F.E., 'Continuity and change in the urban house: developments in domestic space organisation in seventeenth-century London', *Comparative Studies in Society and History*, 28:3 (1986), pp. 558–90.
Bynum, W.F., and V. Nutton (eds), *Theories of Fever from Antiquity to the Enlightenment* (London: Wellcome Institute for the History of Medicine, 1981).
Byzantine Palaces in Istanbul (Istanbul: Istanbul Archaeological Museums, 2010).
Calvi, G., 'L'oro, il fuoco, le forche: la peste napoletana del 1656', *Archivio Storico Italiano*, 139:3 (1981), pp. 405–58.
Caneva, G., M. Cutini, A. Pacini and M. Vinci, 'Analysis of the Colosseum's floristic changes during the last four centuries', *Plant Biosystems*, 136:3 (2002).

Cantor, D. (ed.), *Reinventing Hippocrates* (Aldershot: Ashgate, 2002).

Carré, A., and L. Cifuentes, 'Girolamo Manfredi's *Il perché*: I. The *Problemata* and its medieval tradition', *Medicina e Storia*, 19/20 (2010), pp. 13–38.

Carré, A., and L. Cifuentes, 'Girolamo Manfredi's *Il perché*: II. The *Secretum secretorum* and the book's publishing success', *Medicina e Storia*, 19/20 (2010), pp. 39–58.

Carrera, E., 'Anger and the mind–body connection in medieval and Early Modern medicine', in E. Carrera (ed.), *Emotions and Health, 1200–1700* (Leiden: Brill, 2013), pp. 95–146.

Carrera, E. (ed.), *Emotions and Health 1200–1700* (Leiden: Brill, 2013).

Carroll, P.E., 'Medical police and the history of public health', *Medical History*, 46:4 (2002), pp. 461–94.

Carter, J.F.M., *Nicholas Ferrar, His Household and His Friends* (London and New York: Longmans, 1892).

Castelli, D., 'Il 'De conflagratione di Simone Porzio: la collazione delle tre edizioni, un volgarizzamento e il ms. Phill.12844 dell'HRC di Austin', *Rinascimento Meridionale*, 3:1 (2012), pp. 81–104.

Castiglione, C., 'Peasants at the palace: wet nurses and aristocratic mothers in Early Modern Rome', in J. Sperling (ed.), *Medieval and Renaissance Lactations –Images, Rhetorics, Practices* (Burlington: Ashgate, 2013), pp. 79–99.

Castiglione, C., *Accounting for Affection: Mothering and Politics in Early Modern Rome* (Basingstoke: Palgrave, 2015).

Cavallo, S., 'Health, hygiene and beauty', in M. Ajmar-Wollheim and F. Dennis (eds), *At Home in Renaissance Italy* (London: V&A Publications, 2006), pp. 174–87.

Cavallo, S., 'Secrets of healthy living. The revival of the preventative paradigm in late Renaissance Italy', in E. Leong and A. Rankin (eds), *Secrets and Knowledge in Medicine* (Aldershot: Ashgate, 2011), pp. 191–212.

Cavallo, S., and T. Storey, *Healthy Living in Late Renaissance Italy* (Oxford: Oxford University Press, 2013).

Cavazzini, P. (ed.), *Agostino Tassi (1578–1644): Un Paesaggista tra Immaginario e Realtà* (Rome: Iride per Terzo Millenio, 2008).

Churchill, W., *Female Patients in Early Modern Britain: Gender, Diagnosis, and Treatment* (Farnham: Ashgate, 2012).

Ciancio, L., *Le Colonne del Tempo: il Tempio di Serapide a Pozzuoli nella Storia della Geologia, dell'Archeologia e dell'Arte (1750–1900)* (Florence: Edifir, 2009).

Clericuzio, A., *Elements, Principles and Corpuscles: A Study of Atomism and Chemistry in the Seventeenth Century* (Dordrecht: Kluver, 2000).

Clericuzio, A., 'Chemical medicine and Paracelsianism in Italy, 1550–1650', in M. Pelling and S. Mandelbrote (eds), *The Practice of Reform in Health,*

Medicine and Science. Essays for Charles Webster, 1500–2000 (Aldershot: Ashgate, 2005).
Clericuzio, A., 'Chemical medicines in Rome: Pietro Castelli and the vitriol debate, 1616–1626', in M.P. Donato and J. Kraye (eds), *Conflicting Duties: Science, Medicine and Religion in Rome, 1550–1750* (London: Warburg Institute, 2009), pp. 281–302.
Cocco, S., *Watching Vesuvius: A History of Science and Culture in Early Modern Italy* (Chicago: University of Chicago Press, 2013).
Coffin, D.R., *Gardens and Gardening in Papal Rome* (Princeton: Princeton University Press, 1991).
Cohn, S.K., *Cultures of Plague: Medical Thinking at the End of the Renaissance* (Oxford: Oxford University Press, 2010).
Collingwood, R.G., *The Idea of Nature* (Oxford: Oxford University Press, 1945).
Conforti, M., 'Subterranean fires and chemical exhalations: mineral waters in the Phlegraean Fields in the Early Modern age', in D. Boisseuil, J. Coste and M. Nicoud (eds), *Le Thermalisme. Histoire d'un Phénomène Culturel et Médical* (Paris: CNRS éditions, 2015), pp. 123–36.
Conforti, M., S. Marinozzi and V. Gannaniga, 'Delle arie, acque e luoghi: igiene e sanità pubblica a Roma nell'opera di Giovanni Maria Lancisi', *Roma Moderna e Contemporanea*, 13:1 (2005), pp. 115–32.
Cook, H.J., 'Good advice and little medicine: the professional authority of Early Modern English physicians', *Journal of British Studies*, 33:1 (1994).
Cook, H.J., 'Institutional structures and personal belief', in A. Cunningham and O.P. Grell (eds), *Religio Medici. Medicine and Religion in Seventeenth Century England* (London: Scholar Press, 1996), pp. 91–114.
Cotton, J.H., 'Benedetto Reguardati: author of Ugo Benzi's *Tractato de la conservatione de la sanitade*', *Medical History*, 12:1 (1968), pp. 175–89.
Cressy, D., *Birth, Marriage, and Death: Ritual, Religion, and the Life-Cycle in Tudor and Stuart England* (Oxford: Oxford University Press, 1999).
Crisciani, C., and G. Zuccolin (eds), *Michele Savonarola: Medicina e Cultura di Corte*, Micrologus 37 (Florence: SISMEL Edizioni del Galluzzo, 2011).
D'Amelia, M., 'Becoming a mother in the seventeenth century: the experience of a Roman noblewoman', in A.J. Schutte, T. Kuehn and S. Seidel Menchi (eds), *Time, Space, and Women's Lives in Early Modern Europe* (Kirksville: Truman State University Press, 2001), pp. 223–44.
Daiken, L., *The Lullaby Book* (London: Edmund Ward, 1959).
Dannenfeldt, K.H., 'Sleep: theory and practice in the late Renaissance', *The Journal of the History of Medicine and Allied Sciences*, 41:4 (1986), pp. 415–41.
Daston, L., and K. Park, *Wonders of the Order of Nature, 1150–1750* (New York: Zone Books, 2001).

Daston, L., and G. Pomata (eds), *The Faces of Nature in Enlightenment Europe* (Berlin: BWV-Berliner Wissenschafts-Verlag, 2003).

Daston, L., and M. Stolleis (eds), *Natural Law and Laws of Nature in Early Modern Europe: Jurisprudence, Theology, Moral, and Natural Philosophy* (Aldershot: Ashgate, 2008).

Daston, L., and F. Vidal (eds), *The Moral Authority of Nature* (Chicago: University of Chicago Press, 2004).

Daybell, J., *Women Letter-Writers in Tudor England* (Oxford: Oxford University Press, 2006).

Daybell, J., *The Material Letter in Early Modern England: Manuscript Letters and the Culture and Practices of Letter-Writing, 1512–1635* (Basingstoke: Palgrave, 2012).

De Pompeis, V., *La Maiolica Italiana di Stile Compendiario* (Milan: Allemandi, 2010).

De Vivo, B. (ed.), *Volcanism in the Campania Plain. Vesuvius, Campi Flegrei and Ignimbrites* (Amsterdam: Elsevier, 2006).

Di Filippo Bareggi, C., *Il Mestiere di Scrivere: Lavoro Intellettuale e Mercato Librario a Venezia nel Cinquecento* (Rome: Bulzoni, 1988).

Dietler, M., and I. Herbich, 'Habitus, techniques, style: an integrated approach to the social understanding of material culture and boundaries', in M.T. Stark (ed.), *The Archaeology of Social Boundaries* (Washington, London: Smithsonian Institution Press, 1998), pp. 232–63.

Dixon Hunt, J., 'The sign of the object', in Lubar and Kingery (eds), *History from Things*, pp. 293–8.

Dizionario Biografico degli Italiani, www.treccani.it/biografie/.

Douglas, M., *Purity and Danger: An Analysis of Concepts of Pollution and Taboo* (London: Routledge, 2001).

Duden, B., *Woman Beneath the Skin: A Doctor's Patients in Eighteenth-Century Germany* (Cambridge, MA: Harvard University Press, 1991).

Eamon, W., *Science and the Secrets of Nature. Books of Secrets in Medieval and Early Modern Culture* (Princeton: Princeton University Press, 1994).

Ehrlich, T., *Landscape and Identity in Early Modern Rome: Villa Culture at Frascati in the Borghese Era* (Cambridge: Cambridge University Press, 2002).

Ekirch, R., *At Day's Close: A History of Night time* (London: Phoenix, 2005).

Elliott, B., 'The world of the Renaissance herbal', *Renaissance Studies*, 25:1 (2011).

Elmer, P., 'Medicine, religion and the puritan revolution', in R. French and A. Wear (eds), *The Medical Revolution of the Seventeenth Century* (Cambridge: Cambridge University Press, 1989), pp. 10–45.

Emch-Dériaz, A., 'The non-naturals made easy', in R. Porter (ed.), *The Popularization of Medicine, 1650–1850* (London: Routledge, 1992), pp. 134–59.

Evenden, D., *The Midwives of Seventeenth Century London* (Cambridge: Cambridge University Press, 2000).

Everson, J.E., 'The melting pot of science and belief: studying Vesuvius in seventeenth-century Naples', *Renaissance Studies*, 26:5 (2011), pp. 691–727.
Fagiolo dell'Arco, M., *Jean Lemaire Pittore 'Antiquario'* (Rome: Ugo Bozzi, 1996).
Favier, R., 'Penser le changement climatique au siècle des Lumières', in D. Lamarre (ed.), *Climat et risques: changements d'approches* (Paris: Tec & doc, 2008), pp. 9–24.
Fildes, V.A., *Breasts, Bottles, and Babies: A History of Infant Feeding* (Edinburgh: Edinburgh University Press, 1986).
Fildes, V.A., 'The English wet-nurse and her role in infant care 1538–1800', *Medical History*, 32:2 (1988), pp. 142–73.
Fildes, V.A. (ed.), *Women as Mothers in Pre-Industrial England* (London: Routledge, 1990).
Filippini, N.M., 'The church, the state and childbirth: the midwife in Italy during the eighteenth century', in H. Marland (ed.), *The Art of Midwifery: Early Modern Midwives in Europe* (London: Routledge, 1993), pp. 152–75.
Fiocco, C., and G. Gherardi, *Museo d'Arti Applicate. Le ceramiche*, vol.1, *Musei e Gallerie di Milano* (Milan: Electa, 2000).
Fisher, T., 'What we touch touches us: material affects and affordances', *Design Issues*, 20:4 (2004), pp. 20–31.
Fissell, M., 'Readers, texts and contexts. Vernacular medical works in Early Modern England', in R. Porter (ed.), *The Popularisation of Medicine 1650–1850* (London: Routledge, 1992), pp. 72–96.
Fissell, M., 'The marketplace of print', in Jenner and Wallis (eds), *Medicine and the Market*, pp. 108–32.
Fissell, M., 'Women, health, and healing in Early Modern Europe', *Bulletin of the History of Medicine*, 82:1 (2008), pp. 1–17.
Fissell, M., 'Popular medical writing', in J. Raymond (ed.), *The Oxford History of Popular Print Culture*, vol. 1, *Cheap Print in Britain and Ireland to 1660* (Oxford: Oxford University Press, 2011), pp. 418–31.
Frigo, D., *Il Padre di Famiglia: Governo della Casa e Governo Civile nella Tradizione della 'Economica' tra Cinque e Seicento* (Rome: Bulzoni, 1985).
Furdell, E. Lane, *Publishing and Medicine in Early Modern England* (Rochester, NY: University of Rochester Press, 2002).
Gage, F. 'Exercise for mind and body: Giulio Mancini, collecting and the beholding of landscape painting in the seventeenth century', *Renaissance Quarterly*, 61:4 (2008): pp. 1167–1207.
Gage, F. *Painting as Medicine in Early Modern Rome: Giulio Mancini and the Efficacy of Art* (University Park, PA: Penn State University Press, 2016).
García-Ballester, L., 'On the origins of the "six Non-Natural things" in Galen', in *idem*, *Galen and Galenism* (Aldershot: Ashgate, 2002), pp. 105–15.
Geertz, C., 'Thick description: toward an interpretative theory of culture', in *The Interpretation of Cultures* (New York: Basic Books, 1973).

Gell, A., *Art and Agency. An Anthropological Theory* (Oxford: Oxford University Press, 1998).
Gentilcore, D., 'The organisation of medical practice in Malpighi's Italy', in D. Bertoloni Meli (ed.), *Marcello Malpighi: Anatomist and Physician* (Florence: Olschki 1997), pp. 75–110.
Gentilcore, D., *Food and Health in Early Modern Europe. Diet, Medicine and Society 1450–1800* (London: Bloomsbury, 2015).
Getz, F.M., 'Charity, translation and the language of medical learning in medieval England', *Bulletin of the History of Medicine*, 64:1 (1990), pp. 1–17.
Gibson, J.J., 'The theory of affordances', in R. Shaw and J. Brausford (eds), *Perceiving, Acting and Knowing: Toward an Ecological Psychology* (New York: John Wiley & Sons, 1977), pp. 127–43.
Gil-Sotres, P., 'The regimens of health', in M.D. Grmek (ed.), *Western Medical Thought from Antiquity to the Middle Ages* (Cambridge, MA: Harvard University Press, 1998), pp. 291–396.
Glayser, N., and S. Pennell (eds), *Didactic Literature in England 1500–1800: Expertise Constructed* (Aldershot: Ashgate, 2003).
Goldthwaite, R., 'The economic and social world of Italian Renaissance maiolica', *Renaissance Quarterly*, 42:1 (1989), pp. 1–31.
Golinski, I., *British Weather and the Climate of Enlightenment* (Chicago: University of Chicago Press, 2007).
Goodman, D., 'Designing an education for young ladies', in *idem, Becoming a Woman in the Republic of Letters* (Ithaca: Cornell University Press, 2009), pp. 63–160.
Gowing, L., 'Secret births and infanticide in seventeenth-century England', *Past & Present*, 156:1 (1997), pp. 87–115.
Gowing, L., *Common Bodies: Women, Touch and Power in Seventeenth-Century England* (New Haven: Yale University Press, 2003).
Gowing, L., ' "The twinkling of a bedstaff": recovering the social life of English beds 1500–1700', *Home Cultures*, 11:3 (2014), pp. 275–304.
Green, M., *Making Women's Medicine Masculine: The Rise of Male Authority in Pre-Modern Gynaecology* (Oxford: Oxford University Press, 2008).
Grendler, P., *Schooling in Renaissance Italy: Literacy and Learning, 1300–1600* (Baltimore: Johns Hopkins University Press, 1989).
Grendler, P., 'Form and function in Italian Renaissance popular books', *Renaissance Quarterly*, 46:3 (1993), pp. 451–85.
Grieco, A., 'Food and social classes in late medieval and Renaissance Italy', in J.L. Flandrin and M. Montanari (eds), *Food: A Culinary History* (New York: Columbia University Press, 1999), pp. 302–12.
Grigioni, C., 'Documenti: serie faentinA. I Calamelli maiolicari di Faenza', *Faenza*, 4–5:22 (1934), pp. 143–53.

Groppi, A., 'La sindrome malinconica di Lucrezia Barberini D'Este', *Quaderni Storici*, 129:3 (2008), pp. 725–49.

Groppi, A., 'La malinconia di Lucrezia Barberini D'Este', in F. Cantù (ed.), *I Linguaggi del Potere nell'Età Barocca*, vol. 2, *Donne e Sfera Pubblica* (Rome: Viella, 2009), pp. 197–227.

Guerrini, A., 'Newtonianism, medicine and religion', in O.P. Grell and A. Cunnngham (eds), *Religio Medici. Medicine and Religion in Seventeenth-Century England* (Aldershot: Ashgate: 1996), pp. 293–312.

Guerrini, A., 'Health, national character and the English diet in 1700', *Studies in History and Philosophy of Biological and Biomedical Sciences*, 43:2 (2012), pp. 349–56.

Habel, D. M. '*When All of Rome was Under Construction*': *The Building Process in Baroque Rome* (University Park, PA: Penn State University Press, 2013).

Hamling, T., *Decorating the Godly Household: Religious Art in Post-Reformation Britain* (New Haven, London: Yale University Press, 2010).

Hamling, T., 'Old Robert's girdle: visual and material props for Protestant piety in post-reformation England', in Martin and Ryrie (eds), *Private and Domestic Devotion in Early Modern Britain*, pp. 135–63.

Handley, S., 'From the sacral to the moral: sleeping practices, household worship and confessional cultures in late seventeenth-century England', *Cultural and Social History*, 9:1 (2012), pp. 27–46.

Handley, S., 'Sleepwalking, subjectivity and the nervous body in eighteenth-century Britain', *Journal for Eighteenth-Century Studies*, 35:3 (2012), pp. 305–23.

Handley, S., 'Sociable sleeping in Early Modern England, 1660–1760', *History*, 98:39 (2013), pp. 79–104.

Handley, S., *Sleep in Early Modern England* (New Haven: Yale University Press, 2016).

Harley, D., 'The theology of affliction and the experience of sickness in the godly family, 1650–1714: The Henrys and the Newcomes', in O.P. Grell and A. Cunningham (eds), *Religio Medici: Medicine and Religion in Seventeenth-Century England* (Aldershot: Scholars Press, 1996), pp. 273–92.

Harvey, K. (ed.), *History and Material Culture. A Student's Guide to Approaching Alternative Sources* (London, New York: Routledge, 2009).

Hellinger, L., and J.B. Trapp (eds), *The Cambridge History of the Book in Britain*, vol. 3, 1450–1557 (Cambridge: Cambridge University Press, 2008).

Henderson, J., 'The Black Death in Florence: medical and communal reactions', in S. Bassett (ed.), *Death in Towns. Urban Responses to the Dying and the Death 1000–1600* (Leicester: Leicester University Press, 1992), pp. 136–50.

Hill, C., 'The spiritualization of the household', in *idem*, *Society and Puritanism in Pre-revolutionary England* (London: Secker & Warburg, 1964), pp. 382–416.

Horstmanshoff, M., H. King and C. Zittel (eds), *Blood, Sweat and Tears: The Changing Concepts of Physiology from Antiquity into Early Modern Europe* (Leiden, Boston: Brill, 2012).

Howard, S., 'Imagining the pain and peril of seventeenth-century childbirth: travail and deliverance in the making of an Early Modern world', *Social History of Medicine*, 16:3 (2003), pp. 367–82.

Hunt, M., *The Middling Sort: Commerce, Gender, and the Family in England, 1680–1780* (Berkeley: University of California Press, 1996).

Hunter, M. (ed.), *Robert Boyle Reconsidered* (Cambridge: Cambridge University Press, 1994).

Hurren, E., 'Cultures of the body, medical regimen, and physic at the Tudor court', in T. Betteridge and S. Lipscomb (eds), *Henry VIII and the Court: Art, Politics and Performance* (Farnham: Ashgate, 2013), pp. 65–90.

Ingold, T., *The Perception of the Environment: Essays in Livelihood, Dwelling and Skill* (London, New York: Routledge, 2000).

Ingold, T., 'Bringing things to life: creative entanglements in a world of materials', NCRM Working Paper #15 (Realities / Morgan Centre, University of Manchester, July 2010).

Ishizuka, H., ' "Fibre body": the concept of fibre in eighteenth-century medicine, c.1700–40', *Medical History*, 56:4 (2012), pp. 562–84.

Jacob, W.M., *Lay People and Religion in the Early Eighteenth Century* (Cambridge: Cambridge University Press, 1996).

Jankovich, V., *Reading the Skies. A Cultural History of English Weather, 1650–1820* (Chicago: University of Chicago Press, 2000).

Jarcho, S., 'The "Epidemia Rheumatica" described by Lancisi (1711)', in C.E. Rosenberg (ed.), *Healing and History. Essays for George Rosen* (New York: Science History, 1979), pp. 51–8.

Jedin, H., *Girolamo Seripando. Sein Leben und Denken im Geisteskampf des 16. Jahrhunderts*, 2 vols (Würzburg: Rita-Verlag, 1937).

Jenner, M.R.S., 'The politics of London air: John Evelyn's Fumifugium and the restoration', *The Historical Journal*, 38:3 (1995), pp 535–51.

Jenner, M.R.S., 'Bathing and baptism: Sir John Floyer and the politics of cold bathing', in K. Sharpe and S. Zwicker (eds), *Refiguring Revolutions: Aesthetics and the Politics of Cold Bathing* (Berkeley: University of California Press, 1998), pp. 197–216.

Jenner, M.R.S., and P. Wallis, 'The medical marketplace', in *Medicine and the Market in England and its Colonies, c. 1450–1850* (Basingstoke: Palgrave, 2007), pp. 1–23.

Jones, P.M., 'Medicine and science', in Hellinger and Trapp (eds), *The Cambridge History*, pp. 433–48.

Jones, P.M., 'Medical literacies and medical culture in early modern England', in Taavitsainen and Pahta (eds), *Medical Writing*, pp. 30–43.

Joutsivuo, T., *Scholastic Tradition and Humanist Innovation. The Concept of Neutrum in Renasissance Medicine* (Helsinki: The Finnish Academy of Science and Medicine, 1999).

Jütte, R., 'The social construction of illness in the Early Modern period', in J. Lachmund and G. Stollberg (eds), *The Social Construction of Illness* (Stuttgart: Steiner, 1992), pp. 23–38.

Kavey, A., *Books of Secrets: Natural Philosophy in England, 1550–1660* (Urbana and Chicago, IL: University of Illinois Press, 2007).

Keiser, G.R., 'Practical books for the gentleman', in Hellinger and Trapp (eds), *The Cambridge History*, pp. 470–94.

King, H., 'Female fluids in the hippocratic corpus. How solid was the humoral body?' in P. Horden and E. Hsu (eds), *The Body in Balance* (New York, Oxford: Berghan, 2013), pp. 25–52.

Kingery, W.D. (ed.), *Learning from Things: Method and Theory of Material Culture Studies* (Washington, London: Smithsonian Institution Press, 1996).

Knappett, C., *Thinking through Material Culture: An Interdisciplinary Perspective* (Philadelphia: University of Pennsylvania Press, 2005).

Kümmel, W.F., 'The morbis aulicis: on diseases found at court', in V. Nutton (ed.), *Medicine at the Courts of Europe 1500–1837* (London: Routledge, 1990), pp. 15–48.

Lane Ford, M., 'Importation of printed books into England and Scotland', in Hellinger and Trapp (eds), *The Cambridge History*, pp. 179–201.

Lane Ford, M., 'Private Ownership of printed books', in Hellinger and Trapp (eds), *The Cambridge History*, pp. 205–28.

Lane Furdell, E., *Publishing and Medicine in Early Modern England* (Rochester, NY: University of Rochester Press, 2002).

Laroche, R., *Medical Authority and Englishwomen's Herbal Texts 1550–1650* (Aldershot: Ashgate, 2009).

Latour, B., 'Where are the missing masses? A sociology of a few mundane artefacts', in W.E. Bijker and J. Law (eds), *Shaping Technology / Building Society: Studies in Sociotechnical Change* (Boston: MIT Press, 1992), pp. 225–58.

Latour, B., 'The Berlin key or how to do words with things', in P.M. Graves Brown (ed.), *Matter, Materiality and Modern Culture* (London, New York: Routledge, 2000), pp. 10–21.

Leong, E., 'Medical recipe collections in seventeenth-century England: knowledge, gender and text' (DPhil thesis, University of Oxford, 2005).

Leong, E., 'Making medicines in the Early Modern household', *Bulletin of the History of Medicine*, 82:1 (2008), pp. 145–68.

Leong, E., and S. Pennell, 'Recipe collections and the currency of medical knowledge in the Early Modern "medical marketplace"', in Jenner and Wallis (eds), *Medicine and the Market*, pp. 133–52.

Levenson, J.A. (ed.), *Circa 1492: Art in the Age of Exploration, Washington, DC: National Gallery of Art, 1991* (New Haven, London: Yale University Press, 1991).

Lubar, S., and D. Kingery (eds), *History from Things: Essays on Material Culture* (Washington, London: Smithsonian Institution Press, 1993).

MacDonald, M., *Mystical Bedlam: Madness, Anxiety and Healing in Seventeenth-Century England* (Cambridge: Cambridge University Press, 1981).

Mack, P., *Heart Religion in the British Enlightenment, Gender and Emotion in Early Methodism* (Cambridge: Cambridge University Press, 2008).

Mack, P., 'The unbounded self: dreaming and identity in the British Enlightenment', in A.M. Plane and L. Tuttle (eds), *Dreams, Dreamers and Visions. The Early Modern Atlantic World* (Philadelphia: University of Pennsylvania Press, 2013), pp. 207–25.

Maclean, I., *Logic, Signs, and Nature in the Renaissance: The Case of Learned Medicine* (Cambridge: Cambridge University Press, 2002).

Maclean, I., 'The medical republic of letters before the Thirty Years War', *Intellectual History Review*, 18:1 (2008), pp. 15–30.

Maclean, I., *Scholarship, Commerce, Religion: The Learned Book in the Age of Confessions, 1560–1630* (Cambridge, MA: Harvard University Press, 2012).

Maclehose, B., 'Fear, fantasy and sleep in medieval medicine', in E. Carrera (ed.), *Emotions and Health*, pp. 67–94.

Marin, B., 'La topographie médicale de Naples de Filippo Baldini, médecin hygiéniste au service de la Couronne', *Melanges de l'Ecole française de Rome. Italie et Méditerranée*, 101:2 (1989), pp. 695–732.

Martin, C., *Renaissance Meteorology* (Baltimore: Johns Hopkins University Press, 2011).

Martin, J., and A. Ryrie (eds), *Private and Domestic Devotion in Early Modern Britain* (Farnham: Ashgate, 2012).

Marttila, V., 'New arguments for new audiences: a corpus-based analyses of interpersonal strategies in Early Modern English medical recipes', in Taavitsainen and Pahta (eds), *Medical Writing*, pp. 135–57.

McCleery, I., 'Wine, women and song? Diet and regimen for royal well-being (King Duarte of Portugal, 1433–1438)', in S. Katajala-Peltomaa and S. Niiranen (eds), *Mental (Dis)Order in Later Medieval Europe* (Leiden: Brill, 2014), pp. 177–96.

McCray Beier, L., *Sufferers and Healers: The Experience of Illness in Seventeenth-Century England* (London: Routledge, 1987).

McLaren, D., 'Marital fertility and lactation 1570–1720', in M. Prior (ed.), *Women in English Society 1500–1800* (London: Methuen, 1985), pp. 22–53.

McTavish, L., 'Maternity', in A.M. Paska and K.A. McIver (eds), *Ashgate Research Companion to Women and Gender in Early Modern Europe* (Farnham: Ashgate, 2013), pp. 173–93.

Merchant, C., *The Death of Nature: Women, Ecology, and the Scientific Revolution* (London: Harper & Row, 1980).

Mikkeli, H., *Hygiene in the Early Modern Medical Tradition* (Helsinki: Finnish Academy of Science and Letters, 1999).

Milani, M., 'How to attain immortality living one hundred years, or, the fortune of the *Vita Sobria* in the Anglo-Saxon world', in M. Milani, G. Critser and H. Fudemoto (eds), *Writings on the Sober Life: The Art and Grace of Living Long* (Toronto: University of Toronto Press, 2014), pp. 183–213.

Milani, M., 'Introduction to Cornaro', in Milani, Critser and Fudemoto (eds), *Writings on the Sober Life*, pp. 3–71.

Miller, D., *Material Cultures: Why Some Things Matter* (London: UCL Press, 1997).

Millers, G., ' "Airs, waters and places" in History', *Journal of the History of Medicine*, 17:2 (1962), pp. 129–40.

Minuzzi, S., 'Il medico Tommaso Giannotti Rangone (1493–1577) nell'economia della cura, ovvero un trionfo di libri, segreti e *regimen sanitatis*', *Medicina e Storia*, N.S., 1/2013, pp. 29–66.

Murr, S. (ed.), *Gassendi et l'Europe (1592–1792)* (Paris: Vrin, 1997).

Neuburger, M., *The Doctrine of the Healing Power of Nature Throughout the Course of Time* (New York: privately printed, 1932, originally published in German in 1926).

Newton, H., *The Sick Child in Early Modern England, 1580–1720* (Oxford: Oxford University Press, 2012).

Newton, H., ' "Nature concocts & expels": the agents and processes of recovery from disease in Early Modern England', *Social History of Medicine*, 28:3 (2015), pp. 445–64.

Newton, H., *Misery to Mirth: Recovery from Illness in Early Modern England* (Oxford: Oxford University Press, forthcoming).

Niccoli, O., ' "Menstruum quasi monstruum": monstrous births and menstrual taboo in the sixteenth century', in E. Muir and G. Ruggiero (eds), *Sex and Gender in Historical Perspective* (Baltimore: Johns Hopkins University Press, 1990), pp. 1–25.

Nicoud, M., *Les régimes de santé au Moyen Âge: naissance et diffusion d'une écriture médicale (XIIIe–XVe siècle)* (Rome: Ecole Francaise de Rome, 2007).

Niebyl, P.H., 'The Non-Naturals', *Bulletin of the History of Medicine*, 45:5 (1971), pp. 486–92.

Nutton, V., 'John Caius and the Linacre tradition', *Medical History*, 23:4 (1979), pp. 373–91.

Olagüe de Ros, G., 'La epidemia europea de gripe de 1708–1709', *Dynamis*, 1:1 (1981), pp. 51–86.

Paniagua, J.A., 'El regimen sanitatis ad regem Aragonorum y otres presuntos regimens arnaldiana', in *Studia Arnaldiana. Trabajos en torno a la Obra Medica de Arnau de Vilanova s.1240–1311* (Barcelona: Uriach, 1994), pp. 335–84.

Park, K., 'Nature in person: medieval and Renaissance allegories and emblems', in Daston and Vidal (eds), *The Moral Authority of Nature*.

Park, K., *Secrets of Women: Gender, Generation, and the Origins of Human Dissection* (New York: Zone Books, 2006).

Pelliccia, G., 'Scuole di catechismo e scuole rionali per fanciulle nella Roma del seicento', *Ricerche per la Storia Religiosa di Roma*, 4:1 (1980), pp. 237–68.

Pelling, M., 'Nurses and nursekeepers: problems of identification in the Early Modern period', in M. Pelling (ed.), *The Common Lot: Sickness, Medical Occupations and the Urban Poor in Early Modern England* (London: Longman, 1998), pp. 179–202.

Pennell, S., 'Mundane materiality, or, should small things still be forgotten? Material culture, micro-histories and the problem of scale', in Harvey (ed.), *History and Material Culture*, pp. 173–91.

Peterson, T.V., 'Introduction: cultural and historical interpretation through nontextual material', *Historical Reflections*, 23:3 (1997), pp. 259–67.

Petrucci, A., *Scrittura e Popolo nella Roma Barocca, 1585–1721* (Rome: Quasar, 1982).

Plebani, T., *Il Genere dei Libri. Storie e Rappresentazioni della Lettura al Femminile e al Maschile tra Mediovevo e Età Moderna* (Milan: Franco Angeli, 2001).

Pollock, L.A., 'Childbearing and female bonding in Early Modern England', *Social History*, 22:3 (1997), pp. 286–306.

Pomata, G., 'Menstruating men: similarity and difference of the sexes in Early Modern medicine', in V. Finucci and K. Brownlee (eds), *Generation and Degeneration: Tropes of Reproduction in Literature and History from Antiquity through Early Modern Europe* (Durham, NC: Duke University Press, 2001), pp. 109–52.

Pomata, G., 'Sharing cases: the *Observationes* in Early Modern medicine', *Early Science and Medicine*, 15:3 (2010), pp. 193–236.

Pomata, G., 'Observation rising: birth of an epistemic genre, 1500–1650', in L. Daston and E. Lunbeck (eds), *Histories of Scientific Observation* (Chicago: University of Chicago Press, 2011), pp. 45–79.

Poole, W., *The World Makers: Scientists of the Restoration and the Search for the Origins of the Earth* (Oxford: P. Lang, 2010).

Porter, R., 'The patients' view: doing medical history from below', *Theory and Society*, 14:2 (1985), pp. 175–98.

Porter, R. (ed.), *The Medical History of Water and Spas* (London: Wellcome Institute for the History of Medicine, 1990).
Prown, J., 'Mind in matter: an introduction to material culture theory and method', *Winterthur Portfolio*, 17:1 (1982), pp. 1–19.
Rak, M., *Napoli Gentile: la Letteratura in Lingua Napoletana nella Cultura Barocca, 1596–1632* (Bologna: Il Mulino, 1994).
Rankin, A., 'Exotic materials and treasured knowledge: the valuable legacy of noblewomen's remedies in Early Modern Germany', *Renaissance Studies*, 28:4 (2014), pp. 533–55.
Rather, L.J., 'The "six things Non-Naturals". A note on the origins and fate of a doctrine and a phrase', *Clio Medica*, 3 (1968), pp. 337–47.
Ray, M., *Daughters of Alchemy. Women and Scientific Culture in Early Modern Italy* (Cambridge, MA: Harvard University Press, 2015).
Read, S.L., ' "Thy Righteousness is but a menstrual clout": sanitary practices and prejudice in early modern England', *Early Modern Women: An Interdisciplinary Journal*, 3:1 (2008), pp. 1–25.
Ribouillault, D., *Rome et ses Jardins: Paysage et Pouvoir au XVIe Siècle* (Lassay-les-Châteaux: CTHS and Institute National d'Histoire de l'Art, 2013).
Richards, J., 'Useful books: reading vernacular regimens in sixteenth-century England', *Journal of the History of Ideas*, 73:2 (2012), pp. 247–71.
Riley, J., *The Eigtheenth-Century Campaign to Avoid Disease* (London: MacMillan, 1987).
Rinne, K., 'Urban ablutions: cleansing Counter-Reformation Rome', in M. Bradley and K. Stow (eds), *Rome, Pollution and Propriety: Dirt, Disease and Hygiene in the Eternal City from Antiquity to Modernity* (Cambridge: Cambridge University Press, 2012), pp. 182–201.
Risse, G.B., 'In the name of Hygieia and Hippocrates: a quest for the preservation of health and virtue', in G.B. Risse (ed.), *New Medical Challenges during the Scottish Enlightenment* (Amsterdam, New York: Brill, 2005), pp. 135–69.
Roggero, M., 'L'alphabétisation en Italie: une conquête féminine', *Annales Histoire, Sciences Sociales*, 56:4 (2001), pp. 903–26.
Roodenburg, H., 'The maternal imagination. The fears of pregnant women in seventeenth-century Holland', *Journal of Social History*, 21:4 (1988), pp. 701–16.
Rosen, G., *From Medical Police to Social Medicine: Essays on the History of Health Care* (New York: Science History, 1974).
Röthlisberger, M. *Claude Lorrain: The Paintings*, 2 vols (New Haven: Yale University Press, 1961).
Rublack, U., 'Pregnancy, childbirth and the female body in Early Modern Germany', *Past & Present*, 150:1 (1996), pp. 84–110.
Rublack, U., and P. Selwyn, 'Fluxes: the early modern body and the emotions', *History Workshop Journal*, 53:1 (2002), pp. 1–16.

Rusnock, A.A., *Vital Accounts: Quantifying Health and Population in Eighteenth-century England and France* (Cambridge: Cambridge University Press, 2002).

Russell, S., 'Girolamo Mercuriale's *De arte gymnastica* and Papal health at the Villa Pamphilj, Rome', in A. Arcangeli and V. Nutton (eds), *Girolamo Mercuriale: Medicina e Cultura nell'Europa del Cinquecento* (Florence: Leo S. Olschki Editore, 2008), pp. 182–83.

Ryrie, A., 'Sleeping, waking and dreaming in Protestant piety', in Martin and Ryrie (eds), *Private and Domestic Devotion*, pp. 73–92.

Ryrie, A., *Being Protestant in Reformation Britain* (Oxford: Oxford University Press, 2013).

Salmon, M., 'The cultural significance of breastfeeding and infant care in Early Modern England and America', *Journal of Social History*, 28:2 (1994), pp. 247–69.

Sarasohn, L.T., ' "That nauseous venomous insect": bedbugs in Early Modern England', *Eighteenth-Century Studies*, 46:4 (2013), pp. 513–30.

Schoenfeldt, M., *Bodies and Selves in Early Modern England: Physiology and Inwardness in Spenser, Shakespeare, Herbert, and Milton* (Cambridge: Cambridge University Press, 1999).

Schofield, R., 'Did mothers really die? three centuries of maternal mortality', in L. Bonfield et al. (eds), *The World We Have Gained . Histories of Population and Social Structure* (Oxford: Basil Blackwell, 1986), pp. 230–60.

Shapin, S., 'How to eat like a gentleman: dietetics and ethics in Early Modern England', in C.E. Rosenberg (ed.), *Right Living: An Anglo-American Tradition of Self-Help Medicine and Hygiene* (Baltimore: Johns Hopkins University Press, 2003), pp. 21–58.

Shapin, S., and S. Schaffer, *Leviathan and the Air-Pump: Hobbes, Boyle, and the Experimental Life* (Princeton: Princeton University Press, 1985).

Sharpe, W.D., 'Thomas Linacre 1460–1524: an English physician scholar of the Renaissance', *Bulletin of the History of Medicine*, 34 (1960), pp. 233–56.

Sherman, W., *Used Books: Marking Readers in Renaissance England* (Philadelphia: University of Pennsylvania Press, 2009).

Siraisi, N., *History, Medicine and the Traditions of Renaissance Learning* (Ann Arbor, MI: University of Michigan Press, 2007).

Siraisi, N., *Communities of Learned Experience: Epistolary Medicine in the Renaissance* (Baltimore: Johns Hopkins University Press, 2014).

Skuse, A., 'Wombs, worms and wolves: constructing cancer in Early Modern England', *Social History of Medicine*, 27:4 (2014), pp. 632–48.

Slack, P., 'Mirrors of health and treasures of poor men: the uses of the vernacular medical literature of Tudor England', in C. Webster (ed.), *Health Medicine and Mortality in the Sixteenth Century* (Cambridge: Cambridge University Press, 1979), pp. 238–73.

Smith, L.W., 'Reassessing the role of the family: women's medical care in eighteenth-century England', *Social History of Medicine*, 16:3 (2003), pp. 327–42.

Smith, L.W., 'The relative duties of a man: domestic medicine and France, ca. 1670–1740', *Journal of Family History*, 31:1 (2006), pp. 237–56.

Smith, L.W., 'The body embarrassed? Rethinking the leaky male body in Eighteenth-Century England and France', *Gender & History*, 23:1 (2011), pp. 26–46.

Smith, P., 'Making things: techniques and books in early modern Europe', in P. Findlen (ed.), *Early Modern Things 1500–1800* (London: Routledge, 2012), pp. 173–203.

Smith, V.S., 'Cleanliness: idea and practice in Britain, 1770–1850' (PhD thesis, University of London, 1985).

Smith, V.S., *Clean. A History of Personal Hygiene and Purity* (Oxford: Oxford University Press, 2007).

Solomon, M., *Fictions of Well-Being. Sickly Readers and Vernacular Medical Writing in Late Medieval and Early Modern Spain* (Philadelphia: Penn Press, 2010).

Sparey, V., 'Identity-formation and the breastfeeding mother in Renaissance generative discourses and Shakespeare's "Coriolanus"', *Social History of Medicine*, 25:4 (2012), pp. 777–94.

Spinage, C.A., *Cattle Plague. A History* (New York: Kluwer, 2003).

Stahnisch, F.W., 'The Tertium Compartionis of the Elementa Physiologiae – Johann Gotfried von Herder's conception of "tears" as mediators between the sublime and the actual bodily physiology', in Horstmanshoff, King and Zittel (eds), *Blood, Sweat and Tears*, pp. 595–629.

Steger, B., 'Cultures of sleep', in A. Green and A. Westcombe (eds), *Sleep. Multi-Professional Perspectives* (London, Philadelphia: Jessica Kingsley, 2012), pp. 68–85.

Stevens Crawshaw, J., 'Families, medical secrets and public health in Early Modern Venice', *Renaissance Studies*, 28:4 (2014), pp. 597–618.

Stobart, A., 'The making of domestic medicine: gender, self-help and therapeutic determination in household healthcare in south-west England in the late seventeenth century' (PhD thesis, Middlesex University, 2008).

Stobart, J., *Sugar and Spice: Grocers and Groceries in Provincial England, 1650–1830* (Oxford: Oxford University Press: Oxford, 2012).

Stolberg, M., *Experiencing Illness and the Sick Body in Early Modern Europe* (London: Palgrave Macmillan, 2011).

Stolberg, M., 'Sweat. Learned concepts and popular perceptions, 1500–1800', in Horstmanshoff, King and Zittel (eds), *Blood, Sweat and Tears*, pp. 503–22.

Stolberg, M., ' "You have not good blood in your body". Oral communication in sixteenth-century physicians' medical practice', *Medical History*, 59:1 (2015), pp. 63–82.

Storey, T., 'Italian books of secrets database: study documentation', https://lra.le.ac.uk/handle/2381/4335.

Styles, J., 'What were cottons for in the early Industrial Revolution?' in G. Riello and P. Parthasarathi (eds), *The Spinning World. A Global History of Cotton Textiles* (Oxford: Oxford University Press, 2009), pp. 307–26.

Suhr, C., 'Regimens and health guides', in I. Taavitsainen and P. Pahta (eds), *Early Modern English Medical Texts: Corpus Description and Studies* (Amsterdam, Philadelphia: John Benjamins, 2010), pp. 111–18.

Sullivan, E., 'The watchful spirit: religious anxieties towards sleep in the notebooks of Nehemiah Wallington (1598–1658)', *Cultural History*, 1:1 (2012), pp. 14–35.

Sullivan, E., 'Emotions in history: A review essay', *Cultural History*, 2:1 (2013), pp. 93–102.

Taavitsainen, I., and P. Pahta (eds), *Medical Writing in Early Modern English* (Cambridge: Cambridge University Press, 2011).

Te Hennepe, M., 'Of the fisherman's net and skin pores. Reframing conceptions of the skin in medicine 1572–1714', in Horstmanshoff, King and Zittel (eds), *Blood, Sweat and Tears*, pp. 523–48.

Thomas, K., 'Cleanliness and godliness in Early Modern England', in A. Fletcher and P. Roberts (eds), *Religion, Culture and Society in Early Modern Britain: Essays in Honour of Patrick Collinson* (Cambridge: Cambridge University Press, 1994).

Tilley, C., *Metaphor and Material Culture* (Oxford: Blackwell, 1999).

Tilley, C., 'Ethnography and material culture', in P. Atkinson et al. (eds), *Handbook of Ethnography* (London: Sage, 2001), pp. 258–72.

Torrance, J. (ed.), *The Concept of Nature* (Oxford: Clarendon Press, 1992).

Torrini, M., 'Un episodio della polemica tra "antichi" e "moderni": la disputa sulla macerazione dei lini nel Lago di Agnano', *Bollettino del Centro di studi vichiani*, 5:1 (1975), pp. 56–70.

Tucker, N., 'Mothers, babies and lullabies', *History Today*, 34:9 (1984), pp. 40–6.

Van Dam, F., 'Permeable boundaries: bodies, bathing and fluxes: 1135–1333', in *Medicine and Space: Body, Surroundings and Borders in Antiquity and the Middle Ages* (Leiden: Brill, 2007), pp. 117–49.

Van Der Eijk, P.J., *Medicine and Philosophy in Classical Antiquity: Doctors and Philosophers on Nature, Soul, Health, and Disease* (Cambridge: Cambridge University Press, 2005).

Van Der Lugt, M., 'Neither ill nor healthy: the intermediate state between health and disease in medieval medicine', *Quaderni Storici*, 136:1 (2011), pp. 13–46.

Verbeek, P., *What Things Do: Philosophical Reflections on Technology, Agency, and Design* (Philadelphia: Pennsylvania State University Press, 2005).

Verbeek, P., and Kockelkoren P., 'The things that matter', *Design Issues*, 14:3 (1998), pp. 28–42.

Von Sandrart, J., *Der Teutschen Academie zweyter Theil*, as translated in M. Röthlisberger, *Claude Lorrain: The Paintings*, 2 vols (New Haven: Yale University Press, 1961).

Von Tippelskirch, X., *Letture Femminili in Italia nella Prima Età Moderna* (Rome: Viella, 2011).

Walsham, A., *Providence in Early Modern England* (Oxford: Oxford University Press, 2003, first publ. 1999).

Wear, A., 'Making sense of health and the environment in Early Modern England', in A. Wear (ed.), *Medicine in Society: Historical Essays* (Cambridge: Cambridge University Press, 1992), pp. 119–47.

Wear, A., 'The popularization of medicine in Early Modern England', in R. Porter (ed.), *The Popularisation of Medicine 1650–1850* (London: Routledge, 1992), pp. 17–41.

Wear, A., 'Fear, anxiety and the plague in Early Modern England: religious and medical responses', in J.R. Hinnells and R. Porter (eds), *Religion, Health, and Suffering* (London: Kegan Paul International, 1999).

Wear, A., *Knowledge and Practice in English Medicine* (Cambridge: Cambridge University Press, 2000).

Wear, A., 'Puritan perceptions of illness in seventeenth century England', in R. Porter (ed.), *Patients and Practitioners: Lay Perceptions of Medicine in Pre-Industrial Society* (Cambridge: Cambridge University Press, 2002, first publ. 1985), pp. 55–99.

Wear, A., 'Place, health and disease: the airs, waters, places tradition in Early Modern England and North America', *Journal of Medieval and Early Modern Studies*, 38:3 (2008), pp. 443–65.

Wear, A., 'The prospective colonist and strange environments: advice on health and prosperity', in K. Oslund, N. Brimnes, N. Thode Jensen and C. Folke Ax (eds), *Cultivating the Colony: Colonial States and their Environmental Legacies* (Athens, OH: Ohio University Press, 2011), pp 19–46.

Weatherill, L., *Consumer Behaviour & Material Culture in Britain, 1660–1760*, 2nd edn. (London: Routledge, 1996).

Webster, C., *The Great Instauration: Science, Medicine and Reform 1626–1600* (London: Duckworth, 1975).

Webster, C., 'Paracelsus. Medicine as popular protest', in A. Cunningham and O.P. Grell (eds), *Medicine and the Reformation* (London, New York: Routledge, 1993), pp. 57–77.

Weisser, O., 'Grieved and disordered: gender and emotion in Early Modern patient narratives', *Journal of Medieval and Early Modern Studies*, 43:2 (2013), pp. 247–74.

Weisser, O., *Ill Composed. Sickness, Gender, and Belief in Early Modern England* (New Haven: Yale University Press, 2015).

Westcombe, A. (ed.), *Sleep. Multi-Professional Perspectives* (London, Philadelphia: Jessica Kingsley, 2012).

Wilson, A., 'The perils of Early Modern procreation: childbirth with or without fear?' *British Journal of Eighteenth Century Studies*, 16:1 (1993), pp. 1–19.

Wilson, A., *The Making of Man-Midwifery: Childbirth in England, 1660–1770* (London: UCL Press, 1995).

Wilson, A., *Ritual and Conflict: The Social Relations of Childbirth in Early Modern England* (Farnham: Ashgate, 2013).

Withey, A., *Physick and the Family: Health, Medicine and Care in Wales, 1600–1750* (Manchester: Manchester University Press, 2011).

Wrightson, K., 'Infanticide in earlier seventeenth-century England', *Local Population Studies*, 15 (1975), pp. 10–22.

Wrigley, R., 'Infectious enthusiasms: influence, contagion and the experience of Rome', in C. Chard and H. Langdaon (eds), *Transports: Travel, Pleasure, and Imaginative Geography, 1600–1830* (New Haven: Yale University Press, 1996), pp. 75–116.

Wrigley, R., *Roman Fever: Influence, Infection and the Image of Rome, 1700–1870* (New Haven: Yale University Press, 2014).

Zmora, A.S., 'Schooling in Renaissance Pistoia: community and civic humanism in small-town Tuscany', *The Sixteenth Century Journal*, 34:3 (2003), pp. 761–77.

Zorach, R., *The Virtual Tourist in Renaissance Rome: Printing and Collecting the 'Speculum Romanae magnificentiae'* (Chicago: University of Chicago Press, 2008).

Blogs

Anders, E., http://remedianetwork.net/2014/11/07/locating-convalescence-in-victorian-england/ (accessed 20 February 2015).

Index

EU authorised representative for GPSR:
Easy Access System Europe, Mustamäe tee 50,
10621 Tallinn, Estonia
gpsr.requests@easproject.com

www.ingramcontent.com/pod-product-compliance
Ingram Content Group UK Ltd.
Pitfield, Milton Keynes, MK11 3LW, UK
UKHW061932100926
8556IPUK00007B/879
* 9 7 8 1 5 2 6 1 1 3 4 7 4 *